KT-146-919

Reflections on Midwifery

NAPIER UNIVERSITY LIBRARY

3 8042 00411 2817

Reflections on Midwifery

Mavis J. Kirkham PhD RGN RM Cert Ed
Professor of Midwifery
University of Sheffield
Sheffield

Elizabeth R. Perkins PhD Cert Ed
Research, Training and Development Consultant
Nottingham

Baillière Tindall
London   Philadelphia   Toronto   Sydney   Tokyo

hQ160

co

Baillière Tindall   24–28 Oval Road
London NW1 7DX

The Curtis Center
Independence Square West
Philadelphia, PA 19106-3399, USA

Harcourt Brace & Company
55 Horner Avenue
Toronto, Ontario, M8Z 4X6, Canada

Harcourt Brace & Company, Australia
30–52 Smidmore Street
Marrickville, NSW 2204, Australia

Harcourt Brace & Company, Japan
Ichibancho Central Building, 22-1 Ichibancho
Chiyoda-ku, Tokyo 102, Japan

© 1997 Baillière Tindall
Chapter One © Gay Lee

This book is printed on acid-free paper

All rights reserved. No part of this publication may be
reproduced, stored in a retrieval system or transmitted, in any
form or by any other means, electronic, mechanical, photocopying or
otherwise, without the prior permission of W B Saunders Company Ltd,
24–28 Oval Road, London, NW1 7DX, England

A catalogue record for this book is available from the British Library

ISBN 0-7020-2125-3

Typeset by Paston Press Ltd, Loddon, Norfolk, UK.
Printed and bound in Great Britain by WBC Book Manufacturers, Bridgend,
Mid Glamorgan.

NAPIER UNIVERSITY LIBRARY

AC /	/	ON
LOC	BHMK	SUP
co	618.2 KIRR	
CON		PR

Contents

Contributors

Pauleene L. Hammett BSc(Hons) RGN RM MTD DipN(Lond)
> The Nightingale Institute, King's College London, Cornwall House, 1 Waterloo Road, London SE1 8WA

Brooke V. Heagerty PhD (Women's History)
> Independent Researcher and Writer, 2447 N. Artesian, 2nd Floor, Chicago, IL 60647, USA

Mavis J. Kirkham PhD RGN RM Cert Ed
> Professor of Midwifery, ScHARR, University of Sheffield, 3 Regent Street, Sheffield S1 4DA

Gay Lee SRN RM BA MMedSci
> Job-Share Clinical Midwife, Guy's and St Thomas's Hospital Trust, Lambeth Palace Road, London SE1 7EH

Euranis Neile SRN RM ADM PGCEA MEd   Northern and Yorkshire Regional Research Fellow
> Midwife Teacher, University of Hull, East Riding Campus, Beverley Road, Willerby, Hull HU10 6NS

Elizabeth R. Perkins PhD Cert Ed
> Research, Training and Development Consultant, 11 Exton Road, Sherwood, Nottingham NG5 1HA

Helen Stapleton SRN SCM MNIMH MSc
> Research Midwife, ScHARR, University of Sheffield, 3 Regent Street, Sheffield S1 4DA

Judith Unell BA(Hons) PhD
> Independent Social Research Consultant, 52 Main Street, Calverton, Nottingham NG14 6FN

Diane Walters
> Doula/Birth Companion and Childbirth Educator, 60 Nottingham Road, Belper, Derbyshire DE56 1JH

INTRODUCTION

Mavis J. Kirkham and Elizabeth R. Perkins

In the UK in recent years, and particularly since the publication of the Winterton report (Winterton, 1992) and *Changing Childbirth* (DoH, 1993), there has been considerable impetus to improve midwifery care. Many projects have sought to improve the client's childbearing experience and often also to improve the midwife's skill and job satisfaction. This impetus is very cheering, but there is a danger of trying to implement ideas that are still slogans rather than fully analysed concepts. Without analysis, there is insufficient conceptual basis on which to build strategic plans and little sense of strategic priorities in the face of cuts in funding. Within this analysis there is a particular need to examine the ironies, dilemmas and sometimes contradictions within our endeavours. We have discussed these issues for some time within our meetings for mutual research supervision. At the same time we have become aware of several studies which give insight into these issues, by researchers thinking about the dilemmas at the heart of the current practice of midwifery. The bringing together of these researchers and practitioners led to this book, written by five midwives, two social researchers, one historian and one doula, a combination giving not only deep commitment to the maternity service but also sufficient analytical distance to allow real consideration of its present dilemmas.

THE PAST

In order to understand our present we need to understand how we came to be here. Brooke Heagerty's contribution (Chapter 4) is important in showing the social forces at work in the early moves to professionalize midwifery. Patterns can be seen which continue long after the situations which made them necessary. At the beginning of the twentieth century midwives were oppressed both as women in a male-dominated world and as members of an occupational group which could only continue to exist by subservience to doctors. These midwives internalized the values of the dominant group and went on themselves to scapegoat midwives who threatened the status quo, and thus added to the oppression of women in their care who came from less powerful social groups. This may have been inevitable in the past, but this cannot excuse the continuance of such oppression in our present culture and with the level of educational opportunity now open to midwives. Midwives need to be aware of the inequalities in the service we offer to women and our lack of knowledge surrounding the needs and care of women from ethnic minorities (see Chapter 6).

Knowledge of our past can also help our awareness of parallels in past or present experience. Powerholders change, and it could be that we are now oppressed by Taylorite managerialism (see Chapter 8) as we were in the past by medicine. This is a phenomenon affecting the whole of society, not just midwifery; but as educated midwives, with a strong tradition behind us and close alliance with the women we serve, we are well placed to consider it. Ironically, the forefront of managerial thought has long since found Taylorism to be a barren philosophy (even on production lines and certainly in human services), just as medicine is finding a purely mechanical model insufficient to explain human functioning. It is sadly not unusual for the National Health Service to implement obsolescence.

CULTURE AND CULTURAL CHANGE

The wider culture has changed in recent years. The changing powerbase of different occupational groups provides a good example, as does our multicultural society and the position and voice of women. All these have had a profound effect upon midwifery, as have more subtle yet equally profound changes. Technological advance and the aims of control which a technical culture makes possible have changed birth and midwifery. Sophisticated monitoring is now usually expected before a pregnancy can be seen as provisionally normal. Helen Stapleton (Chapter 3) considers the impact of technocratic change in terms of the gap between the expert and the insignificant (m)others. Such changes increase the challenges of being 'with women' while also having a widening range of technical proficiencies. The rise of the doula movement (Chapter 5) suggests that midwives are not always able to meet these challenges.

Nor is this only a matter of external expertise. Our society is one of self-surveillance: we each 'keep an eye on' our weight and monitor ourselves against many other indicators of health and social status. Likewise with our practice; risk management and quality control can raise standards but may also induce uniformity and add to the worrying list of things a midwife could get wrong.

We also have the pressures of the market economy, where childbearing women become health-care consumers (an ironic description for those engaged in the ultimate productive process); all is costed, and value for money is virtue. These things are not bad but agendas can conflict. Recent developments have inspired midwives to improve their service and it is perhaps not surprising that midwives become weary, faced with pressures to cut costs while they themselves remain committed to radically improving the quality of service. This is alongside the practical dilemmas inherent in offering client choice within evidence based practice with measurable healthcare outcomes.

Cost effectiveness means having the minimum input to achieve an agreed health outcome. But recent developments have inspired midwives to improve care and hence outcomes for mothers and babies. Cost effectiveness can, therefore, feel like meanness to midwives in National Health Service practice who are constantly trying to improve their practice while managers are trying to prune their resources. In contrast, there is a generosity of spirit in statements from countries where midwifery has recently emerged or re-emerged. Barrington writes of midwifery in Canada:

> *Continuous care, involving generous commitments of time, allows a midwife to gather a store of impressions that will substantiate future intuitions and actions. Her familiarity with the norms of mother and baby enables her to notice deviations from these norms immediately.*
>
> *(Guilliland and Pairman, 1995)*

Pelvin speaks of New Zealand:

> *For it is in the relationship between women and midwives as they go through the childbearing process together that the message of value and worth is given. It cannot be given by strangers mouthing words – it is given by the midwife's commitment to the woman and the process she is involved in.*
>
> *(Guilliland and Pairman, 1995)*

Words such as 'generosity' and 'commitment' are not used in the market place of the National Health Service. This is ironic as there is ample evidence of very long-term health gains from commitment and generosity in support for childbearing women and of changes in the organization of care increasing midwives' commitment to their clients (Oakley *et al.*, 1996). Yet the maternity services are hedged in by short-term funding and budgets covering the brief timespan of maternity care in which long-term health gains cannot yet be manifest. Birth stories echo through lifetimes (see Chapter 9).

This is not the first time midwives have faced great change. Thus midwives are accomplished in keeping their heads down and doing their best. Battling on in this way has led to a real danger of losing a sense of midwifery's own identity.

SELF-VALUING

Midwives need to value themselves more highly. They have a long tradition of being 'with women', one which goes back well beyond the traditions of obstetricians and managers. The principles of good midwifery built up over the years are worth asserting, not just for the good of the profession but for the sake of the women it serves. Transforming practice is not simply a matter of faith in midwifery values, but it is not likely to happen in ways that midwives would like if they do not themselves believe that their principles are important. The high-level alliance between women's campaigning groups and the midwifery profession which resulted in *Changing Childbirth* shows the possibilities for transforming the debate, at least, when these principles are asserted with confidence.

Building this confidence, and using it to change practice, is in part a matter of recovering a sense of the richness of midwifery traditions. Brooke Heagerty, in Chapter 4, shows the links between working-class midwives and the poor communities they served, and their unwillingness to accept the views of the ladies of the Midwives' Institute about the one true way to develop midwifery. The Association of Radical Midwives and the various independent midwifery practices have roots in past traditions as well as, one hopes, a future.

It is also useful to recognize that there are traditional roots for the many legitimate ways to learn and develop. Originally training came from apprenticeship and experience. Structured courses now represent the most obvious way of learning, but these should not be seen as superseding the older ways. In this book a number of the authors argue for more sharing of experience between midwives and more opportunity to reflect together. Valuing one's own experience, thinking about it and discussing it with other practitioners, is the bedrock of professional development – how this is arranged is, logically, a secondary affair.

Midwives who value themselves will find it easier to see themselves as a valuable professional resource, both to the women they care for and to the health services as a whole. Such a resource needs maintaining in decent condition, not treated like butter to be smeared across the surface of the maternity services so thinly that it almost disappears. Schemes that rely on staff who sacrifice their family life to their patients may last a few years, until the dedication turns to burn-out and the midwives leave to save their relationships or their sanity. The rhetoric of continuity of care needs to include a concern for continuity of the service. One of the most satisfied users of maternity services I have encountered delayed her pushing in order to be delivered by the midwife who delivered both her and her husband. Midwives who really know the families in their care and develop the service they give are of great value. Sadly, new ideas have often been allowed to sweep through the service in such a way as to sweep away the thinking practitioners who pioneered the very innovations being introduced. Thus dedicated community midwives may be seen to mourn the introduction of team midwifery and independent midwifery is threatened as we implement many of the practices which independent midwives pioneered. Midwives will need to point this out, to themselves, to one another and to their managers the need for continuity of the service, and ignore any suggestions that this is simply unprofessional whinging. As one of the documents produced by the Health At Work in the NHS initiative points out:

> *Whinging is not the alibi of the lazy. Whinging is a committed workforce in pain.*   *(OPUS, 1996)*

A workforce in pain will not work well.

SELF-DEVELOPMENT

Building a sense of self-value is both a consequence and a condition of a willingness to develop oneself. Many of the chapters in this book point to features of current midwifery practice where staff need to extend the range of situations they can handle. This has less to do with clinical skill than with emotional tolerance of other ways of thinking and other ways of doing things, though there are skills and knowledge to be learnt here as well. Giving good care to women from minority ethnic groups, for example, does not just involve finding an interpreter or learning enough Urdu to say 'don't push'! It also requires a willingness to learn about different cultural understandings of pregnancy, childbirth and new motherhood, and about different practical living conditions, and to adapt midwifery practice accordingly – as Euranis Neile shows clearly in Chapter 6.

Even specific skills require a surrounding set of appropriate attitudes before they can be well used. Pauleene Hammett's chapter on debriefing, for example (Chapter 7), provides an account of a specific skill which will be new to many readers, though the idea that women might benefit from talking about their labours will strike chords with most experienced staff. Midwives developing debriefing as part of their practice will need to learn specific skills, but also will need the capacity to listen to a mother's story of the birth of her baby without persistent impulses to defend midwifery practice – their own, their colleagues' or that of the institution in which they work. Explanations may be needed, but they have to be timed to suit the mother, not inserted to head off criticism. Many people can sense when they are dealing with a professional who cannot handle negative feedback, and will censor themselves accordingly; they and the profession may be impoverished as a result.

One reason why staff find negative feedback hard to handle is that they may be receiving too much of it already. This is a good example of a much broader truth – you can't give what you haven't got. It is well recognized within the management literature that caring for staff is a prerequisite for them caring for others. There are good examples of private sector initiatives which incorporate this understanding (Hampden-Turner, 1994). For example, British Airways started a new approach to management with their cabin staff, whose job it was to make aircraft passengers feel well looked after and comfortable:

> *You free the cabin staff to give the best service they can, on the assumption that this is what they really want ... With set procedures and standard techniques you actually force them to give bad service – not tailored to the person, not responsive to unforeseen events. We had to build up their confidence that they could make decisions and could use flexible and ingenious means to fulfil the superordinate goal of satisfying customers. We had them express feelings about their jobs, set personal goals and re-examine all their relationships so that they would be seen as whole people, not just roles.*
> *(Mike Bruce, British Airways human resources department, quoted by Hampden-Turner, 1994)*

The health services applications are obvious. If no one tells you that you are doing a good job, it is hard to praise others, even when praise for courage and endurance could transform a woman's view of her labour. Similarly, it is hard to give choices to clients if you yourself have little choice in the way you do your job. It may not even be possible to protect clients' choices, if your freedom of manoeuvre is restricted enough. Helen Stapleton, in Chapter 3, provides an extended discussion of the restriction of choice for both mothers and midwives which can result from overprotective institutional policies. Midwives must work on empowering themselves before they can usefully talk about empowering mothers – this is both a psychological and a practical truth.

FLEXIBILITY

Midwives who value themselves and their colleagues and develop their emotional range can offer far more flexible care to their patients. Gay Lee, in Chapter 1, suggests four models of relationships between mothers and midwives, and argues for the possibility of choice for both mothers and midwives, since both groups would benefit from a range of options. These models would cover both the National Health Service and the independent sectors. Women's needs vary considerably, and there are examples in this book of women wanting both large and small variations from 'normal' service practice. Women who are enthusiasts for home birth or who refuse antenatal screening tests worry some professionals; those who are enthusiasts for elective induction worry others. Women from minority ethnic groups are faced with a service, which may recognize few of their concerns and has difficulty even understanding, let alone meeting their needs. Now that hospitals are used to the idea of partners being present at the birth, some women are choosing to bring an additional lay supporter, the doula. In Chapter 5 Mavis Kirkham and Diane Walters discuss the troubling implications for midwifery practice – for is it not the midwife's role to support women in labour? Freeing the maternity services to work well in all these circumstances may seem a daunting task.

Yet not all women's choices need be seen as so difficult; there are other desires which can be easier to meet. In Chapter 2 Elizabeth Perkins and Judith Unell describe mothers' responses to a new team midwifery scheme, and show the range of simpler choices that mattered to their informants. For example, women liked having a wide choice of antenatal appointments at the surgery, not just one session, so that they could fit their checks around their other commitments. These mothers' concept of 'delivery by a known midwife' was much less demanding than that used by many professionals; they valued being welcomed in the labour ward by someone they had already met, and wanted to see their delivery midwife on one of the postnatal home visits, to talk over the birth. For professionals who are confident enough to give up the notion that there is one right way to run a service, it is possible to start with the small things and work from there; flexibility can thus become a habit of mind which can be applied in more complex situations with more security.

CHOICE AND CONTROL

'Client choice' is a phrase much used since the publication of *Changing Childbirth*. Yet 'consumer' choice is limited to the services on offer, so the service providers who extol choice also define the choices available. A woman cannot opt to give birth in the now closed general practitioner unit or be delivered by a midwife employed by another health-care trust. Choice is also limited by resources on both sides. A woman wanting to be sure of continuity of midwifery care may book an independent midwife only if she knows of one and can pay for that service. Choices are not equally available to all; many non-English speaking women are not aware of any choices, and even if the options available could be translated they may not include care which is appropriate to their culture and beliefs.

Choice is an unsophisticated concept which assumes that there are clear options to choose between, and implies that choosers should live with the results of their choice. Technology and organizations create pressures around choice. How real is choice in antenatal screening when a woman declining such screening may feel herself blamed if her child is handicapped? Nor can technology answer the mother's central question, 'Is my baby all right?' or, if a handicap is diagnosed, 'How will that affect the baby's quality of life?' Present choices will be viewed from the future as well as the present, and subsequent events may press parents to revisit and reinterpret past choices. Present choices will also limit future options. Stories are fashioned and refashioned if life is to have coherence. Thus individual paths through the childbearing year may be a more appropriate picture than choice, since choice can imply a 'shopping list' of separate items. Rather than a set of options, maternity care should consist of one or more continuing relationships where caregivers have to balance the opening up of horizons and possibilities with support and companionship for clients on their path.

Similarly with control: a sense of control of self and carers is linked with positive outcomes for childbearing women (Green, Coupland and Kitzinger, 1989), and workers sense of control of the work process is generally agreed to enhance their work. Yet in midwifery there is a contradiction between these two needs for control which obscures larger issues. We often see midwives controlling and thereby damaging women's experience and women striving for the self-control needed to present themselves as good patients. Yet, while labour can be surgically pre-empted and contractions can be chemically augmented, none of us can control labour. Midwives need to facilitate women's sense of control of carers and setting, to make possible for all concerned a sense of trust and safety in respect for physiological processes. Here again flexibility, self-value and confidence are essential.

IMPROVING THE SERVICES

There has been a real commitment to improving midwifery care in recent years. Research and development have grown, and several chapters in this book describe how care can be improved, others give us food for thought as to how improvements can be made. Dilemmas are also highlighted.

The Winterton report (Winterton, 1992) and *Changing Childbirth* (DoH, 1993) have changed the language used to discuss maternity services. Different values are inherent in the new language. Midwives sought real change and from that followed closer relationships with clients, different allegiances and changes in interprofessional relationships. If clients are to be involved in decision-making about the care, the professional decision-making must rest with clinical midwives providing that care. We have therefore seen real efforts to devolve decision-making in some places (e.g. Warwick, 1996), and acute discomfort in others. We may now be seeing *Changing Childbirth* slipping down the list of funding priorities, but efforts towards implementation have focused our attention on issues which cannot now be ignored. In this sense, while there are threats to our service, we can be said to have broken the mould of silent subservience. In order to progress, midwives need the openness to be receptive, the space to reflect, room to play with ideas and the support which makes us brave enough to debate in these threatening open spaces. This book is our contribution to the debate which is now possible – though never comfortable.

REFERENCES

Barrington E (1985) *Midwifery is Catching.* Toronto: NC Press.

[DoH] Department of Health (1993) *Changing Childbirth.* Report of the Expert Maternity Group. London: HMSO.

Green J, Coupland VA & Kitzinger JV (1989) *Great Expectations: a prospective study of women's expectations and experiences of childbirth.* Cambridge: Child Care and Development Unit, University of Cambridge.

Guilliland K & Pairman S (1995) *The Midwifery Partnership: a model for practice.* Wellington, New Zealand: The Victoria University of Wellington

Hampden-Turner C (1994) *Corporate Culture.* London: Piatkus.

Oakley A, Hickey D, Rajan L & Rigby AS (1996) Social support in pregnancy: does it have long-term effects? *Journal of Reproductive and Infant Psychology* **14** (1): 7–22.

OPUS (1996) *Organisational Stress: Planning and Implementing a Programme to Address Organisational Stress in the NHS.* London: Health Education Authority.

Pelvin B (1990) Midwifery: the feminist profession. *Proceedings of New Zealand College of Midwives National Conference* held in Dunedin, August 1990.

Warwick C (1996) Leadership in midwifery care. *British Journal of Midwifery* 4(5): 229.

Winterton N (1992) *Maternity Services*. Second report of the House of Commons Health Committee (The Winterton report). London: HMSO.

1

The concept of 'continuity' – what does it mean?

Gay Lee

This chapter focuses on continuity – one of the key concepts in the maternity services today – and one of the least well understood. Continuity of care, caring and carer – what do they mean?

The first section of the chapter summarizes the report *Changing Childbirth* (DoH, 1993) and looks at the key words describing continuity as they are used in the report. The next section looks at how researchers and service providers have used these terms, and at evidence of their meaning and value at various stages of maternity care. A model of continuity and quality of care is then developed. This leads to the suggestion that the concept of continuity distracts us from other issues of quality which we need to concentrate on. It also distracts us from the wider political issues undermining choice and control for women. The implications of the model are then discussed for midwives, mothers and maternity services. Finally, four vignettes of successful and unsuccessful communications between women and 'known' and 'unknown' midwives are used to illustrate the points made above.

UNDERSTANDING THE CONCEPTS WE USE

In midwifery it is important to know what we are talking about. We discuss 'concepts' often without being aware of doing so, even though they are the theoretical backbone of good practice.

Denise Polit and Bernadette Hungler describe a concept as 'an abstraction based on observations of certain behaviours or characteristics (e.g. stress, pain)' (Polit and Hungler, 1993). Taking this further, Rosamund Bryar (1995, p. 26) says of a concept that it is 'the label given to classes of ideas and things in the world and part of the process of learning involves the development of the understanding of concepts'. So concepts are not reality itself, but are a way of referring to many different types of reality by naming them and thus producing mental images that can be agreed and shared with others, at least to some extent. Concepts used in research, and applied in the context of service development, need to be more rigorously defined than is often the case in ordinary life.

By putting concepts together, models can be built. Denise Polit and Bernadette Hungler say that a model is 'a symbolic representation of concepts or variables and interrelationships among them' (Polit and Hungler, 1993). Rosamund Bryar (1995, p. 21) says further that models 'provide a framework for understanding and developing practice, for guiding actions... and identifying research questions'. Thus models can be seen as ways of organizing information in a coherent way in order to make sense of it and develop it further.

'Continuity of care' and 'continuity of carer' are terms that are on many midwives' lips today, but these concepts are ill-defined and poorly researched. One of the main messages of the *Changing Childbirth* report is how important continuity of care and carer are, yet there was very little examination of the concepts before its publication and no conceptual models of care were developed for testing.

THE *CHANGING CHILDBIRTH* REPORT

Changing Childbirth and the concept of continuity

Continuity of carer is seen as being one of the fundamental principles underpinning woman-centred care (p. 14*). The terms used in *Changing Childbirth* to denote continuity are 'named midwife', 'team midwifery' and 'midwifery group practice'. The report is summarized in Box 1.1.

The report says that 'every woman should be given the name of an individual midwife who works locally to whom she can go for advice and help throughout her pregnancy' (p. 5). She 'should know one midwife who ensures continuity of her midwifery care – the named midwife' (second indicator of success; p. 70). It seems that continuity of (midwifery) *care* is synonymous with continuity of (midwifery) *carer*, but what 'knowing' means is undefined.

A summary of the work of the Institute of Manpower Studies (IMS, 1993) is quoted. It researched the number of units implementing team midwifery in England and Wales and attempted to define parameters for a team:

- the team should have no more than six midwives
- each should have a defined caseload
- each should provide total care to each woman
- at least 50% of the women should know their delivery midwife
- the team should operate in whichever places the woman requires care – hospital or community (p. 15).

Changing Childbirth acknowledges that in order to know the labour midwife, continuity is likely to be lost antenatally, as the woman may meet 'up to eight midwives' and this may be 'a price worth paying' (p. 15). However, the report says that 'there is no substitute for a known and trusted professional supporting [the woman]' and suggests that appropriate care can be enhanced 'through a one-to-one relationship with a named professional' (p. 13). The words 'midwife' and 'professional' are used interchangeably, and 'trusted'

---

* The page numbers in parentheses in this section refer to the *Changing Childbirth* report (DoH, 1993).

Box 1.1 A Summary of *Changing Childbirth*

The Expert Maternity Group was set up by the Department of Health to take forward the work of the House of Commons Health Committee which reported on the maternity services in 1992 (the Winterton report). This said that a medical model of care was not applicable to childbirth and that women should have more choice in maternity care, especially over place of birth. The group had no remit to include major socioeconomic factors in its brief. It collected evidence from individuals, maternity units and consumer health organizations and a very little from published studies. It commissioned a survey of consumer views by MORI Health Research (MORI, 1993).

The views and recommendations of the Expert Maternity Group are set out in Part 1 of the report (DoH, 1993). The basic principle underlying Part 1 is that *maternity care should be woman-centred* with the focus on the needs of women and their families. (The expression that is associated with *Changing Childbirth*, 'continuity, choice and control', is not actually used in the report.)

Women's needs include:

- having access to information
- being able to make choices, especially over place and management of birth
- being involved in decision-making and being in control
- having accessible, sensitive, community-based services with emphasis on the needs of disabled women
- being involved in planning and monitoring of services
- having safe care (emotionally as well as physically)
- having continuity of care and carer

There should be:

- effective and efficient use of resources
- more appropriate involvement of general practitioners
- full use of midwifery skills and knowledge
- use of obstetric skills primarily where parturition is complex
- recognition of the training role of senior house officers
- appropriate training for other staff
- research-based and regularly audited clinical practice
- evaluation of new services for effectiveness and acceptability

These recommendations are incorporated into a set of objectives, action points for purchasers and providers, and a list of indicators of success which should be achieved within 5 years. These are:

1. All women should be entitled to carry their own notes.
2. Every woman should know one midwife who ensures continuity of her midwifery care – the named midwife.
3. At least 30% of women should have the midwife as the lead professional.
4. Every woman should know the lead professional who has a key role in the planning and provision of her care. *continued overleaf*

Box 1.1 *Continued*

5. At least 75% of women should know the person who cares for them during their delivery.

6. Midwives should have direct access to some beds in all maternity units.

7. At least 30% of women delivered in a maternity unit should be admitted under the management of the midwife.

8. The total number of antenatal visits for women with uncomplicated pregnancies should have been reviewed in the light of available evidence and the guidelines of the Royal College of Obstetricians and Gynaecologists.

9. All front-line ambulances should have a paramedic able to support the midwife who needs to transfer a woman to hospital in an emergency.

10. All women should have access to information about the services available in their locality.

Part 2 of *Changing Childbirth* is a 'survey of good communications practice'. In comparison with the much-quoted Part 1, the second part is little mentioned. Yet, as the introduction states, 'good communications are an essential part of good... practice and should not be a bolt-on 'extra''. This second part sets out basic principles of good communication and focuses on examples of good practice in the maternity services.

and 'known' are used together, although neither is defined. Elsewhere (p. 41) the report says that teamwork between midwives, obstetricians and paediatricians ought to be 'clarified, enhanced and encouraged'.

Midwifery group practices are considered a possible solution to the problem of too many carers. However, the only qualities ascribed to them in *Changing Childbirth* are that 'they aim to provide a high degree of support and continuity mainly through a single midwife for each woman' (p. 15). This is acknowledged to be an unknown in terms of practicalities and is now being evaluated (e.g. Page et al, 1995).

Continuity of carer is necessary 'most particularly during labour' (p. 6) although no evidence for this is given. It is re-emphasized by the fifth indicator of success: 'at least 75% of women should know the person who cares for them during delivery'. However, again 'knowing' is not defined and 'person' replaces midwife. This could be a doctor or even a non-professional labour supporter. 'The woman should be cared for by people who are familiar to her and aware of her plans for delivery' (p. 6). Here more than a one-to-one relationship is implied, and familiarity replaces knowledge and trust as a quality of the relationship.

No references are given for evidence of the importance of continuity of carer. *Changing Childbirth* suggests that 'each maternity unit will need to seek its own models and strategies' for achieving it (p. 16). However, 'Services can be reorganized, roles and responsibilities altered, but we are convinced that the most fundamental change that needs to occur is one of attitude on the part of some caregivers' (p. 12).

Questions which need to be answered are:

- How many and what kind of professionals can be involved before continuity is impaired?

- What does it mean to 'know' and 'trust' the person or people involved in care and how, if at all, are these concepts linked with 'familiar faces'?
- What is the relationship between continuity of carer and the attitudes of caregivers? How does restructuring care systems affect relationships?

Changing Childbirth is an influential document on which definitive action to change maternity services is being taken. It discusses a key concept which this brief analysis suggests has not been well thought out. The next section looks at ways in which the concept of continuity has been defined and used by others.

CONTINUITY OF CARE, CARING AND CARER

Patricia Murphy-Black (1992, 1993) sees 'continuity of care' as having two aspects: 'continuity of caring' and 'continuity of carer'. 'Continuity of caring' refers to care focused on the mother as an individual, which is underpinned by a shared *philosophy of care* on the part of the carers. Over the years it has taken various forms, such as birth plans and the midwifery process. Continuity of carer is an organizational concept, aimed at minimizing the number of carers involved with individual women, and has taken the form of 'domino' schemes, patient allocation in wards and, more recently, team midwifery.

The King's Fund Centre (1993), quoted in *Changing Childbirth*, suggests continuity of care is a philosophy of consistency of policies, practices and individualized care plans, best achieved through a 'spectrum of continuity' of carer (not necessarily only midwives), since one-to-one care is unrealistic. The woman builds up a 'relationship of trust' with her carers. Continuity in labour is seen as very important.

Jane Sandall (1995a), for the purpose of her research, defined continuity of care as 'a woman developing a relationship of trust with two or three carers throughout her pregnancy, birth and postnatal period, one of whom will be the named midwife'. Thus continuity of care is seen here to be about a relationship with a carer.

There are no standard definitions to be found. In particular, it is not always clear when 'continuity of care' is referring to the processes of care (activities that incorporate philosophies and attitudes and that develop relationships), or organizational structures designed to produce continuity of carer (and which also involve relationships).

In this chapter the processes of care are referred to as '*continuity of caring*' and the continuity of personnel within the structures of care as '*continuity of carer*'. The systems of care in which both these processes and structures involve continuity are referred to as '*continuity of care*'.

Continuity of carer is organized in a variety of ways, some of them overlapping:

- team midwifery
- midwifery group practices
- caseloads
- the named midwife

Team midwifery

The term 'team midwifery' was refined by the Institute of Manpower Studies (IMS, 1993) and quoted in *Changing Childbirth* (as above). Ian Seccombe and John Stock said:

> *There is no single accepted definition ... the central idea is that a small team of midwives takes responsibility for the majority of care of individual women, before, during and after the birth ... it is seen as a partial solution to providing continuity while accommodating a range of practical difficulties.*
> *(Seccombe and Stock, 1995)*

Teams can involve other health professionals. The three Royal Colleges of Midwives, Obstetricians and Gynaecologists, and General Practitioners (RCOG, RCM, RCGP, 1992) describe care as 'best structured ... as an equilateral triangle with the pregnant woman at the centre' of obstetric, midwifery and general practitioner care.

Regarding the midwifery aspect of the care, the central questions seem to be:

- How many midwives constitute a team?
- To how many women should they give care?
- What is the basis of the relationship between the midwives and mothers?

To help answer these questions, teams seem to be evolving into 'group practices' and 'caseloads'.

Midwifery group practices and caseloads

Denis Walsh (1995) described the group practice model as a group of about six community-based midwives, with a geographically based caseload. He feels this is a more fitting term than 'team'. His own group practice of six or seven midwives is the basic unit for audit, quality assurance, peer support, and autonomy of organization and practice. The midwives set their own standards, specifying the frequency with which mothers and midwives should meet. There is a named midwife for each woman. Thus each midwife has a caseload which is shared with the rest of the group. Only 10% of mothers will have intrapartum continuity. However, 'although the degree of continuity of carer is compromised, especially intrapartum, we believe *it is still a meaningful expression of individualised care antenatally and postnatally*' [my italics] (Walsh, 1995).

Like Denis Walsh, Heather Bower (1993), in her research on the implications of team midwifery for midwives, found that most of her subjects perceived 'personal caseloads' as meaning care given predominantly by one midwife but shared with the rest of the team, not with one other person.

The National Childbirth Trust said of caseloads:

> *When a midwife carries a caseload she is the primary care provider of midwifery care (the named midwife) during pregnancy, birth and the early postnatal days for an agreed number of women [in hospital or the community].*
> *(NCT, 1995)*

Each midwife would have:

> *... a reciprocal arrangement with a partner to ensure continuity of care ... when she cannot be available. Those carrying a caseload may form a group practice with midwife colleagues for ongoing support and peer review.*
> *(NCT, 1995)*

[See also Flint (1993)].

Lesley Page (Duff and Page, 1995) says her 'one-to-one' midwifery practice (an example of a caseload practice as defined by the National Childbirth Trust) 'describes the *relationship* between a midwife and a woman' with emphasis on individuality and equality in the relationship. Partnerships of two midwives who share a caseload are organized in larger group practices to provide practical back-up but also for similar reasons to those given by Denis Walsh (Page et al, 1995). Thus the structure of the 'one-to-one' scheme supports the process of a relatively intense relationship.

To summarize, the term 'midwifery group practice' can be used synonymously with 'team' but is more often used to refine the team concept by placing more emphasis on the idea of 'caseloads'. Caseloads can be taken by one or two midwives, with back-up spreading outwards in intensity from a partner to whole group support, with a corresponding variety of relationships between women and midwives.

The named midwife

The Patient's Charter and Maternity Services leaflet (DoH, 1994) says, 'you should be told the name of the midwife who will be responsible for your midwifery care'. *The Named Midwife* leaflet from the Patient's Charter Group (1991) says, 'the ultimate test of the named midwife concept is that the woman is able to say who her midwife is'.

In contrast to these literally meaningless statements, Caroline Flint (1995) suggested that 'being and becoming the named midwife' involves a personal and cosy 'relationship of trust' between the midwife and the mother.

As mentioned above, Denis Walsh (1995) incorporated the named midwife concept into specific standards for continuity of carer. This means the woman must meet the named midwife at booking and be seen by her at least once during the puerperium.

One service describes itself as having a 'named team' rather than a named midwife (Stock and Wraight, 1993), a caseload being assigned to a team not an individual.

So the 'named midwife' – like the other concepts behind 'continuity' – is an idea developed by professionals. It does not necessarily have any meaning to the consumer of maternity services. It can be just a name, a relationship with varying parameters or part of a structure with standards. It has even been applied to a group rather than an individual midwife.

Knowing the midwife

Kate Jackson (1994) suggested that 'knowing' in the sense of 'we've met before' could evolve, via more sophisticated service delivery, into the possibility of 'knowing' being a relationship of trust with a small group of midwives, with care from one of them in labour.

Many studies have defined the word 'know' for the purposes of research or audit in terms of whether the mother has met the midwife before (for example, Gready et al, 1995; Farquhar et al, 1996). In my own small evaluation of community team midwifery care (Lee, 1993), I asked the women to say what 'knowing the midwife' meant to them. The responses showed that a majority attached a specific quality and implied value to it, such as:

- 'the midwives are like friends'
- 'in labour she knows you as a person, not as a patient'
- 'if you have a problem they won't treat you as if you're stupid'

The midwives too, when asked the equivalent question, placed emphasis on the quality of the encounter.

For Caroline Flint (1993, 1995), to 'know' is to have a warm friendship with a named midwife, and the 'one-to-one' midwifery practice seems to offer the same perspective.

Rosemary Currell (1985) referred to a 'special caregiver', who could be a general practitioner, or a community, labour or postnatal midwife with whom the mother had a special relationship, deeper than that developed through meeting once or twice. In her study some women regretted not having this caregiver in labour, despite receiving good care. She speculated as to whether this relationship is to do with the carer's ability to focus on the individual woman and solve her particular problems rather than the fact that she was known.

It may be that 'knowing' is actually related to an *opportunity* to form a relationship, of which time is only one complex dimension, referring not only to numbers of meetings but the length of time of each meeting. Gillian Meldrum (personal communication) suggested that intrapartum continuity with an antenatal carer may not be important because there is usually time during labour for a midwife and mother to get to know each other sufficiently well for both to feel satisfied. Similarly, Patricia Murphy-Black's research (1993) showed that, in a unit where the mothers did not previously know the labour midwives, they 'felt it was easy to get to know them'.

These aspects are summarized in Box 1.2.

Box 1.2   Knowing the midwife

'Knowing' has been used as a quantitative concept related to previous 'meetings'. However phrases such as 'a familiar face' or 'a midwife who is not a stranger' (IMS, 1993) can be used to describe either numbers of meetings, length of time acquainted or the quality of communication. 'Knowing' can also be approached by asking: what does it mean for mother and midwife to know each other? The quality of the relationship may not be directly related to time but does seem to involve trust and perhaps other, unresearched qualities involving good communication.

The importance of continuity of carer

In the context of the implementation of *Changing Childbirth*, studies involving continuity are now beginning to accumulate. There are the inevitable problems of interpretation and comparison with each other because of the lack of rigorous definitions used and different research designs. This chapter concentrates on some that look at continuity of carer.

Women's satisfaction with continuity of carer

Some studies look directly at the relationship between satisfaction and continuity of carer. The Expert Committee which produced *Changing Childbirth* commissioned a MORI poll of women who had recently had a baby (MORI, 1993). Of those interviewed, 19% mentioned some aspect of 'continuity of care' when asked what would matter most to them in terms of care if they went through pregnancy and birth again. This was the most frequently rated category and was unprompted. However, it was still mentioned by a minority of women. The summary report did not – could not – detail what the 'continuity of care' category meant to individual respondents, and its importance appeared to be contradicted in other parts of the survey.

Findings may be clearer where the researcher specifies the meaning of 'continuity'. Sometimes a statement defining it is placed in a list of care items for mothers to prioritize. For example, Drew et al (1989) found that the following were the first three in a mean ranking of the importance of specific aspects of maternity care in a survey of 183 women:

- a healthy baby
- the doctors talking in a comprehensible way
- having questions answered by staff

Being attended by the same midwife throughout pregnancy was ranked 21st. No question was asked about intrapartum continuity. However, the list was compiled from preliminary interviews with 15 women on the basis of preferences voiced. It must be assumed that continuity of carer in labour was not considered important by them.

In my own study (Lee, 1993), findings relating to continuity of carer from the women's perspective were contradictory. Out of 32 women questioned, 26 had previously met their labour midwife and all but one were satisfied or very satisfied with this. They felt 'more comfortable' knowing their midwives but also said they would prefer care from a 'good, unknown' midwife than a 'known, neutral' one.

When asked to rank a list of ideal elements of care they would choose from a system of maternity care, 'knowing the labour midwife' was the most important. Yet when asked to rank ideal qualities they wanted in a midwife, the women placed the quality 'the midwife is known to you' much further down a list of qualities. A possible explanation for these contradictions is discussed later.

Morag Farquhar and colleagues' study of mothers' views of a team midwifery scheme (and non-team control schemes) showed that women felt they had 'formed a relationship' with their midwives if, antenatally, they had met no more than two of them (Farquhar et al, 1996). This group of women were statistically the most satisfied with their antenatal care and were actually in one of the control groups, not the team scheme. However, those receiving team antenatal care were the most likely to say that it was not very important to see the same midwife for all antenatal care. Perhaps this reflected their expectations of seeing many midwives in order to know their intrapartum caregiver.

Having previously met the labour midwife made a large majority of women feel more at ease. However, if they had not met her before, an equally large majority said it 'did not affect them one way or the other'. Since a third of the team women did not meet known midwives for labour but presumably expected to, those expectations did not appear to affect their views. However, because an actual experience of knowing the midwife did appear to meet with women's approval, the authors suggested that delivery by a known midwife could be regarded as 'the icing on the cake'.

Broadly the same results were obtained for postnatal care at home – knowing the community midwife was again 'the icing on the cake'. The authors suggested that 'the focus of continuity throughout pregnancy *and* childbirth and the postnatal period may be misguided' [authors' italic].

It has been suggested by Shapiro et al (1983) that the reason for high satisfaction levels with maternity services is that women's wants, desires and preferences have been so manipulated by those in positions of power that they do not realize their own needs. In other words, expectations are low. *Changing Childbirth* obviously aims to change this.

Maurice Porter and Sally MacIntyre suggested that low expectations may be due to the 'welfare orientation' of the National Health Service (Porter and MacIntyre, 1984). This may also be a reason for high satisfaction levels with care, regardless of the various types of antenatal care offered in their study; women just don't expect a 'free' service to provide anything better. They also suggest another reason might be 'a preference for familiar rather than novel care arrangements' because only when an innovation had actually been experienced was it rated more positively than a familiar system. This could also be an explanation for the findings of Morag Farquhar and her colleagues above. If so, the implications are that predicting reactions to as yet unknown innovations in care is unlikely to produce useful information and that people's innate conservatism will lead them to approve of any (reasonable) system of care provided they have sampled it personally.

My own anecdotal evidence from talking to colleagues is that it is women's increasing expectations of intrapartum continuity and the difficulty of consistently meeting them which is causing *some* of them dissatisfaction and disappointment when it is not achieved. Have women been given unrealistically high expectations which are only 'the icing on the cake' (Farquhar et al, 1996) and – especially in the context of increasingly limited resources and the practical limitations of providing 24-hour on-call facilities – are they so important?

Continuity of carer and other outcomes of care

Some studies find positive clinical outcomes are associated with good continuity of carer without directly asking participants' views about continuity and without showing a causal connection (e.g. Flint and Poulengeris, 1987; Lester and Farrow, 1989). In fact, Caroline Flint (1991) said of her 'Know Your Midwife' study, 'it is not known how much the observed effects of this style of ... care were due to the enthusiasm, personality and efficiency of the midwives'.

Claudia Martin (1990) found that women who always saw the same caregivers in pregnancy were more likely to be satisfied with information they were given and were more able to discuss things than those who saw different staff each time, and this was associated with satisfaction with care. This association of good communication with continuity was not claimed in the context of intrapartum care.

In a survey of over 850 women, conducted by the National Childbirth Trust (Gready et al, 1995), those who felt their midwife or doctor had 'got to know them' antenatally were significantly more likely to say that they had enough information and felt fully involved in decision-making, compared with those who did not feel known. Of those who knew their carer in this way, 90% felt involved in decision-making in comparison with 82% who felt involved but did not know their carer. This percentage difference is not great, so perhaps the actual significance of this aspect of 'knowing' is unimportant.

In the same study, labouring women who had previously met their doctor or midwife were significantly more likely than those who had not to experience similar positive communications with caregivers. However, whether they had previously met them or not, getting to know them prior to labour was *felt* to be unimportant by a majority of women questioned. This is strikingly similar to the results of Morag Farquhar and colleagues' study above.

Continuity of carer at different stages of care

In order to attain the goal of a known labour caregiver, antenatal continuity of carer may be sacrificed because in order to know the labour midwife, all the midwives in a team or group practice will need to be known (e.g. Flint and Poulengeris, 1987; Lee, 1993; Farquhar et al, 1996).

There is some evidence that continuity of carer may be important antenatally (e.g. Martin, 1990; Melia et al, 1991; Lee, 1993; Hemingway et al, 1994; Farquhar et al, 1996). There seems to be less work done on the value of postnatal continuity of carer both within the postpartum period and spanning the intrapartum and postnatal stages. However, some studies show it may have some importance (e.g. Melia et al, 1991; Lee, 1993; Gready et al, 1995).

Midwives' views of continuity of carer

Looking at the relative importance of continuity for midwives at different stages of care, two-thirds of the 12 midwives interviewed in my research (Lee, 1993) felt it was more important to get to know someone well antenatally and postnatally (yet not deliver her) than to deliver a woman they had met but did not know well.

In her interviews with midwives working in settings with various degrees of continuity of carer, Jane Sandall (1995a) found that the 'inability [of midwives] to develop meaningful relationships with women [was] a source of frustration and stress. The type of caseload... either enhanced or reduced the opportunities to 'know' women'. In some cases the stress was compounded by a commitment to an unattainable ideal of continuity.

Debbie Quinney (personal communication) suggested that continuity of carer for hospital-based staff means 'bumping into' the familiar faces of women, whereas for midwives in continuity of carer schemes, relationships with women become the important part of the continuity of carer concept.

Perhaps these last two examples illustrate that midwives' expectations about what kinds of relationships they should develop with mothers may influence their satisfaction with them. Others have found that a team philosophy is considered a reasonable substitute for one-to-one care (e.g. Bower, 1993). Similarly, Judith Dymond and Karen Tonkin said of their team midwifery scheme that it 'gives us the best opportunity to encompass our philosophy of care', and 'mothers really feel a sense of belonging which must be of psychological benefit' (Dymond and Tonkin, 1995).

The value of continuity of care is summarized in Box 1.3.

Four perspectives on continuity of carer

Caroline Flint (1993) used a slogan, repeated throughout her book which is 'get to know her'. It lies at the heart of the meaning of continuity and yet it is ambiguous as to whether the midwife should get to know the woman, or the woman the midwife. This exhortation can be viewed not only from these two perspectives but from two other dimensions also

---

Box 1.3   A summary of the evidence for the value of continuity of carer

From the women's perspective there is still a lack of research, and of opportunities to compare results of studies which have been done. Positive 'hard and soft' outcomes, other than satisfaction with continuity of carer, may be a better way to measure its value, but how quality of care is related to continuity of carer is still unclear. There is also a need to differentiate the value of continuity at the three stages of maternity care. Antenatal continuity may be the aspect to concentrate on.

Women's expectations play a part in their views. Traditionally, low expectations lead to high satisfaction rates with maternity care, and some evidence suggests that even with high expectations of intrapartum continuity of carer, most women's needs are satisfied without it. However, it is appreciated when available so perhaps familiarity breeds content. Also some women's expectations seem to play a large part in their degree of satisfaction with care, and for them intrapartum and postpartum continuity may be more than the 'icing on the cake'. How far can and should maternity care systems cater for these women?

The midwife's view of what continuity of carer means, and the quality of the relationship she develops with women, will vary depending on the type of system she is working in. Whatever the system, a midwife's view of her relationship with a woman she cares for will be different from the woman's views of that relationship because their roles and investment in the relationship are so different. So 'knowing' a woman will mean something very different from 'knowing' a midwife.

(Figure 1.1). This diagram is a model designed to organize the concept of continuity of care into a hopefully coherent and useful framework. It could be tested by various research methods and if necessary changed in the light of new evidence, but it is a start in tackling some unanswered questions, some of which have never been asked.

The model shows what 'knowing' each other means to two groups of participants in maternity care (midwives and mothers). There is a midwife's view and a mother's view. Each has a perspective on two aspects of 'knowing': on the idea of 'the midwife knowing the mother' and 'the mother knowing the midwife'. Thus there are four perspectives, represented by four quadrants – two for women and two for midwives.

Most mothers' primary concern is with individual encounters with professionals within the system. Midwives focus on the system in which they work, as well as holding views about their relationships with mothers. I believe there are – very broadly speaking – two types of midwives. Two systems of care are incorporated into the diagram, each including features which would best fit with the views of the midwives in those two quadrants. The arrows placed centrally on the diagram indicate which system of care each group of mothers is also likely to prefer.

The midwife represented in quadrant 1 focuses primarily on how the mother knows her and so, indirectly, on the quality of her own care for the mother. She is not so concerned about her own relationship with the mother. She will prefer to work in the care system of quadrant 1. The midwife represented in quadrant 2 focuses on her knowledge of the mother – on her own relationship with her – rather than on the mother's view of that relationship. She will prefer to work in the care system of quadrant 2.

There are also two types of mothers. One is concerned primarily that the midwife

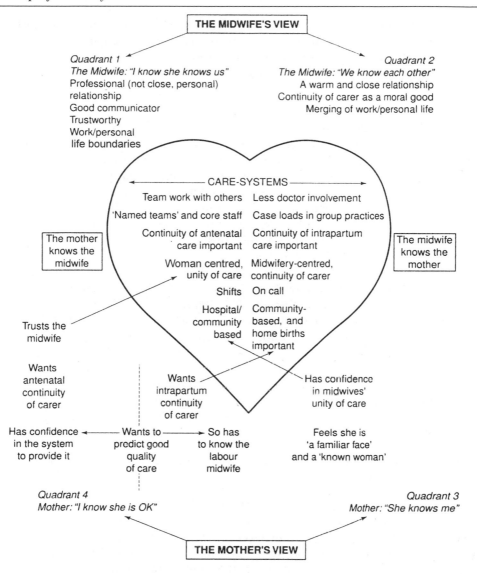

Figure 1.1 Four perspectives on continuity of care – a model.

knows her. Those mothers – in quadrant 3 – will be attracted to the system represented in quadrant 1. Some in quadrant 4 will want to know the midwives in ways that resonate with the view of midwives in quadrant 1 and so they will also be attracted by that system of care. However, a number of quadrant 4 mothers may focus on their relationship with 'their' midwife as the only way of knowing that they will get good care. They will prefer the more personalized care system in quadrant 2.

Needless to say, not all mothers and all midwives will fit neatly into these categories, but I suggest that most mothers and midwives will exhibit enough typical tendencies to fit one of the quadrants. Similarly, the two care systems are not rigid categories but represent tendencies on a spectrum of care.

The objective of these categorizations is to produce a model that will contribute to the further development of workable systems of maternity care. These types of systems do exist, but they are not necessarily in tune with the people who participate in them. Mothers and midwives need to be consciously matched with the systems which operate best for them.

Quadrant 1: 'I know she knows us'

This phrase tries to express the confidence of the midwife that the woman knows for herself that she will get good care, even if more than one midwife is involved. The relationship between mother and midwife has boundaries that probably exclude close friendship, but the midwives and women involved do not aspire to this. The midwife will be competent and trustworthy, a good communicator and able to make good professional relationships fast. This puts women at their ease and is a source of pride for the midwife who is happy with short-term relationships but still prefers to meet a woman several times, especially during pregnancy.

The midwife sees the mother as the individual focus of her care. This is a woman-centred model rather than a midwifery-centred model of care. There is 'unity' of care rather than 'continuity' of carer (Currell, 1985, 1990) (Box 1.4). Care would be given in a team situation, rather than as part of a one-to-one caseload practice. It could also be given by 'core' midwives and those in a traditional hospital or community service. Any structure that maximizes these care processes would be a good one. It could incorporate general practitioners and obstetricians. Patricia Murphy-Black's concept of 'continuity of caring' is useful here – a common philosophy of care, which the woman should understand (Murphy-Black, 1992). Attitudes are an important ingredient in successful care, as emphasized in *Changing Childbirth* and similar things have been said about nursing. Stephen Wright said:

> The named-nurse initiative will work only where nurses are able to use it as a medium to express sincere compassionate caring for another. *(Wright, 1995)*

In fact a named midwife is not a crucial part of the system if continuity of caring is effective. A 'named woman' may be more apt (Lee, 1995). This term emphasizes the individualized focus implicit in a woman-centred philosophy of care, whereas the 'named midwife' concept could be interpreted as putting the midwife at the centre of care. On the other hand, a 'named team' (Stock and Wraight, 1993) which works well together and whose members trust each other may also be a useful concept.

Continuity of carer would be likely at the antenatal and postnatal stages rather than intrapartum, where, if the quality of care is good – and the woman can confidently predict that it *will* be (Lee, 1993, 1994) – continuity of carer may not be necesssary (although during labour itself the number of caregivers should probably be minimized). A shift system rather than an on-call system is therefore possible, and consequently the midwives may feel their personal lives are less disrupted. They would have clear boundaries between work and home life.

It was suggested earlier that antenatal continuity of carer may be important because care is needed over several months. Thus teams could organize themselves to minimize the number of caregivers in pregnancy, thus possibly setting up a modified 'caseload' system at this stage of care.

Box 1.4 Unity of care

Rosemary Currell (1985, 1990) contrasts 'continuity of care' with the concept of 'unity of care'. *Continuity of care* describes the organization of the work of professionals and is not a description of the nature or quality of care. *Unity of care* describes a quality of care which is woman-centred, individualized and holistic.

She develops the 'unity of care' theme by briefly describing a type of relationship discussed in detail by Alistair Campbell (1984) in the context of nursing, involving 'companionship' and 'mutuality'.

Companionship:
The physical presence of a carer who accompanies another person on a journey (but only for a while) and who:
- helps with difficult aspects of that journey by 'sensing the need' of the other, even though this may be a challenge because of cultural differences or difficulties in 'getting on' together
- is sufficiently detached to allow the other to gain self-knowledge, in order to make appropriate decisions and be free to change *in his or her own way*: so being cared for rather than managed

Mutuality:
- Reciprocation with trust and confidence in the carer (words used over and over again by women describing good midwifery care)
- An opening up by 'the other' to receiving help from a professional – who encourages this because their skills and knowledge include 'empathetic understanding' (Rogers, 1967)

Empathy:
- Being able to put oneself in another's shoes, to view the world as if from their perspective but without losing the detachment which comes precisely from not being that other. This gives the ability to appropriately answer the questions: 'What is this person really saying?' and 'What is the meaning behind the words?'. It is about 'being with woman'.

Quadrant 2: 'We know each other'
This phrase attempts to encapsulate the warm and close relationship where the 'midwife is both friend and professional' (Flint, 1995). The 'named midwife' has a counterpart in the 'named mother'.

This relationship is seen as morally good and therefore continuity of carer is seen as a moral imperative. It is epitomized by phrases such as 'a cohesive philosophy of care. . . was no substitute for a known and trusted professional' (a quotation from *Changing Childbirth*) or 'Each time I read the report I am struck by the deep human wisdom which underlies the messages conveyed . . . changes we implement should create systems which support this spirit – a spirit of life-enhancement' (Page, 1992). Lesley Page is here referring to the Winterton report (Winterton, 1992) which preceded *Changing Childbirth*. This is a philosophy of continuity of carer rather than of unity of care, evolving from an enthusiasm and energy rooted in a deep concern about the way midwifery has become more and more subservient to the medical model of childbirth.

The system of care would be community-based and well integrated with local hospitals but with an emphasis on home births. Involvement of general practitioners and obstetricians would be discouraged. There would be an on-call rather than a shift system. Caseload midwifery with named midwives, working with partners within group practices, would be the best system to deliver this type of care. Continuity of intrapartum care would be emphasized because childbirth is seen as an important life experience and support from a loving partner as vital – both professional and non-professional.

Attitudes and approaches of midwives in this quadrant are crucial and the structure of care would aim to maximize their potential for forming close personal relationships with women and with colleagues. Their work is an important focus for their lives but this could cause overwork and overinvolvement, and sometimes possessiveness towards a woman (Sandall, 1995a; Sykes, 1994) and even dependency.

Rosamund Bryar (1995) said that 'to be a midwife is to use the self, the person who is the midwife, in the ... care of women and their families'. The midwives in quadrant 2 are very clinically and interpersonally skilled. However, it may be that in emphasizing the use of the self in this context, there is a danger that a medical model of care is being replaced with a midwife-centred rather than a woman-centred one (Fraser, 1995).

Quadrant 3: 'She knows me'
The phrase 'she knows me' attempts to summarize the confidence the mother has that the midwife knows what care she needs, through a commitment to a philosophy of consistent and individualized care, and because she has some knowledge of the mother's own particular needs. The phrase signifies approval of care and implies a good relationship, but her knowledge of the midwife may (only) be described as familiarity.

The system for providing this kind of care has been described within quadrant 1. Perhaps the 'named woman' (Lee, 1995) is also appropriate here, as illustrated by Claire Metcalfe (1983) in her study of changes in the method of organizing maternity care. Mothers were asked to explain what they meant by 'individualized care'. What was emphasized was:

> ... *the pleasant friendly nurse who remembered to call the mother by her name and did not try to 'fob' her off when she had a problem ... being cared for by ... friendly ... midwives who communicate well with each other, is just as likely to make her feel she is being treated as an 'individual' as is receiving all her care from the same ... midwife. [However] the majority of mothers did enjoy having the same ... midwives coming back to care for them.*   (Metcalfe, 1983)

Quadrant 4: 'I know she is OK'
This phrase tries to emphasize the security the woman feels that the midwife will look after her well. Thus the women in this quadrant feel their knowledge of the midwife is important, but this security can take two forms.

One subgroup of women in quadrant 4 will be confident that the system will provide good midwives, especially during labour. The results of my research (Lee, 1993) suggested that if antenatal care was perceived to be good, women could predict that intrapartum care by the same midwives would also be good, and fear of the unknown would be removed. Knowing the midwife might also enhance the perception of the quality of care. In this way the perception of the concepts of 'continuity' and 'quality' of that care could be confused. However, if the system is understood to be a good one, perhaps knowing individual midwives within it is not essential.

The reality for the woman is the brevity of the relationship. It will last for 9 months at most, centred on her particular needs during this time. For the woman there is continuity with 'midwifery' rather than with midwives. Thus the midwife is familiar and trusted but the mother does not have to know her name. Perhaps the relationship is best described by Claire Metcalfe (1983) in the last part of the quotation above. However, there is a second subgroup in quadrant 4 for whom personal knowledge of the midwife is more important, especially for labour, in a way that can be seen as a mirror image of the view of the midwives in quadrant 2. These women want a more intimate, intense relationship for an emotionally important day, with someone they know will give the care they want. This may be because they are not confident the system will give them this or because they feel personally vulnerable. In order to predict they will get good-quality care they feel they need continuity of carer.

Continuity as a distraction from the issue of good-quality care

Sheila Hunt and Anthea Symonds, in their book *The Social Meaning of Midwifery* (Hunt and Symonds, 1995), typify a view commonly held by midwives and commentators on the maternity services today. They argue that improving continuity of carer will give the mother more choice and control over her maternity care. However, I have argued that continuity of carer is not crucial to the provision of good-quality care and that 'unity' of care is more important to most mothers and most midwives. In saying this I am not denying that particular types of continuity of carer are preferable to no continuity; but by concentrating energy on finding systems to increase continuity, we are missing out on other ways of developing relationships with women which will increase the choice and control they have over their lives.

Suzanne Tyler (1994) argued that we are in danger of focusing continuity of carer schemes on women who already do reasonably well out of our health and welfare systems. The mothers who benefit least are the poor, the young and members of ethnic minorities – those who suffer greatest ill-health, poor nutrition and worst access to welfare benefits. Midwives should become more aware of the political and economic causes of these problems, the implications being that they can begin to educate themselves – and so women too – about these things. Understanding is the basis for action upon them. Suzanne Tyler cites examples of good practice in this field: a drug project, a young mothers' project and Ann Oakley's research on social support in pregnancy (Oakley et al, 1990). I would argue that these and projects such as the Newcastle Community Midwifery Project (Davies and Evans, 1991) are good examples of unity of care, which is not only about listening empathetically and dealing with emotional troubles and the physical problems of pregnancy: it is also about beginning to help women see that, if they can learn to gain more choice and control over this transient phase of their lives, they can begin to do it in their wider social world. Suzanne Tyler ends by saying:

> *Midwives must become more socially and politically aware, to work to make quality maternity care a*
> *reality for every woman.*   *(Tyler, 1994)*

John Mason (1995) goes further and argues that *Changing Childbirth* is a strategy for maternity care which appears to emphasize key neglected groups but ignores the 'long-term requirements for public health' – problems such as nutritional deficiency, infant morbidity (both of which make breast-feeding a political issue), and psychological and social stress. The concept of individual choice denies the fact that many people have no choice. Values of trust and co-operation are eclipsed by the culture of commerce and competition in today's NHS. Thus 'choice' refers to 'consumer choice' in the sense of: 'Shall I buy a dress from Gap or Next?' 'Shall I have my baby in hospital X or Y?' This level of choice does not help a woman with no money to buy a dress in the first place. If the two hospitals she can choose from lack the resources to employ enough midwives to give her attentive or even safe care, then the reality is no choice at all.

Perhaps there is also a real danger here that the emphasis on continuity of carer will mean midwives being held accountable for aspects of care which are politically beyond their control. Jan Savage (1995) discusses the same possible dangers with the 'named nurse' concept.

Perhaps the South East London Midwifery Group Practice offers a model of unity of care within a social and political context. It is a one-to-one caseload practice with an emphasis on community involvement and development. It has its own base in a poor inner-city area where it has a high profile and is in close proximity to other services and community facilities. It positively discriminates in favour of disadvantaged mothers. It is committed to running antenatal and postnatal groups and, through these, creating community networks of mutual support by mothers who are becoming more confident in decision-making and control through their maternity experiences. Continuity of carer is very good and clinical outcomes and satisfaction rates excellent.

While information about the practice (Demilew, 1994; South East London Midwifery Group Practice, 1994) does not focus on the quality of relationships between mothers and midwives, its structure and philosophy makes it likely that the emphasis is on unity rather than continuity of care. Is it this aspect or one-to-one care that is the successful ingredient?

In summary, I believe that to devote our energies to creating one-to-one relationships to 'empower' women focuses too much on the closeness of the relationship and distracts from wider issues. These issues include the problem of how to provide unity of care which, while satisfying the immediate emotional and practical needs of mothers, also addresses the real political world in which we live and work, in order to enhance the possibility of real choice and therefore control.

The medical model of health and maternity care self-evidently decreases the power of women. Our emphasis on continuity of carer is in danger of creating the 'midwifery model' mentioned earlier which does little to increase women's power and control. A truly 'women-centred' model of care would de-emphasize continuity of carer and examine other ways of being 'with women'.

THE IMPLICATIONS FOR WOMEN

A mother does not focus on the *system* of care. Strictly speaking she does not even 'want' continuity of care: she wants *good* care. She needs to understand the system only in so far as she needs to know how good care can be delivered to her. In this sense, continuity of care and carer are qualities, not quantities, of care. When discussing choices with the mother, continuity of caring and the different ways of achieving it need to be explored. Through this exploration the concept of continuity can be presented to her. By making these ideas explicit, women will become more knowledgeable, and some may be motivated to become involved with planning and monitoring of services.

I suggested earlier that many women's desire for continuity of carer stems at least in part from a desire to be able to predict her future (good) care by a (known) midwife, because she is unlikely to be able to control her care in any other way. If complete continuity is impractical or undesirable, then explaining to women the processes of care and alternative structures available to give it will enhance her confidence that she will receive good care regardless of knowing the carer.

THE IMPLICATIONS FOR MIDWIVES

The future of continuity of carer schemes is seriously threatened by the practical problems arising from the need for the constant availability of a 'known' midwife and the psychological stresses of the lack of control midwives have over their personal lives when operating an on-call system. This is documented by increasing anecdotal as well as research evidence (Bower, 1993; Lee, 1993; Stock and Wraight, 1993; Sandall, 1995b).

Jane Sandall (1995b) quoted evidence that 'midwives were trading off increased autonomy and job satisfaction with greater intrusion into their personal lives and increased demands for flexible work hours'.

Others, too, have perceived that providing continuity of carer is a balancing act, not only in terms of professional versus personal life but in terms of other advantages and disadvantages of the work (e.g. Lee, 1993; Wright, 1994; Wraight, 1995). In not providing continuity of carer, midwives may lose the professional satisfaction and clinical expertise gained from providing all three stages of maternity care. They may lose the sense of completion of a 'story' if they do not see a woman from the beginning of her pregnancy through the birth, to the end of postnatal care. A reasonable balance for some might be in working in the system of quadrant 1 of the model in Figure 1.1. Other midwives may choose to work in the system described in quadrant 2. The crucial point is that midwives as well as women *should* have a choice; and they *can*, because I do not believe their choices need reduce the choices of women.

IMPLICATIONS FOR PRACTICE

The implications of this chapter for service development are:

- Every maternity unit should have a policy of explaining not only their structures but also their processes of care to all mothers.
- The model of care outlined here, which has been extrapolated from existing evidence, needs to be examined by others and tested by further evaluation, audit and research. It assumes that women and midwives are different in their needs and in the importance attached to their differing expectations of the maternity services.

The model is therefore made up of a patchwork of smaller models which can fit together, in contrast to the blanket philosophy behind *Changing Childbirth*.

• If the model is confirmed by others to be a coherent and useful way of organizing information on continuity, then a majority of women are likely to choose a structure approximating to a hospital-based or community-based midwifery team. There will not be a guarantee of intrapartum continuity of carer although there will be some degree of antenatal continuity. A majority of midwives will be happy to work in this type of structure where unity of care is the basis of the service philosophy, incorporated into the processes of care.

• A minority of women and midwives will want to be part of a caseload practice, where one-to-one care with a partner within a group practice is the aim. This should be a choice available in most units and should *not* be considered to be the top of an elitist, two-tier system.

By providing structures of care and processes which take account of the individual needs of women, it should be possible to 'match up' those needs with those of midwives who work in the service.

VIGNETTES

The following are four stories loosely based on my own experiences which try to show that, whether or not there is continuity of carer, 'unity' of care (Box 1.4) is a more important consideration when judging its quality. These stories attempt to demonstrate companionship, mutuality and empathy – or the lack of it.

Bad continuity

It was Mary's first baby and third postnatal day. Joyce, her 'caseload' midwife, was visiting her at home. She had done most of her antenatal care and had delivered her, but this was the first time she had seen her since the birth. Joyce was looking forward to a debriefing session but she found Mary in floods of tears.

'Oh, Joyce, I just can't get her latched on properly! My nipples are so sore and I feel as if we've both been awake the whole night. What shall I do? I don't feel I can try any longer though I know it's important for her health and I *know* that everyone should be encouraged to breast-feed because of the baby milk companies... *but why am I worrying about all this now? I've got enough on my plate!' She gave a hollow laugh, 'Here am I – a member of the Baby Milk Action Group and I don't even want to breast-feed! I hate it and I thought it would be such a wonderful feeling!'*

Joyce was shocked and felt like crying herself. What on earth had gone wrong with her partner Judy's visits? All that effort she, Joyce, put in antenatally! Her group practice strongly supported breast-feeding and made every effort to encourage it, and all used the same research-based guidelines to educate women. She felt very warm and sympathetic to Mary's predicament. She was her *midwife and she was* determined *to help her.*

'Come on Mary. I'll make you a nice cup of tea and we'll try again. Don't cry – it'll all come right in the end. Everyone can breast-feed if they want to and don't give up. We won't give up, will we?' She eyed Mary encouragingly.

Mary dried her eyes, 'You know, Judy actually told me I didn't have to if I didn't want to – that it wasn't the end of the world if I didn't. I was angry with her for saying that but now I feel perhaps there was some truth in it. You know, Joyce, I really don't want to try any more.'

Joyce was speechless. She felt very angry with Judy for betraying their philosophy and, even more, for betraying her partner and for letting Mary down. Mary was her mother and she was determined to undo the damage – it was not too late.

Good continuity

It was Maria's second baby and she was 3 cm dilated and had just been admitted to the labour ward. She had tried to draw a veil over her first labour (abroad) as it had been so awful – long and painful, an epidural that never really worked, and a very efficient but cold and unsympathetic midwife she'd never set eyes on before. But she couldn't stop thinking about that first labour.

She was really pleased to see the team midwife. 'How good to see a familiar face!' she sighed. 'I'm sorry I can't remember your name – I get all your team photos mixed up, but somehow it doesn't seem to matter because I know you're all good. It's such a relief to be able to know you'll get good care!'

'My name's Jean,' smiled the midwife. 'I think we've met a couple of times before. It's your second baby isn't it? I vaguely remember you telling me you had a rough old time with the first. What was it that was so awful?'

Between the contractions which were getting worse, Maria talked through the worst feelings. 'You know, I expected to stay in control of the pain but it took me over and I felt I really let myself down. But anyway – plan B – I thought I'd retain control with an epidural but that didn't work properly! It was too painful to push and so – I felt so humiliated – I had one of those suction cap deliveries. The midwife was OK – she got me through to the end and she was obviously annoyed the epidural didn' t work but she couldn't seem to understand this 'control' thing I had – said I was obsessed and it was just better to get on with it and then forget about it as quick as possible.'

Jean asked whether 'control' was still on her mind with this labour. 'Yes, it really is. What do you think I should do about pain relief? I want to do it myself this time, and in any case I'm scared that the epidural won't work again.'

'Did you try TENS last time?' asked Jean. 'No, I wanted to but she discouraged me – to be honest, I think she didn't knew how to work it. Shall I try it now? I know the big advantage is that you can control it yourself and if I do need an epidural, you'll be there, won't you? I know I can trust you to do your best but – if the worst comes to the worst – you'll help me.'

Jean said she thought that was an excellent plan and she would be there. 'Thanks very much, Jean' said Maria.

Good non-continuity

It was the start of the late shift on the labour ward. Julie's heart sank as she entered the room from which screams were coming. There was no early shift midwife there – she had dashed off to catch her train – leaving only a harassed-looking young male SHO to cope.

The mother's name was Marcia. She was a primip. Julie had been told in report that 'she was an anterior lip with the head still quite high and quite out of control'. Julie thought she looked terrified – and so young – like the lost, wild-eyed young man trying to hold her hand. Julie took a deep breath. Looking deep into Marcia's eyes she said gently and more calmly than she herself felt, 'Marcia, Marcia, it's going to be OK if you just listen to me. I know it's painful and you're tired and frightened, but it will end, I promise you. Just breathe out – breathe out.'

She willed Marcia to look at her. She concentrated on that moment of communication. It worked. Marcia breathed out. 'You will stay with me, won't you?' was all she said, but she continued to breathe more calmly, and so did the rest of the room. The SHO said 'I was just recommending an epidural to Marcia because she's finding it so difficult and she's still got a way to go'.

'I definitely don't want no needles' said Marcia. 'My friend's had terrible backache since she had hers. I'm definitely not – don't make me. I'll do it myself if you stay and hold my hand' – to Julie, not to the young man. Julie

touched his arm and smiled. He relaxed a bit. Julie said, 'I think we'll just keep the epidural on hold and see how we go.' 'Excellent!' said the SHO, feeling he could now leave.

It was a struggle but they all managed. When it was over Julie asked Marcia what she was thinking. Marcia said, 'You know, I'm glad it was you, not that other midwife. She kept telling me not to worry when I asked her questions – as if that *takes away the fear and tells me what I want to know! I didn't know what to expect, I suppose – but it certainly wasn't all that pain... I didn't know what to expect of you midwives either... I had thought that that other midwife was OK but you were much better... but I didn't know that 'til you came in. Funny, really... I got the good and the bad – but* not *the ugly!' she laughed, as she looked at her son. 'By the way, I didn't catch your name. What is it?'*

Bad non-continuity

It was one o'clock and Jill was in the middle of a 'ticking off' (undeserved she felt) by a registrar. She still had two women waiting to see her. The phone rang. 'Er, antenatal clinic, midwife speaking – can I help you?' she said, as she forced herself to concentrate on yet something else – the nervous voice at the other end of the line.

'Yes,' said the voice, 'I wonder if you can help me. I'm five and a half months pregnant and I was bleeding yesterday and I went to my doctor's but he was very busy and he just told me to come up to see you. Anyway it stopped so I didn't bother. I've got two other children you see and it was teatime. But then I got worried this morning and I thought I'd better ring... do you think I'm OK not to come? – I'm so busy... and I haven't bled again today... I hope the baby's OK.'

Jill sighed – not another one! She knew she sounded impatient but people should understand how busy midwives are. Maybe something would be done about staffing then. 'Can I have your name and address, please?' She wrote it down. 'Well, Mia, anyone who bleeds at your stage of pregnancy should come in straight away. You should really have done what the GP said. We have the same rules here. You'd better come now. By the way – can you feel the baby moving?'

Mia said yes she could, but her heart sank. She knew something terrible was likely to be wrong from what the midwife said and yet what could she do? Her mum was ill and she thought her eldest was coming down with it too, and the little one was due out of nursery in half an hour. It was really a bad day to squeeze in something else. She was hoping the midwife would say it was OK not to come – or at least come tomorrow. This pregnancy had been such a problem to her, sometimes she wished it had never happened... poor little mite... was it going to be OK? If only there was someone she could talk to... the midwife sounded so harassed and she had her rules to follow like they all did.

Jill was saying, 'Look, I'm sorry, but you will have to come in to check the baby's OK. The chances are very good that nothing's wrong, but you don't want to take any risks, do you? I know it's difficult, but...' she tailed off. What else could she say? She'd have to cover herself. 'OK,' sighed Mia, 'I'll be up as soon as I can but I'll have to bring the two kids with me.' To herself she thought, 'I hope it's someone else on duty by the time I get there.'

REFERENCES

Bower H (1993) *The Personal and Professional Implications of Team Midwifery.* MA thesis, Warwick University.
Bryar RM (1995) *Theory for Midwifery Practice.* London: Macmillan, ch. 2.
Campbell AV (1984) *Moderated Love.* London: SPCK.
Currell RA (1985) *Continuity and Fragmentation in Maternity Care.* MPhil dissertation, University of Exeter. (Quoted with permission.)

Currell RA (1990) The organization of midwifery care. In: Alexander J, Levy V, Roch S (eds) *Antenatal Care: A Research-based Approach*. London: Macmillan.

Davies J & Evans F (1991) The Newcastle Community Midwifery Care Project. In: Robinson S, Thomson AM (eds) *Midwives, Research and Childbirth*, vol. 2. London: Chapman & Hall.

Demilew J (1994) South East London Midwifery Group Practice. *MIDIRS Midwifery Digest* 4(3): 270–272.

[DoH] Department of Health (1993) *Changing Childbirth*. Report of the Expert Maternity Group. London: HMSO.

[DoH] Department of Health (1994) *The Patient's Charter and Maternity Services*. London: HMSO.

Drew N, Salmon P & Webb L (1989) Mothers', midwives' and obstetricians' views on the features of obstetric care which influence satisfaction with childbirth. *British Journal of Obstetrics and Gynaecology* 96: 1084–1088.

Duff E & Page L (1995) 'One-to-one' a model for all? *Midwives* 108(October): 330–331.

Dymond J & Tonkin K (1995) The benefits of team spirit. *Nursing Times* 91(8): 63–65.

Farquhar M, Camilleri-Ferante C & Todd C (1996) *An Evaluation of Midwifery Teams in West Essex: Final Report*. University of Cambridge, Public Health Resource Unit & Health Services Research Group, Institute of Public Health.

Flint C (1991) Continuity of care provided by a team of midwives – the 'Know Your Midwife' scheme. In: Robinson S, Thomson AM (eds) *Midwives, Research and Childbirth*, vol. 2. London: Chapman & Hall.

Flint C (1993) *Midwifery Teams and Caseloads*. Oxford: Butterworth-Heinemann.

Flint C (1995) Being and becoming the named midwife. In Page L (ed.) *Effective Group Practice in Midwifery: Working with Women*. Oxford: Blackwell Scientific.

Flint C & Poulengeris P (1987) *The 'Know Your Midwife' Report*. Available from 49 Peckarmans Wood, London SE26 6RZ.

Fraser DM (1995) Client-centred care: fact or fiction? *Midwives* 108(June): 174–177.

Gready M, Newburn M, Dodds R & Gauge S (1995) *Birth Choices: Women's Expectations and Experiences*. London: National Childbirth Trust.

Hemingway H, Saunders D & Parsons L (1994) *Women's Experiences of Maternity Services in East London: An Evaluation*. East London and the City Health Authority, Directorate of Public Health.

Hunt SC & Symonds A (1995) *The Social Meaning of Midwifery*. London: Macmillan, ch. 8, pp. 145–150.

[IMS] Institute of Manpower Studies (1993) *Mapping Team Midwifery*. Brighton: IMS.

Jackson K (1994) Knowing your midwife: how easy is it? *British Journal of Midwifery* 2(10): 507–508.

King's Fund Centre (1993) *Maternity Care: Choice, Continuity and Change. Consensus Statement*. London: King's Fund Centre.

Lee GA (1993) *Community Team Midwifery Care: An Assessment of its Value and Meaning for Women and Midwives*. MMedSci research dissertation, University of Sheffield.

Lee GA (1994) A reassuring familiar face? *Nursing Times* 90(17): 66–67.

Lee GA (1995) The named woman? *Midwives* 108(May): 162.

Lester C & Farrow S (1989) *An Evaluation of the Rhondda Know Your Midwife Scheme: the First Year's Deliveries*. University of Wales, College of Medicine, Institute of Health Care Evaluation.

Martin C (1990) How do you count maternal satisfaction? A user-commissioned survey of maternity services. In: Roberts H (ed.) *Women's Health Counts*. London: Routledge.

Mason J (1995) Governing childbirth: the wider view. *Journal of Advanced Nursing* 22: 835–840.

Melia RJ, Morgan M, Wolfe CDA et al (1991) Consumers' views of the maternity services: implications for change and quality assurance. *Journal of Public Health Medicine* 13(2): 120–126.

Metcalfe C (1983) A study of change in the method of organising the delivery of nursing care in a ward of a maternity hospital. In: Wilson-Barnett J (ed.) *Nursing Research: Ten Studies in Patient Care Developments in Nursing Research*, vol. 2. Chichester: John Wiley.

MORI (1993) *Maternity Services Summary Report*. London: MORI Health Research Unit.

Murphy-Black T (1992) Systems of midwifery care in use in Scotland. *Midwifery* **8**: 113–124.

Murphy-Black T (1993) *Identifying the Key Features of Continuity of Care in Midwifery.* University of Edinburgh Nursing Research Unit.

[NCT] National Childbirth Trust (1995) *Midwife Caseloads.* London: NCT.

Oakley A, Rajan L & Grant A (1990) Social support and pregnancy outcome. *British Journal of Obstetrics and Gynaecology* **97**: 155–162.

Page LA (1992) Choice, control and continuity: the 3 'Cs'. *Modern Midwife* July/August: 8–10.

Page LA, Lathlean J, Campbell M, Vail A, Piercy J & Wilkins R (1995) *Progress Report: One-to-one Midwifery Practice.* London: Centre for Midwifery Practice.

Patient's Charter Group (1991) *The Named Midwife: Your Questions Answered.* Department of Health.

Polit DE & Hungler BP (1993) *Essentials of Nursing Research: Methods, Appraisal and Utilization,* 3rd edn. Philadelphia: JB Lippincott.

Porter M & MacIntyre S (1984) What is known must be best: a research note on conservative or deferential responses to antenatal care provision. *Social Science and Medicine* **19**(11): 1197–1200.

[RCOG, RCM, RCGP] Royal Colleges of Obstetricians and Gynaecologists, of Midwives and of General Practitioners (1992) *Maternity Care in the New NHS: A Joint Approach.* London: RCOG, RCM, RCGP.

Rogers CR (1967) *On Becoming a Person: A Therapist's View of Psychotherapy.* London: Constable, ch. 14, p. 284.

Sandall J (1995a) *Achieving Changing Childbirth Indicators of Success: A Multiple Case Study Approach of Organising Midwifery Care.* NHS Research and Development Scientific Basis of Health Services First International Conference.

Sandall J (1995b) Choice, continuity and control: changing midwifery, towards a sociological perspective. *Midwifery* **11**: 201–209.

Savage J (1995) Political implications of the named-nurse concept. *Nursing Times* **91**(41): 36–37.

Seccombe I & Stock J (1995) Team midwifery. In: Page L (ed.) *Effective Group Practice in Midwifery: Working with Women.* Oxford: Blackwell Scientific.

Shapiro MC, Najman JM, Chang A et al (1983) Information control and the exercise of power in the obstetrical encounter. *Social Science and Medicine* **17**(3): 139–146.

South East London Midwifery Group Practice (1994) Independent means. *Nursing Times* **90**(4): 40–42.

Stock J & Wraight A (1993) *Developing Continuity of Care in Maternity Services.* Brighton: Institute of Manpower Studies.

Sykes W (1994) *Forest Midwifery Group Phase I Evaluation.* Forest Healthcare.

Tyler S (1994) Maternity care and the paradox of plenty. *British Journal of Midwifery* **2**(11): 552–554.

Walsh D (1995) The Wistow Project and intrapartum continuity of carer. *British Journal of Midwifery* **3**(7): 393–396.

Winterton N (1992) *Maternity Services.* Second report of the House of Commons Health Committee (Winterton report). London: HMSO.

Wraight A (1995) Organizational styles and patterns of care. In: *Continuity of Care to Meet the Challenge of 'Changing Childbirth'.* Midwifery Educational Resource Pack 3. London: ENB.

Wright B (1994) *Caseload Midwifery at Queen Mary's Sidcup NHS Trust – the Evaluation of a Pilot Scheme Established February 1993.* Queen Mary's Sidcup NHS Trust.

Wright S (1995) The named-nurse initiative: what is the point? *Nursing Times* **91**(47): 32–33.

FURTHER READING

Malin N & Teasdale K (1991) Caring versus empowerment: considerations for nursing practice. *Journal of Advanced Nursing* **16**: 657–662. This article considers the difference for patients between being able to simply predict or actually control events during episodes of illness, and how this is influenced by the way nurses present information to them. They present information differently depending on whether they believe they have an empowering or caring role.

Tschudin V (1989) *Beginning with Empathy: A Learner's Handbook.* Edinburgh: Churchill Livingstone. This short book is a simple and practical way to begin to learn how to be more empathetic in relationships with others.

Berg M, Lundgren I, Hermansson E et al (1996) Women's experience of the encounter with the midwife during childbirth. *Midwifery* **12**: 11–15. This article describes a qualitative study which found that the 'presence' of the midwife was central to a positive encounter for the woman. Being 'present' involved treating the woman as an individual, enabling her to have a trusting relationship with the midwife, and supporting and guiding her on her own terms.

2

Continuity and choice in practice: a study of a community-based team midwifery scheme

Elizabeth R. Perkins
Judith Unell

This chapter is based on an evaluation of one particular team midwifery scheme in the UK. A description of the practical and academic context of the evaluation is followed by a look at the scheme itself and professional reactions to it. The findings of the main study, the views of women who had their maternity care under the scheme, are discussed in relation to choice and continuity, and the different interpretations which can be put on these much-used words. The chapter closes with a section on the implications for midwifery practice.

In 1994 we were asked, as independent researchers, to undertake a study of a new scheme involving three separate health-care trusts. It had been commissioned by purchasers using the principles laid down in the Winterton report (Winterton, 1992), and in fact predated the report *Changing Childbirth* (DoH, 1993). In 1993, when the scheme started, the intention was to introduce the new approach to maternity care gradually, beginning with two geographical areas and adding more as lessons were learned from the initial experience. Application had been made for funding to conduct a comprehensive evaluation including clinical issues, but delays in this process led purchasers and managers to seek an interim report based on the perceptions of the women involved in the first two areas. As discussions about the evaluation progressed, it was decided to extend the initial brief to include a systematic investigation of the opinions of midwives and doctors concerned; strong feelings had been generated by the scheme, both in support of and in opposition to it, and it was felt that the views of both staff and patients should inform the extension of the scheme to a wider area.

THE STUDY IN CONTEXT

Before launching into the findings, it is worth setting this study in its context. It is firmly rooted in the long tradition of studies of women's views of the maternity services (e.g.

Cartwright, 1964, 1979; Graham, 1979; Graham and Oakley, 1981; Oakley, 1979, 1980, 1992; Macintyre, 1982; McIntosh, 1988) which have contributed to the present rethinking of the principles on which it is based. Many of these have been undertaken by sociologists with academic funding and an academic base; they have stimulated further studies by consumer groups like Community Health Councils or the Association for Improvements in Maternity Services (AIMS): see Jones et al (1987) for a review. More recently, midwives have begun their own investigations of the views of their clients. These range from well-meaning enquiries which lack academic rigour but will undoubtedly have taught the investigator a lot, to highly professional research studies which belong in the academic league; the *Midwives, Research and Childbirth* series (Robinson and Thomson, 1989) includes many good examples.

This tradition, with its various strands, has contributed to the growth of interest in consumer satisfaction studies within the health service, which has now become a small industry on its own. In siting this study within that tradition also, we run the risk of trivializing its nature and its conclusions; at an early meeting we were challenged by an obstetrician who feared we would only be interested in asking women whether they liked the wallpaper!

It is true that consumer satisfaction surveys are vulnerable to oversimplification. There are considerable conceptual difficulties in transferring the consumer model from business to the health service (Stacey, 1976; Locker and Dunt, 1978; Calnan, 1988), one of the most crucial being the difficulties in handling the variable of patients' expectations. People who expect very little do not complain about care which professionals deem to be inadequate; Evans (1987) and Porter and Macintyre (1989) provide examples of this problem in broader studies of midwifery care. Statements of satisfaction with the service cannot therefore necessarily be treated as a statement that all is well. It is not surprising to find local studies that gloss over these problems and retreat from them to simple measures of general satisfaction and a heavy emphasis on the quality of the accommodation.

The current Department of Health emphasis on the need to take account of consumer views does make it easier, however, for imaginative health authorities to use scarce resources to commission more serious studies. If research on women's views of the maternity services is the preserve of academics or pressure groups alone, it will reflect their interests rather than those of the service.

THE SCHEME IN OUTLINE

Team midwifery schemes vary considerably and there is no agreed definition (Wraight et al, 1993; Chapter 1). Teams can be responsible for hospital care, community care, or both. In this scheme, teams covered both hospital and community care (with minor exceptions as shown in Box 2.1), and were based in the community, at local health centres. These arrangements replaced the traditional 'shared care' model familiar in most UK settings, where separate groups of midwives provide care in hospital and community settings, and women book with obstetricians for hospital care while also receiving care from their general practitioner (GP) in the community. The new system for maternity care is described in Box 2.1.

Two contrasting geographical areas were chosen. Each area had two community-based

Box 2.1   Team midwifery scheme: the options for pregnant women

From the pregnant woman's point of view, the scheme offered four packages of care, as follows:

Package 1: antenatal and postnatal care in the community, delivery at home by team midwife with GP support.

Package 2: most antenatal and postnatal care in the community, hospital visit for scan (multipara) or initial consultant interview and then scan (primipara), hospital delivery by team midwife, early discharge home, thus most of postnatal care in the community.

Package 3: antenatal care shared between community and hospital, but hospital visits kept to the minimum necessary for the woman's condition, rather than routine; delivery in hospital by team midwife; most of postnatal care in community, depending on discharge date.

Package 4: a specialized package of antenatal care for women with complex needs, provided mostly by hospital staff; delivery in hospital by hospital staff, postnatal care as appropriate.

Women opted for one package at the start of pregnancy, with professional advice, but their package could be changed if their clinical condition warranted this or – at least in principle – simply if they wanted to do so.

Most women could therefore expect to have most of their midwifery care from team midwives, apart from the tiny minority booked for package 4. The exceptions would be:

- hospital antenatal visits
- delivery on occasions when no team midwife was available
- non-planned postnatal care while still in hospital (team midwives visited scheme mothers in hospital as if they were in the community)

A team midwife would provide home assessment for women in labour who were booked for hospital delivery, to advise on the right time to go into hospital.

Women could choose which of the two hospitals they booked for (packages 2, 3 and 4), and were advised which consultant to book with (packages 3 and 4).

---

midwife teams, with individual staff attached to particular GP practices. The teams consisted of a mixture of community midwives previously based there and hospital midwives who had volunteered to work in this new way. All midwives were responsible for a caseload, drawn from their GP's patients, but continuity of care was to be provided by the team, rather than the individual midwife. There were, on average, seven midwives in each team (six full-time equivalents).

The first area, Ashby, was a small town on the edge of the main city, a primarily white, working-class district with a stable population. The second area, Westcliffe, was a suburb, mainly middle-class but with pockets of poverty; it was also more multiracial than Ashby, though still predominantly white. Two large hospitals in the city served women from either area; both were used in the training of midwifery and medical students. Greenfield Hospital had a larger site and its maternity unit was located in a separate building;

Townsend was one large modern block. Pregnant women from Ashby normally booked into Greenfield Hospital, which was nearest to them and had reasonable public transport links; women from Westcliffe had no predictable loyalties, though Townsend was somewhat nearer.

The key objectives of the scheme were summarized in the draft service specification for maternity services issued by the purchaser in 1992. The objectives relevant to this chapter can usefully be divided into those concerning midwives and those concerning mothers, though the specification was concerned with all professional groups. The new form of service delivery was intended to allow midwives to make fuller use of their midwifery skills, to make midwifery beds available in hospital, and to provide integrated management between the hospital and community parts of the service, leading to less duplication. For mothers, the scheme was intended to provide known professional carers, a choice of type of care, and more information about those choices, and a level of care appropriate to the normality or abnormality of the pregnancy (i.e. more community care for normal pregnancies). Box 2.1 shows the service as it was offered to women.

PROFESSIONAL VIEWS OF THE SCHEME

In principle, the scheme presented a challenge to established ways of working in the maternity services, and thus created considerable ferment among professionals. It was for this reason that the first stage of the evaluation, concentrating on professionals' views, was commissioned; purchasers and managers wished both to consult staff and to obtain an independent assessment of the strength of professional opinion in any particular direction. Accordingly, semistructured individual and group interviews were arranged with the following groups (numbers in parentheses):

- team midwives (13)
- hospital midwives (22)
- community midwives in the areas likely to be incorporated next into the scheme (13)
- midwifery managers responsible for the workings of the new scheme (4)
- GPs in the areas covered by the scheme (13)
- consultant obstetricians in both hospitals (9)

It became clear to us that the scheme divided professionals in a number of complex ways. Although team midwives, as might be expected, were the most positive about the scheme, there were supporters and opponents in all professional groups, and a number of widely differing issues were raised. Some felt that previous efforts to provide better care were being ignored by the new scheme; obstetricians pointed to previous efforts to reduce routine hospital visits for low-risk pregnant women; and hospital midwives at Greenfield felt their previous smaller-scale team scheme had been buried without trace.

Others pointed out the problems the scheme raised for midwives themselves, both professionally and personally; the extension of individual midwives' roles and responsibilities would certainly involve much updating and there were the inevitable concerns about safety in the new framework, a matter that this evaluation was not designed to address. Some professionals were worried about the implications of mothers making choices about care which they would not themselves advise – what if the worst happened as a result? Whose responsibility would a dead or damaged mother or baby be?

In addition, it was recognized that team midwives faced a considerable disruption of their professional and private lives, with the requirement to be 'on call' to go into hospital with women in labour and to stay with them throughout labour if possible. This is a major change from predictable shifts or the normal working day in the community. The early teams in the study areas were a mix of volunteers from the hospitals and those already working in the community. Some of those who worked in hospital or in other community areas, seeing the prospect of team midwifery approaching, had serious misgivings – what were the implications for midwives who could not drive, or who had dependent children and no automatic child-care cover at home? There were also concerns about safety for midwives when home visiting for assessment in labour at night in some of the more unsavoury areas of the city. All these are legitimate areas of concern; several of the contributors to Page's book on group practice in midwifery (Page, 1995) took these problems very seriously as part of the process of making such schemes work.

In assessing the scheme as it worked in practice, professionals tended to say that the extension of choice through the scheme was actually more apparent than real. From this perspective, home delivery had been available before, though with the usual problems of GP cover which the scheme did not change; few women wanted this anyway. There was little difference for most women between package 2 and package 3, since few obstetricians expected frequent hospital visits from low-risk women, and most antenatal care was therefore provided in the community; package 4 had only ever been used once. So what was new?

The issue of continuity of care therefore became the crux of the judgments on the scheme, but was interpreted in very different ways. There were GPs in group practices who described the careful arrangements they made to ensure continuity of care by the woman's chosen GP. One consultant stated bluntly that in his view the only kind of continuity which mattered was that of consultant care. Professionals from many different groups were concerned lest the relationship between community midwife and pregnant woman during antenatal and postnatal care be damaged in the effort to extend it to provide team cover for delivery in hospital.

In every group there were professionals who wondered how much it really mattered to women that they should know the midwife who delivered their baby – surely, said some, it is only important that the midwife should be competent and kind. Others were sure of the importance of the 'known midwife' and felt that the value of providing continuity, by team care, through pregnancy, delivery and postnatal care justified the disruption and 'teething troubles' the scheme inevitably generated. There was also considerable variation in the interpretation of 'delivery by a known midwife' – some thought this could include situations when mother and midwife had only met once, others thought that only a relationship built up through regular contacts really counted.

In all the areas of disagreement about the scheme, professionals tended to support their views by citing 'what women really want'; it was interesting to note that the more restricted were the opportunities for women to talk to the professionals concerned in a relaxed atmosphere, the more dogmatic their views seemed to become. Only one quoted more than anecdotes in support, a midwife who had done an interview survey in her own hospital about women's views of their care. All this unsupported opinion would have convinced us, had this been needed, of the wisdom of purchasers and managers in commissioning an independent study of the views of women who had experienced the scheme at first-hand.

METHODS USED TO INVESTIGATE WOMEN'S EXPERIENCES

The study was designed to give insight into the ways in which women perceived the care they received, and, where appropriate, how it differed from their previous experience. Owing to the complexity of the issues surrounding continuity and choice, it was felt that a small-scale, qualitative approach was required. This was also more appropriate than a large, quantitative survey, given the scale of the resources available and the speed with which findings were required. The purchaser was fully in agreement with this approach. Inevitably, this choice of method exposed the study to questions about the representativeness of its findings, particularly amongst professionals unfamiliar with qualitative research. However, the value of analysing a range of experiences in depth, even though drawn from a small group, was subsequently recognized.

Forty women, 20 from each area, were interviewed in their own home approximately 3–4 weeks after the birth, by a trained interviewer using a semistructured interview schedule. The schedule took women through their experience of pregnancy, birth and postnatal care in chronological order, enquiring at the appropriate times about the scheme's innovations, and including some demographic questions at the beginning and summaries of their views at the end.

The sample was constructed from a list of those who expressed their willingness to be interviewed – 36% of the total deliveries over the study period. This list was obtained with the help of the team midwives, who agreed to hand out a letter explaining the study and asking for a tear-off slip to be returned if a woman was willing to be involved. This system was cheap, but not particularly effective; there was considerable trouble with its administration in Westcliffe, where there was also a lower response rate, despite the expectation of higher rates in middle-class areas.

Despite these difficulties, however, the sample was socially broadly representative of the delivery populations from which it was drawn. Most women were between 25 years and 34 years of age, most had none or one previous child, and employment patterns varied as expected with the area, with Westcliffe having more women with professional or managerial jobs than Ashby. We were not concerned to maximize representativeness, however, but to maximize groups likely to be underrepresented. Efforts were made therefore to include women from ethnic minorities and women in poor material circumstances (indicated initially by the lack of a telephone – four in the delivery sample, all interviewed). Only one ethnic minority woman indicated her willingness to be interviewed (out of seven in the whole delivery population during the study period) and she was included in the study.

The same principles were applied to maternity care issues. The sample was intended to balance parity, with approximately one-third primiparas and two-thirds multiparas, thus giving more scope for women to make comparisons with care in earlier pregnancies. We planned to include any woman who opted for packages 1 or 4 during the study period (in fact none was booked during that time) and to aim for a rough balance of the more popular packages, finally interviewing 22 women who booked for package 2 and 18 for package 3.

WHAT KIND OF CHOICES?

Although the scheme combined attempts to improve choice and continuity, the two are in fact separate issues, and are addressed separately in this chapter. Many professionals were dubious about the extension of choice afforded by the scheme, arguing that the main elements were either in place earlier (choice of hospital, consultant or home delivery if GP cover could be arranged) or were between options that differed little (packages 2 and 3). There were also hesitations about the extent to which choice in this context was meaningful for all women; GPs and midwives would feel obliged to advise against certain choices for women with difficult obstetric histories.

Despite this, more than half the women considered that they had made a completely free choice, and most of the rest had either accepted a strong recommendation based on their individual circumstances and obstetric history, or had been happy to leave the decision to the GP or midwife. Only one woman identified a definite preference on the part of the midwife, and even she felt that she had been free to choose. There seems to have been no problem, therefore, for these women, in combining freedom of choice with professional advice. This sense of choice was explicitly valued by some of the study women:

> *The one I was on was 2. I'd know the midwife and she'd come with me for the birth and it was just a short stay in hospital. I can't remember about the other packages. I didn't pay much attention to them. I knew what I wanted and this package fitted the bill.*   *[Ashby 13]*

> *I'd discussed with my husband what we wanted and I found it was right there. I thought I'd have to fight for it, but it was actually available.*   *[Westcliffe 15, primipara]*

Our study evidence suggests that the professional concerns about choice or the lack of it tend to miss the point as seen by the women we interviewed. We asked about many different aspects of choice in care during pregnancy and childbirth, and it is possible to see these as operating at two different levels:

- Level 1 – explicit choice:
  of GP (within a group practice, or by changing GPs)
  of package of care
  of hospital for delivery
  of consultant
- Level 2 – flexibility:
  balance of GP/midwife care in the community
  clinic or surgery appointment with GP, day or evening
  hospital care for emerging clinical concerns
  change of package

Level 1 choices

On the whole women found the level 1 choices obvious and easy to make. The overwhelming majority of women stayed with the GP they already knew and trusted; everyone said that the choice of package had been straightforward; choice of hospital was made on the basis of previous experience (or that of friends or relatives), and convenience, with only a few opting for the smaller of the two units or asking advice from the midwife. When asked about their criteria for an ideal maternity service, about half the women from Westcliffe, where it was convenient to consider both hospitals, included choice of hospital in their first list, but it became very much less popular as fewer options became available (see below for a full discussion of this issue).

The majority of women in both areas said that they had not been offered a choice of consultant. Within this group, the multiparas said that they had been placed under the same consultant as before, and that they had had little choice last time either. The primiparas had all accepted their GP's choice. Of the 12 women who felt that they had actively chosen their consultant, four had sought guidance from their GP and four specifically requested a consultant who had cared for them before.

> *I wanted Miss X. I'd battled with her over [previous baby] but I thought she was very good and I certainly didn't want to change.* [Westcliffe 16]

One chose on negative grounds:

> *I knew I could say who I didn't want and that was the consultant I'd seen before.* [Westcliffe 20]

Three primiparas had based their choice upon recommendations from friends:

> *I chose Mr Y. I don't know why. I think I'd just heard that he was good.* [Ashby 9]

For most women, choice of consultant was not really an issue; when asked about their priorities for an ideal maternity service, it came very low on the list. This is not very surprising, since our evidence suggests that few GPs offered any information about different consultants' style or practice, so that women had little basis for making a choice.

Level 2 choices

The choices the scheme was explicitly offering were perhaps less important to women than the offer of choice itself, and the flexibility in the system which allowed women to tailor the care to their circumstances and needs. Most of this was to do with the pattern of antenatal care. In Westcliffe, most women were given a clear explanation at the beginning of their pregnancy about how their community antenatal care could be shared between midwife and GP. The vast majority felt that they had a choice about who to see, and – if they opted to see their GP – often a choice of time of day, since they could go to any normal surgery for their antenatal checks. This arrangement was valued both as a choice of professional and because it provided practical assistance in fitting appointments in with work or other child-care. The four who did not perceive a choice, however, were content with the pattern they had.

In Ashby, there was less choice and less widespread explanation. Some women were told early about how their care would be shared between the midwife and GP, but for others, the pattern simply evolved as they attended the antenatal clinics. The balance of care in this area varied between practices; alternating appointments with GP and midwife seemed to be the most common arrangement. Separate appointments with GP and midwife were almost universal in both areas, and these were popular.

Three-quarters of the women in Ashby said that they had not been able to choose whether to see the midwife or the GP. However, this did not seem to be a matter of great moment to them. They simply accepted the pattern that was offered and, in almost all cases, were satisfied with it. When asked if they would have liked to have seen more of their midwife or GP, only one of these women said she would have liked something different. This was someone who clearly did not like her GP and would have preferred not to have seen him at all! The few women in Ashby who felt that they did have a choice over the pattern of care had not felt the need to exercise it. Nonetheless, they were appreciative of the offer of flexibility:

> *It alternated but if I wanted an extra visit to the doctor, I could – there was no strictness about it. It was*
> *very flexible.* [Ashby 12]

The overwhelming majority of women welcomed the reduction of hospital visits from the norm of the traditional pattern, and the improved speed with which necessary visits could be made. Women who had been asked to attend frequently said that they believed this to be because of their particular circumstances, and no one said that there had been too many visits. Many of the multiparas contrasted this pregnancy sharply with earlier ones:

> *It was much better! I had to make sure I took sandwiches and a drink with me when I went to hospital*
> *with David [previous baby]. I went at least four or five times, and wasted the best part of a day each time.*
> *[Ashby 20]*

Antenatal care, when offered primarily in the community, was clearly perceived by women as offering a considerable increase in flexibility over a pattern that included many hospital visits. Despite the general changes in the pattern of antenatal care in this direction which predated the new scheme, two of the women in the study were aware of a considerable difference from current care in other areas:

> *Myself and my husband went to classes and met people from other areas, and they were very envious of*
> *my being in this scheme – they complained about their long hospital visits, having to take time off, etc.*
> [Westcliffe 13]

> *The second [hospital visit] was unnecessary. The first time I had to give all the details about myself, they*
> *had my notes from [previous baby] but they said they couldn't use that. It was ridiculous, having to repeat*
> *it all again.* [Westcliffe 12 (moved into a team midwifery area part way through pregnancy)]

The final element of flexibility in antenatal care offered by the scheme was the opportunity to change packages if this was clinically necessary. No one was actually aware that this had happened, though women recognized changes in their pattern of care which could well have indicated this:

> *I think it probably was [changed] because of the caesarean at the last minute, but I didn't really ask*
> *about the package. I just trusted them to do the best for me.* [Ashby 7]

It is possible that the most important elements of choice for women lie in the flexibility offered to them – from the evidence of this study, to fit in their antenatal care with the rest of their life. Flexibility comes from a mixture of structures and individual willingness to offer small choices. The structure of the scheme put a new emphasis on the community contribution to antenatal care, including taking booking interviews out of hospital. The GPs in Westcliffe gave women a basic framework for antenatal visits and left them to sort out who they would see at any one visit, and therefore what surgery or clinic they would attend.

The willingness to make efforts to accommodate maternity care to everyday life, and to provide such small, ongoing choices, are not confined to antenatal care. Freeley (1995) described graphically the contrast between the flexible, informed care for the whole family (including the 'man who has difficult pregnancies') offered by the team midwives who cared for a woman in her third pregnancy, with the discontinuities and misunderstandings which started when she went into labour with her fourth, in a more traditional system. Perkins (1980a,b) and Kirkham (1983) have both detailed the effective deprivation of choice experienced by ill-informed women and their partners who feel ill at ease in labour with midwives they do not know, in the unfamiliar environment of hospital. While choice and continuity are separate issues, and should be analysed separately, the small choices which often matter most to women may be promoted as successfully by continuity of care as by structures which proclaim choice but cannot actively support it in detail.

CONTINUITY

Our study set out to explore women's perceptions of continuity at all stages of maternity care. It also sought to discover precisely which aspects of continuity mattered most to them. Many of the findings challenged commonly held professional views on this issue.

Antenatal care

Continuity of GP care
There was a high level of continuity of GP care during the antenatal period. All but three of the Ashby women said that they had seen the same GP throughout. Of the remainder, two were registered with a practice where the two partners alternated in taking the antenatal clinics. All the Westcliffe women saw the same GP throughout, except for two who saw another in an emergency or when their GP was on holiday. More than half the women in both areas felt that this continuity had been important to them. This was because they knew the GP well and felt confident about the care that would be given. One woman in Ashby and three in Westcliffe said that it was particularly important to her that her GP was female.

A quarter of women in both areas said that it did not matter to them whether or not they saw the same GP. In three cases in Ashby, this was because they saw the midwives as primarily responsible for their care.

Care by the scheme midwives
Clear messages had been conveyed to most of the women about how their antenatal care would be organized by the scheme midwives. Everyone understood that antenatal care would be provided through the team rather than through a single midwife.

> *When the midwife did the booking she said my midwife would be X, but... it was explained to me that which midwife you get depends on who's on duty at the time.* [Ashby 15]

In both areas, therefore, continuity of care was defined from the beginning in terms of shared responsibility by a group of midwives.

The women were asked how many scheme midwives they had seen in the antenatal period. In Ashby, the largest number was 5 and the lowest was 2, with an average of 3.6. Some women included the midwives they had met at antenatal classes; others mentioned only those who had given personal care. In Westcliffe, the range was between 2 and 10, with an average of 4.0.

The numbers of midwives encountered in the community had risen significantly under the new scheme, although it must be remembered that women would have seen more hospital midwives under the old scheme. Information from the 13 multiparas in Ashby revealed that the average number of community midwives they had seen during their previous pregnancy was just 1.5; the comparable figure for Westcliffe was 2. Nonetheless, all but one of the Ashby women said that the number of team midwives providing care under the new scheme was 'about right'. Only one woman, who saw 5 midwives, felt that too many had been involved. In Westcliffe, one woman, who saw 4 midwives, felt she had seen too few, and two felt that they had seen too many midwives. These were women who estimated seeing 4–5 and 8–10 midwives respectively and could not identify a particular midwife or midwives who had provided most of their care.

> *No names were given, it was 'the Group' or 'the Hazel team', but I got increasingly dissatisfied as I saw someone different every time I went. I was quite rude to some of the midwives.... It turned out that the person I was rude to was from the Sycamore team, but I didn't know that at the time.*
>
> *[Westcliffe 16 (8–10 midwives)]*

This was unusual; women were generally able to name the midwives who had looked after them most. Almost three-quarters of the women in both areas identified a particular midwife. Of the remainder, half named two midwives who had cared for them most and half said their care had been shared equally. This suggests that although the numbers of midwives providing care for each woman has risen overall, there is ample opportunity within the scheme for personal relationships to develop between women and their midwives.

The quality of these relationships is clearly an important issue. In order to shed more light upon it, the multiparas were asked how their relationships with their midwives during this latest pregnancy compared with last time. Two-thirds of the women in Ashby said that their relationship was better this time; all but one of the remainder said it was the same, and the last woman simply said that it was different but did not express a preference either way. None of the women said that they had enjoyed a better relationship with their midwife last time.

In Westcliffe women were less uniformly positive, but there was still a majority (seven) of multiparas experiencing a better relationship this time, with three saying it was the same, and two saying it was better last time (one of these had had a 'domino' delivery, by the midwife who took her antenatal classes.) A messy antenatal period could be redeemed after the birth: even the highly dissatisfied woman quoted above said:

> *It was closer this time, funnily enough.... It all made sense after the birth, but the experience during pregnancy was a shambles.*   *[Westcliffe 16]*

The reasons most often given for relationships being better this time were that the midwives were friendlier and the care was more relaxed:

> *It was more businesslike last time; this time it was like going to see a friend.*   *[Ashby 2]*

While they clearly valued their close relationships with one or two midwives, the women liked the opportunity to get to know others, and felt that this was a significant improvement over last time.

> *I wouldn't say there was any relationship last time at all. This time it was far better because even the midwives in the other doctor's team I'd seen coming out of antenatal classes and they had their photo on the wall. It seemed that they were a lot more involved.* [Ashby 15]

Antenatal visits to the hospital

The average number of visits to hospital for the women was 2.85 in Ashby and 3.75 in Westcliffe. In Ashby, package 2 women attended less often than those registered under package 3. The average number of visits for the former was 1.6 while for the latter it was 5, although this figure was skewed by two women who had an unusually large number of visits. Official records about the women's choice of package in Westcliffe were too unreliable to attempt a similar comparison. Only four women, two from each area, experienced complications that required a hospital stay, and in all cases these were of short duration.

The multiparas in the group were asked to compare their experiences with what had happened in earlier pregnancies. Almost two-thirds of those in Ashby said that they had had more visits last time *and* that those visits had been longer. Of the remainder, one said that both the number and the length of visits had been the same, and one was unable to compare because she had not been in the area at the time. The rest said that they had had the same number of visits last time but that they had been much longer. The emphasis in Westcliffe was that the visits were shorter, rather than less frequent, which is consistent with them having a higher average number of visits than the Ashby women.

How far the movement towards fewer and shorter visits to hospital for these women could be attributed to the new scheme was questionable. For example, it is normal for women to have more visits when pregnant with their first baby. Also, independently of the scheme, there was a trend to provide most care in the community. Furthermore, Patient's Charter targets on waiting times may have had an effect upon the average length of hospital visits. The data from Ashby do, however, suggest that the scheme had accentuated the general trend for women opting to have most of their care in the community.

Whatever the reason, the new pattern was warmly welcomed by the women in the study. It promoted a stronger sense of continuity of care within the community and allowed women to arrange their antenatal care more flexibly to fit in with their working and child-care commitments.

Labour

Labour was the touchstone for assessing the success of the scheme. The new system of antenatal care had been introduced primarily in order to achieve continuity of care into labour and beyond. Unless the scheme could deliver a degree of continuity which was valued by women and which significantly enhanced their experience of giving birth, it would be difficult to justify the financial and human costs of extending the scheme more widely.

Home assessments

Home assessment worked very smoothly. No one had difficulty getting in touch with a midwife initially, and most had at least one visit at home to confirm labour and advise on what to do next; those who did not had either been advised to go straight into hospital without waiting for the midwife to visit, or were booked for induction. This extension of the service was appreciated:

> *Under the old system I'd have gone in early in the day, my children being unnecessarily looked after by a friend. And I'd have sat there all day doing nothing. … It was important to me to know that it was the real thing – saved a lot of organization and aggravation, and embarrassment too!*   *[Westcliffe 1]*

The scheme midwife as a bridge between hospital and community

The role of the scheme midwife as a bridge between the known community and the unknown hospital labour ward was mentioned frequently. Many of the mothers reported pleasure at finding their midwife 'waiting for them at reception' or 'walking down the corridor'. Several mothers with previous children mentioned spontaneously that they had liked not having to report at reception and give details about themselves; the scheme midwife had already done this and they felt expected and welcomed.

Care in labour

The picture of care in labour is much more complicated. The complexity comes from the number of different definitions of continuity that are circulating and the difficulty of applying these to the actual experience as reported by each woman.

The scheme aimed to offer care by a member of the midwifery team, preferably but not inevitably a midwife known to the woman. This tended to be summarized and presented as delivery by a known midwife, but both professionals and women recognize that this will not apply where medical intervention is necessary. Nearly all women in the sample had *care from* a scheme midwife for the whole of their labour.

Where a scheme midwife was present throughout, it was generally the same person, although there were examples of two midwives providing care simultaneously, and of handovers between midwives during early labour (but not at the later, more critical stages). Continuity of care by the scheme midwives through labour was therefore very high. However, just over a third of the women were *delivered by* someone other than a scheme midwife – mostly by hospital doctors following an unanticipated complication. Nonetheless, the continued presence of the midwife was valuable to the women concerned:

> *But it was nice that she was there. I wouldn't have liked it if X had left.*
>
> *[Westcliffe 19 (Caesarean section)]*

The questionnaire was designed around the emphasis within the scheme on delivery by a known midwife, taking into account the various definitions of 'known' which are in circulation. Accordingly, we asked whether women were delivered by a scheme midwife they had met before, and we also asked, through forced choice questions, about the quality of the existing relationship with this midwife, the options ranging from 'a close personal relationship' to 'I hadn't met her before'.

The findings were that only half of the women were delivered by a scheme midwife whom they knew. These figures are, however, skewed by the significant minority who were, in the end, delivered by hospital staff. If the latter are excluded, the picture looks rather different. For example, of the 14 women in Ashby who were delivered by a scheme midwife, all but two had met her before, and six said they had met her regularly during the pregnancy. Most of the remainder said that they had met her more than once. In Westcliffe eight of the 13 women in this category had met their midwife before but only three had seen her regularly during the pregnancy.

With regard to their existing relationship with the scheme midwife who delivered them (once again excluding those delivered by hospital staff), half of the Ashby women said they had a close, trusting relationship, and almost as many said that they had met her and liked her although they did not know her that well. The pattern differed somewhat in Westcliffe where only two said they had a close, trusting relationship, six said that they had met their midwife and liked her although they did not know her that well, and four had not met her at all.

These findings suggest that the scheme was achieving a degree of continuity through antenatal care, labour and delivery, despite in many cases falling short of the 'ideal' of delivery by a well-known and trusted midwife. It must be remembered too that by focusing women's attention upon the person who performed the delivery, the interview did not systematically collect similar information about midwives who had attended throughout labour but who did not deliver the baby. If it had done so, the pattern might well have looked rather different.

What is indisputable is that the scheme was providing an impressive amount of continuous, personal midwife support for women during labour itself. This aspect of the scheme received little attention from the professionals in the earlier phase of the study but it was clearly something which was highly valued by the women. The fact that they were rarely left on their own during labour, and the efforts made by the midwives to see them through the entire experience until they were comfortably settled in the postnatal ward, were remarked upon appreciatively. For the multiparas in the interview group, it was this element of continuous, personal care which most sharply differentiated this labour from previous labours:

> *I had a whole trolley-load of midwives last time and I didn't know any of them.*   [Westcliffe 16]

> *Last time there were more people coming in and out, student midwives and student doctors. It didn't bother me much, but it was better this time – more personal.*   [Ashby 15]

Only one woman forgot the name of any scheme midwife who cared for her in labour, excusing it by reference to the effects of pregnancy on memory; where hospital midwives were involved, the impression was that they had no names to forget! The overriding impression is of care that was given from person to person, rather than from anonymous professional to anonymous patient.

The concept of a 'known' midwife
There was no consensus among the professionals we consulted about the definition of a 'known' midwife. There were broadly two views. Some said that it was a matter of a woman having met her midwife before delivery; others said that it meant a close personal relationship between the two. Both camps claimed that women shared their definition.

In order to find out women's own opinions on this question, the concept was refined into four definitions, graded according to the frequency and closeness of the relationship between woman and midwife. The results showed that many women were content with a very loose definition of a 'known' midwife. Across the two areas, almost half said that it would be enough for a woman to meet her once or twice. This view was challenged, however, by a sizeable subgroup of just under one-third (with a particular concentration in Ashby) who said that it would be necessary for a woman to meet a midwife often and for her to feel that the midwife knew her as a person. Almost all the remainder took the intermediate position that it would simply be necessary to meet the midwife often.

The evidence from this study is that women do want care from a known midwife during labour and that they do want the option of being delivered by a known midwife. However, women are prepared to be more flexible and realistic in their definition of 'known' than are many professionals. While a close existing relationship may be ideal, women appear to derive considerable benefit from being cared for by a midwife with whom they have had some degree of contact during pregnancy. This provides a bridge into an unfamiliar environment; personal care by someone who knows about you from the community; continuity of care which will be broken, if it has to be broken, for human rather than institutional reasons; and, very importantly, not being left alone.

Even those women who had not previously met the scheme midwife who attended them derived comfort from the fact that she came from their own area. Feelings of trust towards the midwives they knew were readily extended to colleagues they did not know. Implicit in this was a belief that all the scheme midwives would be working to similar values and standards.

Postnatal care

Care on the ward

At the time of the interviews, it was the practice for the scheme midwives to provide care on the wards for the women from their areas. The pattern, as expected, was of short hospital stays for most women. Three-quarters of the Ashby women and just over half of those in Westcliffe went home within 48 hours; those who stayed longer did so for the usual mixture of medical and family reasons.

The scheme midwives visited regularly, once a day or more. Only two women had no visit, one because she had given birth in the evening and was discharged the following morning, and the other because of a muddle over discharge arrangements which she solved by going home. One woman in Ashby who had had a caesarean delivery explained that she had been under continuous medical care afterwards and, although the scheme midwives had visited socially, it was the hospital staff who actually looked after her.

Almost all the rest had a good level of continuity, seeing just one or two scheme midwives whom they knew already. Postnatal care on the ward from the scheme midwives had a number of elements. Most women mentioned the usual personal care and postnatal checks for mother and baby. Some also said the midwife had given advice or demonstrations on baby care, and many mentioned with appreciation that the scheme midwives had talked to them, sometimes about the birth but also about other things. Thus the midwives were prepared, when required, to take on the 'debriefing' of women following labour (see Chapter 7).

It was interesting that when asked what the ward staff had done, there was no mention of conversation, and a less frequent mention of practical care or checks. In general, the care given by the ward staff was fairly low-key – for example, providing paracetamol and ice-packs or holding a crying baby. When more active care was given, this appeared to be in response to an expressed need rather than as a matter of routine. This may well have reflected an expectation on the part of the ward staff that the scheme midwife had the anchor role in providing both practical care and emotional support.

All women were asked how important they thought it was to have a scheme midwife visiting them on the wards. There was a clear difference here in the responses of the two groups of women, with half of the Westcliffe women saying it was really important to them, compared with only one-fifth of those in Ashby. Almost half of the Ashby group said that it was nice but that it was really a bonus. Only two women, one from each area, felt that it would have been simpler to have been cared for by the hospital staff.

This element of the scheme was clearly valued by the women but was less critical to them than the care they received at other points. From the perspective of the professionals, ward visiting by the scheme midwives was widely criticized as wasteful of resources and as involving midwives in unnecessary time spent in travelling and parking. A decision to discontinue the visits was in fact taken during the course of the study.

Postnatal care at home
Considerable concern had been voiced by some professionals in the earlier stage of this study about the possibility that the quality of postnatal care in the community was suffering because of the efforts put into arranging delivery by a known midwife. The concept of care by a team, it was argued, inevitably diluted the continuity provided by the single community midwife attached to a GP practice.

The initial results seem at first sight to support the concern, since over half the sample had visits from more than three midwives. Multiple midwife involvement was particularly evident in Ashby where five women had visits from five midwives each, and one woman saw six midwives. The corresponding figures for Westcliffe were that two women saw five midwives, one woman saw six and one woman lost count! The average number of visits was 3.8 for Ashby and 3.5 for Westcliffe, the latter excluding the woman who lost count.

It was clear that such a large number of midwife visitors did stretch some women's tolerance. Six women – three in each area – felt that they had seen too many. However, the remainder of the women said that the number of midwives had been about right, and there seemed to be a readiness to accept that the ideal of having just one or two midwives involved was unrealistic under the new system:

> *It would have been nice to have just the one, but of course it depends on the rota and they were all very*
> *good.* [Westcliffe 5 (four midwives)]

Two factors seemed to be important in women's acceptance of multiple midwife involvement. The first was knowing the midwives concerned. A succession of familiar faces was clearly more acceptable than being visited by strangers. It was striking that a large majority (17) of the Ashby women had met all the midwives who visited and were able to name them individually. The remaining three women, each of whom had four or more midwife visitors, could name all but one – in each case this was a midwife from a different practice. In Westcliffe, however, the women were less likely to be visited exclusively by midwives they had met before. Just under half said they had met and could name all of them.

The second factor was that an element of continuity was achieved through care being provided mainly by a midwife whom the women had seen in pregnancy, or from the midwife who had cared for them during labour, where this was a different person. For several women, the bond with the delivery midwife seemed to be as strong as with the midwife they had known for longer, and a few expressed a preference for the latter providing most of the postnatal care.

Professional concern about continuity focused particularly on the possibility of postnatal depression and the need for mutual trust to explore this. We therefore asked mothers whether they felt they could talk to the midwives about how they felt, and whether there was a particular person they would choose for such issues. All said that they could have talked to the midwives, although most had not felt the need to do so. For those who did feel low, having a particularly sympathetic and well-known midwife to turn to was a lifeline.

> *Yes, especially in the first week I was quite low and hadn't had much sleep and I told the midwife I had shouted at the baby. But she said I was quite normal to feel like that and I wasn't being a dreadful mother; that was really encouraging.* [Westcliffe 7]

Although most women, asked whom they turned to, or would have turned to in need, named either the main antenatal midwife or the delivery midwife, a few chose others they had got to know during the postnatal period or said that they could have confided in all their midwives equally. Having several midwives visiting does offer a choice of confidante.

On the whole, the women were very satisfied with the postnatal care they received within the scheme; it appears to have met their needs, and the results from the study sample dispelled the worst professional fears about discontinuities. Efforts to plan postnatal visiting to include the delivery midwife and reduce the overall number of visiting midwives were likely to be repaid by even higher levels of satisfaction.

WHAT REALLY MATTERS TO WOMEN?

The early interviews with professionals showed the range of views held, often strongly, about what really matters to women about the care they receive. Women's perceived priorities are often used to justify particular professional attitudes and practices. The interview survey provided an opportunity to find out what women themselves believe to be important. Towards the end of the interview, each woman was presented with a list of choices and opportunities available under the scheme (Box 2.2).

The women were first asked to identify *any* of the options in Box 2.2 which they felt mattered to them. Their initial shortlist showed a remarkable similarity in responses between the two areas. Overall, the aspects of care that were identified most frequently as being important were to be visited at home after the birth by a midwife who had provided care throughout pregnancy (option g) and to be delivered by a midwife known during pregnancy (option e). Following close behind were the opportunity to have antenatal care provided mainly in the community (a) and being visited at home by the midwife who had delivered the baby (h).

The women were then asked to refine their initial shortlist by picking out the three aspects which were most important to them. Again, there was an overall consistency between the two sets of responses. When the women's top three nominations were combined, three clear front-runners emerged. These were: having antenatal care mainly in the community (a); being delivered by a midwife who provided care during pregnancy

---

Box 2.2   Options offered

(a) Having my antenatal care mainly in the community
(b) Being able to choose whether I have a home delivery
(c) Choosing which hospital I go to
(d) Choosing which consultant keeps an eye on me
(e) Being delivered by a midwife who looked after me while I was pregnant
(f) Being visited in hospital by a midwife I knew while I was pregnant
(g) Being visited at home after the birth by a midwife who has looked after me from the beginning
(h) Being visited at home by the midwife who delivered me

(e); and being visited at home by a midwife who has provided care throughout pregnancy (g).

These choices underline the importance to women of continuity of midwife care at every stage. In particular, they challenge the assumption which has widespread currency among professionals that women do not mind who delivers their baby so long as the care is competent. It is clear from this study that women do mind a great deal and that they attach great value to the continuity around birth and delivery that the scheme sought to provide. Indeed, when the women were asked to choose the one aspect of care which was of paramount importance, the largest number (15) plumped for being delivered by the midwife who had provided care during pregnancy. Having antenatal care mainly in the community came second, chosen by 11 women.

IMPLICATIONS FOR PRACTICE IN THE MATERNITY SERVICES

This chapter discusses only one team midwifery scheme, developed in a particular context. What general implications does the evaluation have for practice elsewhere? We can offer suggestions of three main kinds: some conclusions from our original report, some comments on the action taken as a result of the study, and some more general thoughts on the translation of new ideas into practice.

Conclusions from our original report

Choices are important to women. Having choices makes it easier for them to manage pregnancy, childbirth and the care of a new baby in relation to their other relationships and responsibilities. Page (1995) summarized research on control and choice, including the link between a sense of control in childbirth and mothers' later emotional well-being. This small-scale study suggested that the choices that bring a sense of control may be clinically trivial, or may be, externally, the same as those that professionals would have made on the woman's behalf. It is important to recognize that these, nevertheless, matter.

Our study supported the view that continuity through labour and delivery is important to women, including the transition from home to hospital; a known midwife is an important element of this support. However, this continuity does not have to be about one-to-one care – it can and did work with a team of six or seven, providing closer relationships could develop with one or two people within it.

Professionals in our study seemed to have a much more exalted definition of the 'known midwife' than the mothers for whom they cared. Most women felt that someone they had met before was a great support in the unknown territory of the hospital, and did not need to know the delivery midwife very well.

Midwives using the more ambitious definition of the 'known midwife' were prone to despair about the possibility of organizing good continuity, whether they worked in one of the teams or not. Midwives working in the area which used the more exacting definition were more worried about their difficulties in organizing continuity in the community, and seemed, from the evidence of the women we interviewed, to be doing it less successfully, both antenatally and postnatally. Schemes of this type would be well advised to build in as low key, practicable essentials:

- ways to see that all women meet the team before birth
- most antenatal care should be delivered by one or two midwives
- arrangements to see that the delivery midwife visits postnatally, as well as the antenatal midwife

Effects on the service

A follow-up discussion with the purchaser 18 months later revealed that the study had made an impact upon the debate within the maternity services, transforming the agenda for discussion. Before the study, there had been much debate about what women really wanted. What the study achieved was to gather up the litter of impressions and anecdotes about women's views that had been floating about within the service and to give shape to them. Although the study was small in scale, its findings about what women really wanted were consistent with the assumptions underlying national policy. Local professionals were thus enabled to move on from a debate about whether these assumptions were valid in their area and focus on the problem of how to develop the service in ways that met women's needs more effectively – a political and organizational problem.

New ideas for practice

Inevitably, new ideas for practice are started by enthusiasts. The ideas circulate, become known in outline to numerous people who have not had time to study them, and some eventually become generally approved, at least in principle. Bandwagons begin to roll. Early efforts to put these ideas into practice are usually staffed by enthusiasts, who are willing to work harder and give up more of their personal life to make them work than most of their peers would choose to do. Second and third stage attempts cannot necessarily rely on this level of dedication; they require different kinds of effort.

The experience of this team midwifery scheme shows the need for clear thinking as well as caring, from field staff and managers. 'Delivery by a known midwife' is a splendid slogan, but it needs careful definition of its two main terms if it is not to make practitioners' lives a misery and handicap the development of the best possible service for women. The difficulties caused to midwives, and to their planning of their work, by pursuing an overambitious definition of the 'known midwife' have been discussed above.

Similar difficulties could be expected to arise at a later stage in the process by failing to examine the term 'delivery'. At the start of our study we were told that the service was routinely monitoring the number of deliveries carried out by 'known midwives'. We therefore asked women questions about who delivered their babies, and how important it was to know the person who did the delivery. We picked up the issue of defining 'knowing' early enough to ask questions about it in the interview schedule; it was not until we started to analyse the data that we realized that 'delivery' too, was ambiguous. Women who had had caesarean or forceps deliveries, necessarily performed by a doctor, were enthusiastic about the comfort they had gained by having 'their' team midwife with them, a person they knew, all the time.

We were asking the wrong question. So was the monitoring process. So could many others, seduced by the appeal of 'delivery by a known midwife'. We should have been asking about care throughout labour by the same person, not about delivery itself, a process whose nature depends crucially on the presence or absence of obstetric complications. Continuity of care will inevitably be underestimated by data based on deliveries, not on care in labour itself. Clear thinking is essential for good practice – and as these examples show, it cannot be delegated to managers, purchasers, or even, heaven forbid, to outside researchers, without diminishing practice in one way or another. Midwives will be well advised to do it themselves.

REFERENCES

Calnan M (1988) Towards a conceptual framework of lay evaluation of health care. *Social Science and Medicine* **27**(9): 927–933.
Cartwright A (1964) *Human Relations and Hospital Care.* London: Routledge & Kegan Paul.
Cartwright A (1979) *The Dignity of Labour? A Study of Childbearing and Induction.* London: Tavistock.
[DoH] Department of Health (1993) *Changing Childbirth.* Report of the Expert Maternity Group. London: HMSO.
Evans FB (1987) *Newcastle Community Midwifery Care Project: An Evaluation Report.* Newcastle Health Authority Community Unit.
Freeley M (1995) Team midwifery, a personal experience. In: Page L (ed.) *Effective Group Practice in Midwifery: Working with Women.* Oxford: Blackwell Scientific.
Graham H (1979) *Problems in Antenatal Care.* Department of Sociology, University of York.
Graham H & Oakley A (1981) Competing ideologies of reproduction: medical and maternal perspectives on pregnancy and birth. In: Roberts H (ed.) *Women, Health and Reproduction.* London: Routledge & Kegan Paul.
Jones L, Leneman L & MacLean U (1987) *Consumer Feedback for the NHS: A Literature Review.* London: King Edward's Hospital Fund.
Kirkham M (1983) Labouring in the dark: limitations on the giving of information to enable patients to orientate themselves to the likely events and time scale of labour. In: Wilson-Barnett J (ed.) *Nursing Research: Ten Studies in Patient Care.* Chichester: John Wiley.
Locker D & Dunt D (1978) Theoretical and methodological issues in sociological studies of consumer satisfaction with medical care. *Social Science and Medicine* **12**: 283–292.
Macintyre S (1982) Communications between pregnant women and their medical and midwifery attendants. *Midwives Chronicle* **95** November: 387–394.
McIntosh J (1988) Women's views of communication during labour and delivery. *Midwifery* **4**: 166–170.
Oakley A (1979) *Becoming a Mother.* Oxford: Martin Robertson.

Oakley A (1980) *Women Confined: Towards a Sociology of Childbirth.* Oxford: Martin Robertson.

Oakley A (1992) *Social Support and Motherhood.* Oxford: Basil Blackwell.

Page L, ed. (1995) *Effective Group Practice in Midwifery: Working with Women.* Oxford: Blackwell Scientific.

Perkins ER (1980a) *Education for Childbirth and Parenthood.* London: Croom Helm.

Perkins ER (1980b) *Men on the Labour Ward.* Leverhulme Health Education Project Occasional Paper no. 22. University of Nottingham.

Porter M & Macintyre S (1989) Psychosocial effectiveness of ante-natal and postnatal care. In: Robinson S, Thomson A (eds) *Midwives, Research and Childbirth,* vol. 1. London: Chapman & Hall.

Robinson S & Thomson A, eds (1989) *Midwives, Research and Childbirth.* London: Chapman & Hall.

Stacey M (1976) The Health Service Consumer: a sociological misconception. *Sociological Review Monograph* **22**: 194–200.

Winterton N (1992) *Maternity Services.* Second report of the House of Commons Health Committee (Winterton report). London: HMSO.

Wraight A, Ball J, Secombe I & Stock J (1993) *Mapping Team Midwifery.* IMS Report no. 242. Brighton: Institute of Management Studies.

3

Choice in the face of uncertainty

Helen Stapleton

For many people the only satisfactory way of speaking about the world is in terms of a series of sharply defined categories, the properties of which are exactly known. Such a procedure has great advantages, but it severely limits our powers of speaking about all the variety that we observe around us.

(J. Z. Young, quoted by Calman, 1996)

The words 'choice' and 'uncertainty' mask a huge range of perceptions which are uniquely personal and not at all easy to tease apart for analysis. In this chapter I have four main objectives: to outline general concepts of choice and risk and to provide alternative models showing how these might be understood; to look at antenatal screening and home birth as specific areas of perceived risk; to examine the process of communication in the transfer of information and the relationship this has with subsequent decision-making; and finally to discuss the implications of these issues with respect to the formulation and implementation of women-centred health policies. This is a broad agenda in which many conflicting viewpoints are raised and for which there are few definitive answers.

There is a wide variation in the meaning of words such as 'choice', 'control', 'risk' and 'uncertainty', all of which are pivotal to this discussion. That there is such ambiguity suggests that topics closely allied to this field of enquiry may be similarly affected. With this in mind, this chapter constantly refers to more complex questions such as how and by whom knowledge is created and accessed; how risk and safety are perceived and evaluated; and how information is prioritized and disseminated. The orientation of this chapter is feminist and woman-centred, but situated within the wider agenda of reproductive health and women's rights. It has been written at a time of massive social change and uncertainty within contemporary society, particularly regarding the prevailing model of health care.

THE INFLUENCE OF CIRCUMSTANCES: VALUING PERSONAL EXPERIENCE

In addition to the referenced literature on the subject, this chapter includes material generated from the research undertaken for my MSc in medical anthropology (Stapleton, 1993). At that time I was in practice as an independent midwife carrying half a caseload while also working part-time as a medical herbalist. Towards the end of my studies, my colleague and I were suspended from midwifery practice. The charges against us concerned infringements to Rule 40; that of practising outside the boundary of normal midwifery practice and of failing to call appropriate medical aid. The limits of choice for both client and midwife in the context of what is considered normal (midwifery) practice were the focus of both the initial disciplinary hearing and our subsequent appearance before the Professional Conduct Committee (PCC) of the UK Central Council for Nursing, Midwifery and Health Visiting. It became apparent that at the heart of the matter were serious conflicts of interest which were not easily resolved by reference to either the Midwives Rules or the Code of Professional Conduct (UKCC, 1993, 1992).

In trying to make sense of the experience, I decided to investigate the embedded meanings in the words 'choice' and 'risk', particularly as they pertained to independent midwives and the women who employed them. Creating a context that facilitated both working through and analysing the painful feelings which surfaced in the months following the incident helped me to resolve and move on from a situation that threatened my integrity. It also gave meaning and purpose to the midwife struggling to stay alive inside me, while facing the possibility of removal from the register. In the event, the suspension was lifted after 3 weeks, and when we finally did both appear before the UKCC(PCC) some 20 months later, although four of the eight original charges were upheld, the case was closed with a recommendation that no further action be taken.

Unless otherwise indicated, all the quotations in this chapter have been taken from my own research. In total, eight clients and six independent midwives agreed to a one-off, tape-recorded interview lasting 90–120 minutes. The tapes were transcribed and analysed from an anthropological perspective using a broadly based grounded theory approach. When referring to my respondents, all of whom were women, I have used fictitious names to preserve their anonymity.

RECENT CHANGES AND THE NEW DEMANDS ON MIDWIVES

The issues raised in this chapter need to be seen within the context of the current reorganization of maternity services in the UK and the emergence of a business management culture within the National Health Service. The language of quality assurance, cost benefit analyses, indicators of performance and success, patients' charters, consumer rights and risk limitation now increasingly directs the provision of health care. Midwives, like many other workers in the industrialized nations, are having to adjust to a working environment which is insecure and unpredictable. It is an unfriendly world in which short-term contracts, threats of litigation, customer complaints, humiliating regrading structures and poor child-care provision militate against employees greeting further change with much enthusiasm. This climate of uncertainty is heightened by what appears to be an ever-increasing array of choices in many areas of life, including those related to health. The associated, but largely unexamined, responsibilities which accompany these developments are central to this discussion.

Although it may appear at first glance that midwifery is undergoing an isolated crisis of confidence regarding the role and scope of contemporary practice, this is not dissimilar to other changes occurring within the wider social framework. As the Nolan Committee revealed, there is a dissatisfaction with the performance of even the highest echelons of British society who have traditionally been shielded from public criticism. The goodwill and trust that the public previously extended to members of the caring professions, the royal family, government ministers and religious leaders, can no longer be assumed. The everyday decisions we make in the workplace are now exposed to a more critical audience who are ever more inclined to take disputes and grievances directly to the law courts. While some individuals and professions may be better protected than others from the effects of litigation, it may be only a matter of time before each one of us is called to account.

In the recent past midwifery was dominated by a biomedical perspective which viewed the events of pregnancy and birth as normal only in retrospect. A number of psychosocial commentaries have exposed deficiencies in this model of care; an exposure which has gradually encouraged the need for a more humane, woman-centred approach. In keeping with many other changes in health-care provision, it has been the collective pressure from consumer groups, rather than the midwifery profession, that must be credited with this achievement. Within the maternity services, the changes demanded by users have been of such a magnitude that huge uncertainty has arisen amongst midwives who have not been allocated any extra resources either to meet the recent government policy recommendations, or to quell the expectations arising from them. Any period of readjustment is normally associated with varying degrees of fear and resistance; it may also be accompanied by a (painful) reframing of identity. If this process is not well supported and safely contained, it may threaten to overwhelm both the individual worker and the employing organization.

Midwives are now required to provide care for women which is not only sensitive to and respectful of their needs, but which also recognizes the authority of the supervisor of midwives and the NHS trust or local employing agency. These demands may not be easy to reconcile, as has been demonstrated by two Hertfordshire midwives who courageously defied the policy of their employing NHS trust which tolerated women choosing to labour in water, but did not permit them actually to give birth there (Reid, 1994). They honoured instead the perfectly reasonable request of their client booked for a home birth, who in the absence of any clinical contraindications, requested to remain in the pool to birth her baby. The midwives were both suspended from duty for disregarding the trust's policy, and subsequently received written warnings before being required to undergo a 3-month period of supervised practice within the unit. The power exercised by NHS trusts and insurance underwriters (rather than our statutory bodies) to define the boundaries of midwifery practice is an alarming but perhaps not altogether unexpected outcome of a service increasingly driven by economic forces rather than by any egalitarian principles governing woman-centred care.

MIDWIVES, WOMEN AMD THE LANGUAGE OF RISK WITH RESPECT TO HOME BIRTH

The manner in which risk (and associated benefit) is perceived and evaluated has a relationship with the degree of uncertainty associated with particular life events. It is a uniquely individual process and one that has a direct relationship with subsequent decision-making, as the way in which the individual has experienced the world will reflect the level of confidence felt when confronting the unknown. If life has essentially been concerned with basic issues of survival, then what constitutes a risky event will be perceived differently in comparison with a person whose needs have been met in a consistent and predictable manner. If we shift the focus away from the individual to examine the ways in which occupational groups gain power, DeVries (1996) has suggested that certain strategies used to reduce (or contain) risk on behalf of client groups may also be of benefit to these same occupational groups. It is no coincidence, he suggests, that the most highly placed members of society in terms of power, prestige and earning capacity are those engaged in either defining the limits of risk (financiers, entrepreneurs and politicians) or reducing the more frightening ones (lawyers, doctors and insurance brokers). It could also be said that these same professional groups maintain their powerful hold by 'creating' risk, by emphasizing the uncertainty associated with particular events – in short, by redefining public risk in keeping with their own value systems and conservative professional traditions.

This is clearly demonstrated in the home birth debate. With a national home birth rate of less than 2%, 'it would appear that the personal bias and preference of those who believe that birth in hospital is safer continues to operate, and it could be argued that the majority of women are still being 'persuaded' to give birth in hospital' (Leap, 1996). I am in agreement with Leap and other midwives who have had considerable experience with home birth and who consistently describe it as the environment in which a woman is most likely to labour normally. Conversely, midwives who are uncomfortable in this domain may (intentionally or otherwise) find their personal anxieties and lack of experience guiding decision-making toward alleviating their own distress rather than helping women arrive at decisions that reflect their needs (Price, 1995). It is certainly not difficult for the midwife to capitalize on the negative conditioning we have all been subjected to with regard to home birth, and if this holds true for us as midwives, then women in our care will need massive reassurance to correct such misinformation. If women are encouraged by health professionals to conceptualize risk superficially in terms of the 'safety of the baby', then in my experience women will usually prioritize this over any other need they may have, including that of birthing in an environment which they perceive as safe and supportive. For an appraisal of the evidence contributing to debate on 'where to be born', Campbell and Macfarlane (1994) and Tew (1990) clearly illustrate the arguments.

All the women in my study had booked for a home birth, a decision which they perceived as affording maximum control and minimal risk over the uncertain events of labour and birth. The more experienced independent midwives encouraged women to be open-minded and flexible about this; that having fixed ideas about the actual place of birth was not appropriate until labour was established. It was only at this point that a more complete 'risk appraisal' could be made which allowed space for the emergence of the woman's own (unpredictable) feelings about whether she still felt safe and comfortable at home, how the events of her labour were unfolding and the reactions of her partner and other birth attendants. Each woman was also told (and subsequently reminded) that when she was in labour, the midwife would come to her home with all the equipment needed to deal with an emergency if she preferred to stay put, but that if she wanted to go to hospital, or it became obvious during her labour that she needed help, then the midwife would go with her and her birth partner(s) into hospital and stay with them. That the actual place of birth is imbued with considerable significance is emphasized by Bettine:

Where the baby would actually be born was very important to me ... if you do even the tiniest bit of reading between the lines, you realize what dangerous places hospitals are and how recent this modern way of childbirth is and that makes you feel much more secure and safe about trying for a home birth ... but I was amazed at other people's reactions; across the board it seemed that I was doing something outrageously foolhardy ... so eventually I stopped mentioning it. [Bettine, client]

My research suggested that there may be differences in the way women perceive risk generally, but that pregnancy added another dimension as illustrated by Jane:

I only came across the word 'risk' in pregnancy, so I had to really think about it because of course they threw that in my face all the time. They frequently said I was 'risking my child'... but as I've got a fairly positive attitude to life and also because I have a spiritual life which holds for beliefs and concepts such as karma, I don't actually believe in risk ... Also, as I don't see my baby as being separate from me, I just can't take on board this idea that it is affected by influences which don't have any bearing on me. We are one unit and we function in unison. [Jane, client]

Why the culture of pregnancy has come to be so inflated with associations of danger and threat is perhaps significant. The suggestion that unnecessary risks were taken in pregnancy which jeopardized their own health or that of their baby, was vehemently denied by the women and midwives participating in my study. They tended to view all choice as beset with ambivalence and uncertainty. Although risk analysis attempts to turn these uncertainties into probabilities, the formal training required to achieve this is also embedded within a heavily culture-bound framework. The final result may simply widen the gap between decisions made by the 'experts' and those made by the 'insignificant others'.

Perhaps because pregnancy has a fixed and definite ending, it is the outcome rather than the entire process which is sometimes given an unwarranted emphasis. This is particularly so in the case of a home birth where this is seen as the safe container for *all* risk, so that the biggest risk of all becomes the possibility of the home birth being sabotaged in some way. This contrasts strongly with the ideology that hospital be seen as the ultimately safe container for all the unpredictable (and inherently) dangerous and risky events that *might* happen. Labour and birth may be seen as the bifurcation point when perceptions of risk change for both mother and midwife; until that point they have been inextricably buried within a wider relationship. Following the moment of transition from woman to mother however, if the outcome does fall short of the (unspoken) expectations, the latter may suddenly switch from being the midwife's advocate to the most devastating critic. The immediate moments before and after birth then, form the axis of congruence for appreciating a whole order of risks which, until that point, Catherine could only describe as having been ...

... held suspended in a kind of bag woven with superstition and dread and hope and prayer and a kind of overarching optimism that it would all be just fine. [Catherine, client]

CONTROLLING RISK: THE TECHNOCRATIC MODEL OF BIRTH AS AN ALTERNATIVE REPRODUCTIVE CHOICE

In contrast to the model of childbirth which embraces what can be described as a 'hands off' or minimalist approach, is what Davis-Floyd has termed the 'technocratic' model.

Although both viewpoints embrace opposing philosophies, 'like all cohesive and hegemonic mythologies, the technocratic model functions as a powerful agent of social control, shaping and channelling individual values, beliefs and behaviours' (Davis-Floyd, 1994, p. 1125). During the course of Davis-Floyd's research to identify and define this technocratic model, 40 American women were interviewed, of whom 32 gave birth in hospital in complete accordance with the beliefs and value systems ascribed to this ideology. They were then compared with eight women who birthed at home in complete opposition to it. The 32 hospital birthers were all highly successful women in the wider commercial world, holding positions wherein they controlled 'valued goods and resources'. They were compared with the home birthers who also defined themselves as successful, but who emphasized an alternative world view. Davis-Floyd points out that while some women place a high value on the notion of surrendering to the natural processes of birth within the familiar environment of their home territory, opposition to this is being voiced by an increasingly powerful and vocal sector. This is evident in the responses of the women opting for a technocratic model of birth who described the attitudes of the home birthers as frightening and irresponsible. In contrast, they perceived hospitals and technology as 'liberating them from the tyranny of biology; as empowering them to stay in control of an out-of-control biological experience' (Davis-Floyd, 1994, p. 1137).

Feminists and anthropologists alike have for some time now interpreted many of the customs associated with reproductive function as primarily an issue of control over women's bodies (Arms, 1981; Kitzinger, 1984; Oakley, 1984; Rothman, 1986; Martin, 1987; Donnison, 1988; Ruddick, 1989; Spallone, 1989; Davis-Floyd, 1992). Although such encroachment has not been without resistance, technology has pervaded our lives to such a degree that it can no longer be considered a fringe model, but one which constitutes the central, inescapable reality of contemporary Western culture. It is not unreasonable to assume that women will increasingly seek options for birth that reflect the totality of the environment in which they feel in control. As women become more visible in business, management and finance – in worlds that reflect what has hitherto been described as a masculine ethos rewarding qualities such as power and domination – we can expect to see new tensions emerging in all of the debates concerning reproductive choice. If, however, the uncertain space where the client and professional meet can be seen as mutually beneficial, then there is potential for both parties to move towards finding alternative but personally meaningful solutions. This would require an emotional and intellectual flexibility which encourages the formulation and exploration of novel ideas. Such a process is not static, nor does it ever reach an end-point. It embraces endless possibilities, each of which holds a hugely liberating potential for enabling people to re-experience change and the attendant anxiety embedded in new situations. Similarly, it allows for paradoxes and conflicting research to be transcended as an attitude is fostered whereby inconsistencies are welcomed because they provoke a further round of questioning.

REFRAMING PERCEPTIONS OF RISKS: LAY VERSUS EXPERT OPINION

Although there is little doubt that childbirth has become a safer journey for both mother and baby, there are competing theories as to why the significant falls in both maternal and perinatal mortality rates have occurred. What is indisputable is that medical control over pregnancy and childbirth has increased to such an extent that women (and midwives?) who do not submit themselves to regulation, may still be regarded as irresponsible mavericks gambling with the health and lives of babies. This view would fit with the wryly expressed comment that 'childbearing is too important to be left to women' (Oakley, 1984, p. 232).

Our lives are not compartmentalized in such a way that it is ever possible to tease out the significance of isolated events from the myriad of influences continuously affecting each one of us. Perceptions of risk are inseparable from how we broadly view the world and the kind of society in which we want to live. An alternative understanding of some factors that influence risk perception has been provided through an analysis of the explanatory models people use to describe local and personal relationships (Kleinman, 1978; Hunt et al., 1989; Atkinson and Farias, 1995). Such an approach facilitates a view of people as social beings with attitudes and beliefs which are formed and re-formed through the relationships they have with one another. In any multicultural society, this will require health policies to reflect a multitude of health-related requirements and expectations. The word 'risk' will invariably hold a variety of meanings for people. This will inevitably generate conflict as to how risk is identified and subsequently contained and managed, in a manner that is sensitive to cultural difference. All of this is to argue against the one-dimensional approach to risk assessment currently favoured by 'experts' in the field. Within this paradigm, the probability of any adverse outcome materializing is measured along a linear reference, despite the lack of evidence that for any given risk, there is *no* single, universal definition or measure that can be applied.

There is an extensive library of material covering decision analysis which I do not intend to duplicate and upon which I am poorly qualified to comment (Tversky and Kahnemann, 1974; Weinstein and Fineberg, 1980; Lindley, 1985; Dowie and Elstein, 1988). Some of the models from which these analyses developed were based on literature pertaining to game theory, the reference lottery originally devised to measure outcome values (Von Neumann and Morgenstern, 1947). In their essay entitled 'Making Difficult Decisions', Lilford and Thornton have similarly outlined a model of decision-making for obstetrics and midwifery which is well referenced to the current literature on the subject (Lilford and Thornton, 1992). My remit here is to explore what could be seen as the more human interface of decision-making: the signs and gestures of an irrational language set apart from the rules and calculations of mathematics. That is not to dismiss the importance and relevance of quantitative research, as much to argue a place for a flexible methodology capable of tolerating a more extensive range of human expression.

In a study that analysed consumer's perceptions of risk, Lisa Saffron asserted that disagreement about risk is inevitable because there is no definition that avoids embedded values, beliefs and assumptions (Saffron, 1993). This is compounded by the scarcity of evidence-based information which might guide such judgments. It is also worth remembering that where non-experts are concerned, '...there is wisdom as well as error in public attitudes and perceptions. Lay people sometimes lack certain information about hazards. However, their basic conceptualization of risk is much richer than experts' and reflects legitimate concerns that are typically omitted from expert risk assessments' (Slovic, 1987). The social values embedded in risk assessment strategies are not infrequently marginalized by the scientific investigative model which insists upon containing or explaining risk factors as if they were visible, tangible entities whose control would result in a better outcome.

CULTURE AND THE 'NATURAL' SUBORDINATION OF WOMEN

It is not possible to discuss the issues of risk and choice without reference to gender differences, visible as they are across the boundaries of social class, health and employment opportunities. Anthropological analyses approach the study of gender from two different but not mutually exclusive perspectives: that of symbolic construction or of social relationship (Moore, 1988, p. 13). Within the context of this chapter, we need to situate women and their carers within a world which has generally proscribed choice for all women and has increasingly tended to view pregnancy and birth not just as a right of passage with all the attendant dangers, but as fraught with such uncertainty as to require constant (medical) surveillance and an ever-increasing readiness to intervene. Ortner (1974) puzzled over what facet of the social hierarchy could possibly be common to every culture such that all cultures seemed to automatically ascribe a lower value to women. Her suggestion was that women everywhere were associated with some aspect of culture which is universally devalued. She proposed that the only thing that expressed that premise was 'nature', in the most generalized sense of the word.

The worlds of 'nature' and 'culture' are generally seen as distinct and in opposition to one another, with that of 'culture' regarded as superior to the natural world. Within this framework, women are traditionally identified or symbolically associated with nature and the underworld of physicality, emotions, loose boundaries and unpredictability. Men, in contrast, are associated with culture and the sanitary, cerebral world of abstract ideas. Since the impetus of culture is to control or to transcend nature, then an obvious consequence will be that women, by virtue of their close affiliation with the latter, will be similarly controlled and constrained. In real life, of course, women are in fact no closer or further away from nature than are men. The intention is rather to isolate and make explicit the cultural variations and subsequent limitations imposed upon them.

This view of women's culturally endemic subjugation has been challenged by a scholarly exposition of the part women played as the outspoken and independent founders and shapers developing the traditional practice of Tantric Buddhism (Shaw, 1994). While I am not suggesting that the practice of Tantric Buddhism is related to midwifery, there is a shared theme of female practitioners attempting to formulate their own rules and resisting the definitions imposed upon them by conservative, patriarchal societies. Historians have generally portrayed Tantric Buddhism as being an oppressive movement in which women were at best marginal and subordinate and at worst humiliated, degraded and exploited. Although perhaps not quite as extremely, midwives have similarly been discounted, and in rewriting history to present women's actual experience, Shaw makes it more possible for women everywhere to similarly formulate and describe their own unique journeys.

Sex, pregnancy and childbirth, in common with all culturally embedded activities (but especially those concerning women's sexuality) are imbued with an element of risk – which from a biomedical perspective is primarily seen in terms of pathology or bodily harm (Gordon, 1990; Maine, 1991; Maine et al., 1995). These activities, and perhaps more importantly their regulation, also pose a threat to the social ordering and the control of women in any society. What is perhaps less obvious is that women have a long history of withstanding or actively resisting such regulation. This has occurred primarily because women have invested other meanings in their ability to bear children, for example that of status, of economic survival, as source of personal power and triumph, for the feelings of personal fulfilment, or for a depth of emotional and psychological satisfaction which is reckoned to be otherwise unattainable.

THE SUBORDINATION OF PARTICULAR WOMEN: THE CASE OF INDEPENDENT MIDWIVES

In relation to childbirth as a particular focus of women's experience, the old nature/ culture division which emphasizes a medical rather than a feminist or socialist interpretation, exposes the process of control and fragmentation which has come to signify birthing within Western societies. Lest the reader be deluded into thinking that life has surely changed for the better, attention is drawn to the following passage taken from a booklet entitled *Consent to Treatment* which conveys a prevailing medical attitude (Beech, 1992):

> *The union does not consider that a maternity patient need give her written consent to any operative or manipulative procedures that are normally associated with childbirth. When she enters hospital for the confinement (sic) it can be assumed that she assents to any necessary procedure including the administration of local, general or other anaesthetic.* (Medical Defence Union (MDU) 1974)

Although this paragraph has been deleted from later editions, it is unlikely that the intervening years have so effortlessly erased the underlying attitudes. A statement that makes such a mockery of the notion of informed consent does little to reassure me about the fact that independent midwives who have made the difficult decision to purchase indemnity insurance cover have few options but to obtain it from the MDU. It seems to me a disheartening indictment of the midwifery profession in the UK that members who have been such visible and vulnerable pioneers for change and choice in childbirth, should now be aligning themselves with such an organization for indemnity cover. I consider this an issue for the entire profession; if we do not have the strength and unity, nor indeed the integrity to publicly (and financially) support innovation amongst our own members, then we remain vulnerable to the same external pressures which have historically been so successful in controlling and limiting our sphere of practice (Heagerty, 1990).

Focusing any discussion on the future of independent midwifery as a viable option in maternity care may be somewhat of an irrelevance in the aftermath of the debacle over vicarious liability insurance. Although some self-employed midwives in the UK have already stopped practising midwifery in any form, what will unfold in the future is not clear. A minority of practitioners will probably continue to work without insurance, while group practices such as the South East London Midwives Group Practice may finally achieve their aim of contracting their services to a local health authority on a more permanent arrangement. The remainder, who pay the annual premium of £10,890 (1997 price), will find their practice espousing less of the independent and more of the private sector ethos, as their clients will increasingly be drawn from the financially comfortable, articulate, middle to upper classes. While I do not mean to imply that this group has less need of independent midwives, I do think that a caseload that excludes social variation inevitably sacrifices its cutting edge for the safe zone of homogeneity. It is also ironic that the women and families whom independent practice initially attracted – those whose voices and choices were ridiculed or marginalized by mainstream maternity services – will be unable to afford the cost of choosing their preferred model of care.

CHOICE: CONSIDERED DECISION, UNFORTUNATE CIRCUMSTANCE OR PERMANENT REGRET?

'Choice' has become something of a vexed word, not only within the world of midwifery but also in the wider arena wherever social policy is informed through gender analysis. The realms in which women are highly visible figures in decision-making processes cover increasingly diverse and complex territory, as is evident from the material introduced in this section. Women are creating alternative models of motherhood, although it cannot always be assumed that these are products of considered choice rather than of unfortunate circumstances. The fact is that lone mothers and their children currently comprise almost 20% of all families with dependent children in Britain, and these numbers have nearly trebled since the 1970s (Haskey, 1994). Although the majority of these single mothers suffer the consequences of being poor and/or young, they are also increasingly visible across the traditional boundaries of social class and sexual orientation (Saffron, 1994). Politicians and the media have focused on this as both cause and symptom of a wider breakdown in the social fabric of modern life, yet until the publication of a timely study (Bortalaia Silva, 1996), very little was known about the actual conditions and consequences of lone motherhood and even less about the role choice has played in this. Through analysis of historical and contemporary factors, lone mothers are seen as a specific category of women with unique needs. Despite being a sizeable group, they generally receive no particular attention from maternity services unless they fall into special service groups set up to address specific (usually health-related) needs, for example teenage mothers or those who smoke, use drugs or drink excessive amounts of alcohol. It is not known how midwives as a group react to single mothers nor whether the care they give is influenced by any (idealized) model they may themselves hold of motherhood, or whether conflict is experienced when pregnant women contradict this ideal. It is not unreasonable, however, to assume that if what the mother rates as important in pregnancy and childbirth is not similar to the values held by the midwife, then the overall quality of care may suffer.

In closely following the recommendations of the Winterton report emphasizing choice for women (and midwives) in maternity care (Winterton, 1992), the remit of *Changing Childbirth* (DoH, 1993) has perforce exposed the deficiencies in the current maternity system. Within this new regime, women are now encouraged to articulate their needs, to even express their opinions about their health and well-being in the (false) hope that there are real options available to them. However, as is increasingly evident in the case of *Changing Childbirth*, where government policy is ratified in the absence of a national financial infrastructure, real choice (and by extension real change) is severely compromised. Midwives meanwhile are in a quandary: potentially liable if clients are not 'fully informed' about the various choices (theoretically) available, but held personally responsible if clients make the 'wrong' choice. Making options available is a deliberate and conscious act; one which encourages participation and a sense of personal authority. Within an egalitarian society, it also means shifting the process of decision-making from professionals to women, but retaining a share of the overall responsibility. This is particularly important in preventing the emergence of a culture of blame and scapegoating. The self-awareness, skill, knowledge and flexibility required to ensure that changes of this magnitude are intelligently managed, should not be underestimated. They demand that higher standards of professional training are made available for midwives 'whose enhanced role has forced obstetricians and general practitioners to rethink their own' (Steer, 1995).

Women themselves offer fascinating perceptions as to why the events of pregnancy and birth sometimes happen the way they do. Many of them speak as if pregnancy afforded them contact with another reality within which there was a greater freedom to draw on material from other dimensions and experiences. I was witness to this when Marta, pregnant with her second baby, booked with my partner and me for a home birth. Although describing herself as 'not fanatical' about home births, she did volunteer her . . .

> *. . . loathing of hospitals and resentment of the inevitable devolution of power to uniformed strangers with whom I've never so much as shared a cup of tea.*   *[Marta, client]*

As 42 weeks of pregnancy was approaching with no signs of labour, we again discussed the implications of postmaturity and the current recommendations to assess and monitor the baby's well-being. Marta flatly and absolutely refused intervention, deciding instead to have an induction on the first day of her 43rd week if still pregnant. She felt her baby was absolutely fine; it was more her own impatience that she felt unable to contain. Much to everyone's profound relief, Marta duly went into labour in the early hours of the day on which the induction was scheduled. A few hours later with labour progressing rapidly and with no outward signs of fetal distress, her baby suddenly died. Although by that stage Marta and her husband were very familiar with the documented risks associated with postmaturity, they had also felt themselves to be somehow personally protected against the possibility of a tragedy occurring. Later that afternoon, Marta transferred to hospital for augmentation as labour had drawn to a standstill.

During the long evening, with her labouring body now set and regulated to autopilot by technology, she began the process of 'making sense' of this pregnancy which had been so different from that of her first child born 2 years earlier. She spoke rather resentfully of . . .

> *. . . the lack of effort this baby had made; how, unlike my first child, it had never responded to any of the family singing or talking or stroking it . . . that it had made no effort to communicate . . . that it just felt as if I had been carrying a dead weight around; although I looked like I was carrying a baby it never, ever, acted like one . . .*   *[Marta, client]*

Marta finally birthed; a beautiful, gentle unfolding of a perfectly formed baby boy. It seemed not at all strange to either herself or her husband that this '*weird thing*' had died while trying to get itself born. Rather, it simply confirmed to them that '*it was never really serious in the first place*'.

One of the concerns illustrated by this account is the degree to which people should be protected by health professionals from making 'inappropriate' choices. As 'medicotechnical' possibilities are often experienced as being strongly compelling, the extent to which choice is perceived as an option rather than as a pressure, is increasingly open to debate (Tymstra, 1989; Bayer, 1994; Wilson, 1993; Lupton et al, 1995). There is evidence, for example, that people find it increasingly difficult to refuse screening tests, especially those of a diagnostic nature, for fear of regretting such a decision at a later date. This is particularly so in the case of a positive diagnosis suggesting a variable degree of impairment and which might have permitted a different outcome had action been effected earlier. The anticipation of negative feelings arising at a later date has been suggested as an important motivational factor in avoiding what has been termed 'decision regret' (Tymstra, 1989). This mechanism has also been proposed as an explanation for the difficulty people experience in refusing the medical technologies 'offered' to them. It has been suggested that it is the responsibility of the practitioner to anticipate, through their sustained interaction with the client, just how sensitive the client will be to subsequent regret in the event of an unexpected outcome (Bell et al, 1988). This presumes the existence of an established relationship with the client concerned, which in reality is often not the case. There is also a need to distinguish between the understandable anguish ensuing as a result of an unfortunate outcome, and the regret for a decision made in good faith, but which was subsequently lamented. This further confounds many of the usual issues raised in discussions concerning choice and risk.

Women and choice in the context of prenatal screening

Research by Sandelowski and Jones (1996) has suggested that choice does not necessarily follow a logical or linear progression; from receipt of information through reflection and the gathering of additional material, to wider discussion up to the point of decision-making. In the case of prenatal screening, they suggested that their respondents had often 'backed into' screening tests rather than actively choosing or refusing such investigations. What is surfacing from this and other research is the extent to which women participate in screening procedures because such tests are perceived and portrayed by professionals as simple, routine and not meriting the seriousness associated with the notion of 'informed consent'. It has been further suggested that the very fact that such examinations are offered 'within the context of the routine, regular and normal' antenatal visit, 'favours consent and militates against refusal' (Sandelowski and Corson Jones, 1996, p. 356). It seems that women who do take up the offer of prenatal screening do so partly because this has become the norm within their social circles, and also to confirm that everything is all right with their baby. My own and colleagues' personal experience is that despite counselling, in the absence of any family history or recent media coverage, clients do not usually anticipate that screening will reveal anything actually wrong with their baby.

In sympathy with these views, the expanding facility of fetal diagnosis is seen as a contraction rather than an expansion of choice. Writers in this field denounce the so-called advances afforded by such programmes as fictional, or indeed 'a mockery of the concept of choice', in the absence of treatment that positively alters the outcome (Rothman, 1986). Seen from this perspective, the very notion of choice is perceived as downright fallacious or at least no better than 'a double edged sword' (Beck-Gernsheim, 1989; Gregg, 1993). Such opinions present a powerful contradiction to the prevailing cultural myth which celebrates advances in genetic screening as entirely progressive occurrences; a stance that (as would be expected) is vigorously invoked in defending the 'ruling interests of the normative order' enshrined in Western obstetrics (Richardson, 1990). The ethos of biomedicine celebrates and incorporates technological achievements, often before determining whether such innovations are either safe or even appropriate. With specific regard to fetal diagnosis, the mere availability of the technology seems to mandate its automatic inclusion into antenatal care, despite the current absence of fetal therapy as a viable alternative to termination. This undermines any serious discussion concerning choice and also calls into question the very concept of informed consent, as prenatal screening has already assumed 'a legal and moral *sine qua non* of both good obstetric care and responsible parenting' (Henifin et al, 1988).

Jane, aged 38, illustrated this conundrum as she recalled the incredulous reaction of a senior registrar at the local hospital. Early in her pregnancy, Jane had arranged a consultation to discuss the antenatal screening choices locally available to her, with specific regard to her age and a family history of a disabling chromosomal disorder. When she ventured to express her reservations about amniocentesis (presented by the senior registrar not as an option to be considered but as an imperative), the response was:

> *'Oh, so you're going to accept whatever you get, then?'... with the implication that I deserved to get a badly handicapped child for which I would then have only myself to blame.* [Jane, client]

She subsequently refused the amniocentesis, enjoyed a perfectly healthy pregnancy and gave birth at home to a baby boy whose normal, healthy appearance was subsequently confirmed by chromosomal analysis. Jane was left feeling rather sceptical about the notion of choice when one's ideology does not conform to the status quo, and as long as power remains vested in the medical profession, she does not hold much hope for real change.

Making unconventional choices; the freedom to play

Suspending judgment throughout the crucial interpretative process of weighing up information and deciding on a particular course of action, requires a flexibility which is paralleled by a willingness to conceptualize and theorize. It has been suggested that it is this capacity to 'conceive of' which facilitates choice and the subsequent process of decision-making. This ability, by which we can understand anything – even the most abstract notions – encourages the freedom to play with inconsistencies; to revel in introspection and entertain the most absurd fantasies. I am reminded of a quotation echoing this sentiment from Krishnamurti, the philosopher and anti-guru:

> *Freedom is not in fragments. A non-fragmented mind, a mind that is whole is in freedom. Freedom of choice denies freedom; choice exists only where there is confusion. Clarity of perception; insight, is the freedom of the pain of choice.* (Krishnamurti, 1995)

An approach that encompassed such elasticity was useful in my own research at a particularly worrying moment when I found myself quite unable to discern a homogeneous pool of beliefs or values to which all participants subscribed. Even when discussing themes such as home birth, with which my respondents might be expected to reflect a consistent opinion, many contradictory theories emerged. It gradually became apparent that even the powerful drive for home birth is not a single set of arguable or coherent processes, but one that is derived from an all-embracing philosophy which may not be available for discussion within the terminology or boundaries of Western logic. Acknowledging the reality of this 'other' lived out (rather than verbalized) existence, requires a constant struggle to reconcile demands from worlds which fundamentally oppose one another and between which no common language currently exists.

LANGUAGE, INFORMATION AND COMMUNICATION: THE EFFECT OF UNEQUAL ACCESS

Effective communication requires clarity of thought, focus of mind, and the necessity of being thoroughly conversant with the subject matter. It remains something of a paradox, however, that wherever words and their diverse meanings are concerned, doubt and confusion are also often highly conspicuous (Brown, 1958; Gallie, 1964; Williams, 1976; Spender, 1980; Tannen, 1991). Intentions are communicated not only through the explicit and conscious use of language, but are also conveyed through an extensive repertoire of bodily gestures. As Kirkham has pointed out, communication cannot be described as 'just part of midwifery care'; it is rather the vehicle by which all else is learnt and upon which relationships are built (Kirkham, 1993). Good communication plays a vital role in determining choice and assisting positively in the decision-making process; in contrast, poor communication heightens uncertainty and effectively serves to conceal available options. Communication is also about exercising conscious choice in the language we use. With particular regard to midwifery, reference has been made to the profusion of commonly used words and phrases which disempower and trivialize women (Bastion, 1992; Leap, 1992). These authors further claim that the language we use indicates not only where the balance of power lies within the relationship, but also reflects our own personal attitudes and the wider ideologies informing midwifery care. Planning or implementing woman-centred care without serious and continuing effort to reconstruct and redefine our language base is a misguided enterprise which we would do well to avoid.

All of this is not to say that words are hopelessly inaccurate descriptors, but rather that meaning must be periodically reviewed. Raymond Williams suggests that we include in this periodic review words with which we are all familiar, but which are value-laden and have more than one meaning (Williams, 1976). He called these 'keywords' and implied that such a list invariably contains phrases that play a significant role in framing our experience both in and of the world. There are many examples within the culture of midwifery: some are listed in Box 3.1. Words or phrases such as these do not convey a clear, unambiguous message but can accommodate a variety of meanings which may simply add to the confusion already created by the use of jargon and technical language.

Even when they were literate and reasonably well-informed on health and social issues, the clients of the self-employed midwives in my study recollected the enormous difficulty of discovering just what options were available to them in pregnancy. Despite the fact that independent midwifery was well established within the four area health authorities in which I conducted interviews, none of the women was informed of this option from

---

Box 3.1   Keywords of significance in midwifery

natural birth	risk	empowerment
informed choice	sexuality	holistic
fully informed	choice	scientific
partners in care	research-based	protocols
guidelines	informed consent	allow
equality	rules	autonomous

inside the establishment. The majority heard of the facility through local networks, but often not until pregnancy was well established, and they had been misled or deliberately lied to about their options for midwifery care. Elaine described this process as:

> … *a real battle, just trying to find out about how to get a home birth organized was one thing, and then when they realized it was my first baby, they threw up all kinds of smoke screens, some of which I later found out just weren't true. I had to do an awful lot of homework before I found out about Independent Midwifery … it was incredibly difficult to get the information and in the end I was just lucky to hear about her. But you've got to find out these things for yourself as it seems nobody is going to tell you.*
>
> *[Elaine, client]*

Melanie described a similar situation in which she remembered:

> … *feeling incredibly resentful that the only way I could find out was to go and dig up the information. I was just following my gut feeling that there must be another way of doing it than through the hospital system, but there was absolutely nothing available in the way of literature, so I had to borrow or buy books … it was difficult because I was a student and didn't have any money but also, you've only got a finite amount of time to find things out … I wished there had been some kind of net to catch me in and give me all the facts and just tell me what options and choices I had at that stage. So I had to consciously go out and say 'right, I am going to have some choice about this …'* *[Melanie, client]*

Both of these accounts illustrate that making information available requires an active commitment on behalf of the health professional. It also demonstrates the need for a multimedia approach to conveying information and that effective mechanisms for monitoring and improving such a service are in place.

There may, however, be more subtle factors inhibiting explicit communication, as Berger seems to imply in his moving account of the life of a country doctor in a solo practice in an isolated, deprived part of England (Berger and Mohr, 1967). Pointing out that there are large sections of the working and lower-middle classes who are inarticulate as the result of wholesale cultural deprivation which has 'denied them the means of translating what they know into thoughts which they can think', he emphasizes these difficulties (*ibid.* p. 99). Although he refers to the 'inarticulateness of the English' as something of a tired but familiar joke, he is also aware of the obstacles this creates in denying people an opportunity for expression. With the intimacy of these 'spoken traditions' long destroyed, many people are now literate in a purely technical sense; much of their emotional and introspective experience remains unnamed, with consequences for both users and providers of maternity services. If Berger's assertions have any current relevance then we have a problem; if this is even partly true for those who have English as a first language, how can we begin to assess the scale of the problem for those whose command of English is rudimentary or non-existent? Taking an active part in decision-making is extremely difficult for those whose grasp of English is poor, because the complexity of assumptions and meanings embedded in any language does not readily translate into the factual data on which contemporary evidence-based approaches rely.

The new charters for health-care services, written in the didactic language of rights and choices, denies the fact that for sizeable populations in the UK, English literacy levels are simply inadequate to take on these new responsibilities. This situation effectively forecloses on the notion of informed decision-making within the context of maternity care. With specific regard to this dilemma, concern has been raised about the launch of the *Informed Choice* leaflets by Midwives Information and Resource Service (MIDIRS)

(Rosser, 1995). Although the egalitarian principle upon which this initiative rests is a welcome change in the delivery of information to consumers, it does not address the fact that the fundamental inequalities which currently inhibit or limit access to health services remain unresolved (Townsend et al, 1988; Davey Smith et al, 1990; McCarron et al, 1994). This is discussed further in Chapter 6.

INFLUENCES ON THE CONSTRUCTION AND IMPLEMENTATION OF WOMEN-CENTRED HEALTH POLICIES

Versatility and fluidity with language is closely associated with power and privilege. Although the opinions of consumer groups did contribute significantly to *Changing Childbirth*, women's health networks have been a relatively recent emergence and subsequently may have had limited influence in shaping health policy. This has been suggested as a reason for the scant regard accorded women's experiences when health policies are formulated and implemented (Ravindran Sundari, 1995). Since the 1980s, pressure groups concerned explicitly with women's health issues have grown. Organizations such as the National Childbirth Trust and the Family Planning Association have made the transition from outsider to insider and are now accorded high legitimacy and status by policy-makers. Other pressure groups referred to by Walt (1994) as 'threshold groups' may be accorded ambiguous status depending on the degree to which their perspective and analysis of problems challenge conventional social welfare analysis.

Walt cites the case of Women's Aid – a pressure group committed to bringing attention to the widespread but hitherto unreported issue of domestic violence and its effect on women and children. Women's Aid workers acted not only as spokeswomen but also as service providers through identifying safe homes (often their own) as refuges for those fleeing abusive male partners, friends or relatives. Although the work of this organization was valued by the 'policy community' of health and allied professionals and local authorities, they did not always accept their feminist analysis of why the violence occurred. In addition to the unpalatable nature of these and similar issues, researchers have further suggested that the general reluctance of women to persist in demanding improvements to health-service provision further militates against the implementation of health reforms, even when these have been ratified (Coney, 1992; Lecky-Thompson, 1995; Plata et al, 1995).

An orientation on women's health issues which primarily concerns itself with the biological functions of contraception, pregnancy, childbirth and related pathologies of the genital tract does not emphasize the central role of women, their status, nor their overall well-being. Furthermore, it does little to challenge the various visible forms of social control exerted over the expression of women's sexuality. Examples that come to mind include the criminalizing of abortion, handcuffing female prisoners in labour, demographically driven population control programmes, female genital mutilation, forced marriages and female infanticide. Although some of these practices may appear as an exotic irrelevance within the humdrum routine of practice in the UK, I am in agreement with other writers who have suggested that the mindset that governs the conditions setting the global agenda for women's health, may not be so very different to that at large in non-Western countries (Maine et al, 1995). Until this is recognized and service delivery is subject to the 'bottom up' transformation in which women as users of health services have the right to determine their own agenda, I suspect that the notion of choice for women, as lauded by policy documents such as *Changing Childbirth*, will remain a contentious issue. Policy process is not a linear transformation from formulation to implementation. Rather it is an interactive, ongoing developmental activity with both of these aspects carrying equal weight in a continuously evolving process.

At a time when public policy is under close scrutiny, the traditional role of the client as perhaps 'the most critical and yet underused resource for improved health care outcomes and cost control' requires urgent review (Chewning and Sleath, 1996, p. 389). The patriarchal biomedical model which has traditionally dominated the manner in which provider–patient relationships are conceptualized and conducted is no longer appropriate. There is now increasing pressure to implement a more participatory model of caring which acknowledges that accountability, decision-making and power are responsibilities to be shared collectively by all parties involved in the delivery and receipt of health care. These new, person-centred models demand skills and attitudes from both health professionals and clients that emphasize a more co-operative, equitable alliance. DiMatteo encapsulates this with her assertion that these relationships require 'a recognition of the need for effective communication, a conscious approach to the therapeutic relationship as a collaboration, and a recognition of the patient's right to choose her own course of action' (DiMatteo, 1994). What remains unresolved is the conflict of who assumes medicolegal responsibility when clients exercise choices that are known by health-care professionals to be associated with adverse outcomes.

CREATING ALTERNATIVE MIDWIFE–CLIENT RELATIONSHIPS

The women who employed the midwives of my study volunteered a desire to foster very different relationships with these chosen midwives; women they regarded as 'reliable, trustworthy, approachable friends and confidantes', to whom they looked for support and protection throughout a journey fraught with uncertainty and threat. They wanted to feel able to defer responsibility for decision-making without the need to operate what one client described as:

> the usual filtering mechanisms required to defend one's integrity from the uniformed stranger, familiar only with the binary systems and values of hospital medicine.

Many of the women recalled previous situations where the ambivalence or negative attitudes of health professionals had impinged upon their ability to even consider the available options. This was especially so in situations described as '*in extremis*' where, without the context of an established relationship of mutual respect and understanding, Catherine spoke of:

> ... being reduced to a thing; discounted as an eccentric with no acknowledgement of me as a vulnerable, terrified, scarcely human, being at the bottom of the heap within the hierarchy of a hospital.
>
> *[Catherine, client]*

This poignant statement hints at the ease with which (institutionalized) professionals may unwittingly expropriate ownership, especially during transition points in women's lives. At such moments, when the body boundaries are weakened and lack the usual protective mechanisms, women are more susceptible to the (malign) influences visited upon them by insensitive care providers (Douglas, 1973; Turner 1984). The structure and mechanics of institutions seem to militate against anything other than the formation of superficial, arbitrary, 'top down' relationships, rather than those specifically chosen, actively developed and requiring a high degree of commitment from both sides for the duration of the engagement. It seems that it is within the context of such relationships that the worries and anxieties which preface most decision-making can surface, be formulated and as far as possible be resolved. The midwives I interviewed thought of the alliances created between themselves and their clients as providing opportunities for mutual learning; a scenario which credited the 'lived interactions, participatory experiences and embodied knowledge' of both parties (Okley and Callaway, 1992). Both parties spoke of the relationship as being of fundamental importance in providing a place of deep trust and security from which decision-making was possible.

Alliances of this nature foster the 'emancipated dialogue', which Habermas suggested typified discussions where neither party seeks to mystify or exploit the other on the basis of technical knowledge or social or language skills (Habermas, 1984, 1986). Although the nature of these exchanges seems a world away from the hard facts and evidence-based information that characterize 'scientific' discussions, there is a new paradigm of science emerging which does not discount our unique, experiential past, but incorporates a feminist ethic into the reshaping of knowledge. It pleads for the rediscovery of the feminine principle not as a gender-based quality but rather as an organizing principle; as a way of seeing the world. Within this context, there is no absolute 'Truth' in which to take refuge, but simply an obligation to uncover 'the most reliable account' and one which emphasizes and values a female perspective (Rose, 1994).

Despite any real evidence supporting the image, midwives, doctors and nurses are still often regarded as model citizens, upholding a code of ethical conduct within which fraud and deceit are anathema. However, in the meeting space between the client and the professional, whether this be the antenatal clinic, the labour ward or the client's home, there may be room for speculating just how much and which particular version of 'the truth' is being told (Higgs, 1985). Even in cases where there are substantial grounds for suspecting the health professional of behaviour ranging from being 'economical' with the truth to concealing pertinent information, or even to deliberately lying, this is not uncommonly justified as being 'in the patient's best interests'. Truth-telling may thus be seen more in terms of good intentions; of honouring the rather crude maxim of 'first do no harm', rather than attending to the real issue of whether clients actually have the necessary and relevant information to make their own decisions.

It appears that the notion of an equitable relationship, supported by core values such as integrity, justice and impartiality, cannot be assumed to be a universal feature governing exchanges between care provider and client. Paradoxically, it seems that without a commitment that does honour the creation of a relationship in which these core values operate, the feelings of powerlessness and fear which surface in the client are likely to interfere with any decision-making processes. From her position as a client, Catherine suggested that this had consequences for both midwives and obstetricians:

> *I tried to get round these feelings (of helplessness and fear) by doing a kind of Masonic handshake through reading the 'right' kind of books and learning the 'right' terminology to describe things correctly; as a way of saying 'Watch out ... I do know a little bit about this ... enough to stop you walking all over me' ... and that's particularly so in childbirth where an essentially natural thing is turned into a*

potential medical disaster ... rather like deciding that every time women have a period they have to go into hospital for a day just to have it checked out ... imagine ... it's the same process ... there's that nice little bit of blood which might just mean the beginning of a major haemorrhage ... it would seem grotesque because it's a common experience for all women ... just like having babies.[Catherine, client]

The element of ordinariness, of everyday familiarity, was a component of the relationship which clients valued as the reliable, stable element enabling both parties to negotiate through the inevitable conflicts arising during such a major life transition as childbirth. It also encouraged the development of an active, collaborative, more realistic partnership which endangered neither the client's autonomy nor the midwife's authority.

The reciprocal nature of this exchange, while tolerant of errors of judgment, did however oblige practitioners to own and admit to actual mistakes. One midwife respondent volunteered that this required a substantial shift in attitude from that engendered by the NHS, where she was frequently reminded that her accountability was primarily directed to the Trust, which dictated her contractual obligations, and The Midwives Rules (UKCC, 1993) guiding professional conduct, rather than to the woman and family in her care. Such a culture encouraged an attitude of watching one's back and avoiding engaging with clients or colleagues in an open and forthright manner. In contrast, the relationship between independent midwife and client required that the professional reveal her own personal agenda and prejudices. This was not without considerable risk to both parties, as the consequences of a major conflict of interest might not be easily resolved. In fact, most disagreements were defused without recourse to outside agencies such as counsellors, lawyers or mediators, although one of the midwives had weathered the experience of having a client terminate her contract late in pregnancy because of unresolvable differences. Continuing to provide support when clients made decisions which could not be defended by research-based evidence or which conflicted with a midwife's personal ideology, was a not altogether unusual event and one that was resolved or accommodated in various ways. As Barbara commented after pondering over the case of a client who insisted on an induction of labour in the absence of any clinical indication:

I didn't try to persuade her out of it although I did try to explain the risks of induction; at the end of the day the choice is hers... we have talked about this quite a lot since as she knows me from her last pregnancy, and this time [the client] was quite upset on my behalf and kept on saying to me, 'you are not happy about this, are you?' ... but I have thought long and hard about it since as I didn't feel comfortable with her decision, but it did occur to me that that's what a lot of midwives are doing all the time; making decisions and choices on behalf of women in their care without any discussion whatsoever as to the pros and cons ... or otherwise manipulating women to make the choices that they [the midwives] feel comfortable with. *[Barbara, midwife]*

CONCLUSION

As midwives, we live in an increasingly sanitized world in which the tyranny of the 'should' and the 'ought', in combination with the rules and regulations of our professional bodies and of the wider society, conspire to keep us safe but not necessarily fulfilled. Perhaps, instead of attempting to judge what is acceptable in terms of individual conduct, we should try instead to define what constitutes an actual or potentially hazardous activity and then ask what society would tolerate as a form of control. Women and midwives are in transition; both parties are moving from an environment where choice has been severely restricted. The pendulum is now in danger of swinging to the other extreme; of encouraging a 'shopping list' mentality where in the name of choice (providing this choice is well documented), midwives are expected to accommodate every wish and whim, no matter how unrealistic it may be. If this situation goes unchecked, we may find that childbirth comes to be seen as the arena for the reparation of all previous (negative) experiences, and that the midwives are to blame if they do not make good this earlier damage. We need instead to consider a broader canvas; that if notions of choice and risk essentially translate into people management, then how does any 'civilised' society impose and evaluate regulatory mechanisms on personal behaviour?

Without access to well-presented, relevant literature in the language of choice, a range of visual aids and frank discussions regarding the subsequent clinical and personal implications, the notion of choice is farcical and any evaluation of risk is made impossible. The continued denial of this fact has repercussions for the integrity of both the midwifery profession and the women it purportedly serves. The motivating forces which devised and are currently engaged in implementing the changes in maternity services arose from deep dissatisfaction amongst both midwives and user groups. I consider it crucially important that while this progressive spirit is to be congratulated and encouraged, other strategies will need to be developed which continue to support such innovation. This wider agenda will articulate the controversial and welcome the disturbance provoked by profound thought, viewing it as a healthy sign of professional development. It will liberate the voice of the feminine within midwifery; a voice which is unafraid to be in disagreement with the establishment as it appreciates that:

> ... to think deeply in our culture is to grow angry and to anger others and if you cannot tolerate this anger you are wasting the time you spend in thinking deeply. One of the rewards of deep thought is the hot glow of anger at discovering a wrong, but if anger is taboo, thought will starve to death.
>
> (DiGiacomo, 1963)

IMPLICATIONS FOR PRACTICE

- Research is needed to establish whether midwives' own internalized and idealized perceptions of motherhood subsequently influence either the range of options women are given or decision-making on their behalf.
- Recognition of the limits to midwives' responsibility with regard to decision-making by clients requires clarification. At present this vulnerability seems to be expressed in ever more detailed record-keeping and incident form-filling to protect midwives from litigation.
- Woman-centred care means fostering an atmosphere where all women – midwives and clients – are encouraged to express their opinions without fear of 'getting it wrong'. In such a culture freed from the fear of blame and retribution, unconventional views are welcomed and seen as a healthy stage in the developmental process.

REFERENCES

Arms S (1981) *Immaculate Deception: A New Look at Women and Childbirth in America.* New York: Bantam.

Atkinson SJ & Farias MF (1995) Perceptions of risk during pregnancy amongst urban women in northeast Brazil. *Social Science and Medicine* **41** (11): 1577–1586.

Bastion H (1992) Confined, managed and delivered: the language of obstetrics. *British Journal of Obstetrics and Gynaecology* **99**: 92–93.

Bayer R (1994) Screening and treating women and newborns for HIV infection: ethical and policy issues. *Reproductive Health Matters* **4**: 87–91.

Beck-Gernsheim E (1989) From the pill to test-tube babies: new options, new pressures in reproductive behaviour. In: Ratcliff KS (ed.) *Healing Technology: Feminist Perspectives*, pp. 23–40. Michigan, USA: University of Michigan Press.

Beech BAL (1992) Women's views of childbirth. In: Chard T, Richards MPM (eds) *Obstetrics in the 1990s: Current Controversies*, pp. 153–167. London: MacKeith.

Bell DE, Raiffa H & Tversky A (1988) In: Bell DE (ed.) *Decision Making: Descriptive, Normative and Prescriptive Interactions.* Cambridge University Press.

Berger J & Mohr J (1967) *A Fortunate Man*, republished 1989. Cambridge: Granta.

Bortolaia Silva E, ed. (1996) *Good Enough Mothering: Feminist Perspectives on Lone Motherhood.* London: Routledge.

Brown R (1958) *Words and Things; An Introduction to Language.* USA: Free Press.

Calman C (1996) Cancer: science and society and the communication of risk. *British Medical Journal* **313**: 799–802.

Campbell R & Macfarlane A (1994) *Where To Be Born: The Debate and the Evidence*, 2nd edn. Oxford: National Epidemiology Unit.

Chewning B & Sleath B (1996) Medication decision-making and management: a client centred model. *Social Science and Medicine* **42** (3): 389–398.

Coney S (1992) *The Unfortunate Experiment.* Auckland, New Zealand: Penguin.

Davey Smith G, Bartley M & Blane D (1990) The Black Report on socio-economic inequalities in health 10 yrs on. *British Medical Journal* **301**: 373–337.

Davis-Floyd RE (1992) *Birth as an American Rite of Passage.* Berkeley: University of California Press.

Davis-Floyd RE (1994) The technocratic body: American childbirth as cultural expression. *Social Science and Medicine* **38** (8): 1125–1140.

DeVries R (1966) The midwife's place: an international comparison of the status of midwives. In: Murray SF (ed.) *Midwives and Safer Motherhood*, pp. 159–175. London: Mosby.

DiGiacomo D (1963) Quoted in: Henry J. *Culture Against Man*, p. 341. New York: Random House (Vintage Books).

DiMatteo MR (1994) The physician–patient relationship: effects on the quality of health care. *Clinical Obstetrics and Gynecology* **37**: 149.

[DoH] Department of Health (1993) *Changing Childbirth.* Report of the Expert Maternity Group. London: HMSO.

Donnison J (1988) *Midwives and Medical Men.* London: Heinemann.

Douglas M, ed. (1973) *Rules and Meanings.* Harmondsworth: Penguin.

Dowie J & Elstein A (1988) *Professional Judgement: A Reader in Clinical Decision Making.* Cambridge University Press.

Gallie WB (1964) *Philosophy and the Historical Understanding.* London: Chatto & Windus.

Gordon L (1990) *Woman's Body, Woman's Right.* New York: Penguin.

Gregg R (1993) 'Choice' as a double-edged sword: information, guilt and mother blaming in a high-tech age. *Women and Health* **20**: 53.

Habermas J (1984) *The Theory of Communicative Action*, vol. 1. *Reason and the Rationalization of Society.* London: Heinemann.

Haskey J (1994) Estimated numbers of one parent families and their prevalence in Great Britain in 1991. *Population Trends* (winter): 5–19.

Heagerty BV (1990) *Gender on Professionalisation: The Struggle for British Midwifery 1900–1936.* PhD thesis, Michigan State University (copy in RCM library).

Henifin MS, Hubbard R & Norsigian J (1988) Prenatal screening. In: Taub N, Cohen S (eds) *Reproductive Laws for the 1990s: A Briefing Handbook,* pp. 129–154. Newark, NJ: Rutgers University Press.

Higgs R (1985) On telling patients the truth. In: Lockwood M (ed.) *Moral Dilemmas in Modern Medicine.* Oxford: Oxford University Press.

Hunt LM, Jordan B & Irwin S (1989) Views of what's wrong: diagnosis and patient's concepts of illness. *Social Science and Medicine* **28** (9): 957–961.

Kirkham M (1993) Communication in midwifery. In: Alexander J, Levy V, Roch S (eds) *Midwifery Practice: A Research-based Approach.* Basingstoke: Macmillan Press.

Kitzinger S (1984) *The Experience of Childbirth.* Harmondsworth: Penguin.

Kleinman A (1978) Concepts and a model for the comparison of medical systems as cultural systems. *Social Science and Medicine* **2**: 85–95.

Krishnamurti (1985) Quoted in *Women's Health Newsletter* September (26): 7.

Leap N (1992) The power of words. *Nursing Times* **88** (21): 60–61.

Leap N (1996) 'Persuading' women to give birth at home – offering real choice? *British Journal of Midwifery* **4** (10): 536–538.

Lecky-Thompson M (1995) Independent midwifery in Australia. In: Murphy-Black T (ed.) *Issues in Midwifery.* Edinburgh: Churchill Livingstone.

Lilford RJ & Thornton JG (1992) Making difficult decisions. In: Chard T, Richards MPM (eds) *Obstetrics in the 1990s: Current Controversies.* London: MacKeith.

Lindley DV (1985) *Making Decisions.* Chichester: John Wiley.

Lupton D, McCarthy S & Chapman S (1995) 'Doing the right thing': the symbolic meanings and experiences of having an HIV antibody test. *Social Science and Medicine* **41** (2): 173–180.

McCarron PG, Davey Smith G & Womersley JJ (1994) Deprivation and mortality in Glasgow: changes from 1980 to 1992. *British Medical Journal* **309**: 1481–1482.

Maine D (1991) *Safe Motherhood: Options and Issues.* New York: Center for Population and Family Health.

Maine D, Freedman L, Shaheed F, Frautschi S & Akalin MZ (1995) Risks and rights: the uses of reproductive health data. *Reproductive Health Matters* November **6**: 40–51.

Martin E (1987) *The Woman in the Body: A Cultural Analysis of Reproduction.* Milton Keynes: Open University Press.

Moore HL (1988) *Feminism and Anthropology.* Cambridge: Polity Press.

Oakley A (1984) *The Captured Womb: A History of the Medical Care of Pregnant Women.* Oxford: Basil Blackwell.

Okley J & Callaway H, eds (1992) *Anthropology and Autobiography.* London: Routledge & Kegan Paul.

Ortner S (1974) 'Is female to male as nature is to culture?' In: Rosaldo M, Lamphere L (eds) *Woman, Culture and Society,* pp. 67–88. Stanford University Press.

Plata IM, Gonzalez VAC & de la Espriella A (1995) A policy is not enough: women's health policy in Colombia. *Reproductive Health Matters* November **6**: 107–113.

Price C (1995) Do midwives really provide choices for women. Presentation at A.C.M.I. 9th Biennial Conference *Knowledge and Wisdom, the Keys to Safe Motherhood.* Sydney, September 1995.

Ravindran Sundari TK (1995) Women's health policies: organising for change. *Reproductive Health Matters* November **6**: 7–11.

Reid T (1994) Delivery dilemma. *Nursing Times* **90** (9): 16.

Richardson L (1990) Narrative and sociology. *Journal of Contemporary Ethnography* **19**: 116.

Rose H (1994) *Love, Power and Knowledge; Towards a Feminist Transformation of the Sciences.* Cambridge: Polity Press.

Rosser J (1995) Informed choice initiative. *MIDIRS Midwifery Digest* **5** (4): 382–384.

Rothman BK (1986) *The Tentative Pregnancy; Prenatal Diagnosis and the Future of Motherhood.* New York: Viking.

Ruddick S (1989) *Maternal Thinking: Towards a Politics of Peace.* Boston: Beacon.

Saffron L (1993) The consumer's perception of risk. *Consumer Policy Review* **3** (4): 213–221.

Saffron L (1994) *Challenging Conceptions; Pregnancy and Parenting Beyond the Traditional Family.* London: Cassell.

Sandelowski M & Corson Jones L (1996) Healing fictions: stories of choosing in the aftermath of the detection of fetal anomalies. *Social Science Medicine* **42** (3): 353–361.

Shaw M (1994) *Passionate Enlightenment: Women in Tantric Buddhism.* Princeton University Press.

Slovic P (1987) Perceptions of risk. *Science* **236**: 280–285.

Spallone P (1989) *Beyond Conception: Elemental Journey through the Labyrinth of Sexuality.* Granby, MA: Bergin & Harvey.

Spender D (1980) *Man Made Language.* London: Routledge & Keegan Paul.

Stapleton H (1993) *Choosing Risk or Risking Choice: A Study of Independent Midwives and the Women who Employ them.* MSc dissertation, Brunel University (copy in RCM library).

Steer P (1995) Education and debate: recent advances (obstetrics). *British Medical Journal* **311**: 1209–1212.

Tannen D (1991) *You Just Don't Understand: Women and Men in Conversation.* London: Virago.

Tew M (1990) *Safer Childbirth? A Critical History of Maternity Care.* London: Chapman & Hall.

Townsend P, Phillimore P & Beattie A (1988) *Health and Deprivation: Inequality and the North.* London: Croom Helm.

Turner B (1984) *The Body and Society.* Oxford: Basil Blackwell.

Tversky A & Kahnemann D (1974) Judgement under uncertainty: heuristics and biases. *Science* **185**: 1124–1131.

Tymstra T (1989) Assessment in health care. *International Journal of Technology* **5**: 207–213.

[UKCC] United Kingdom Central Council for Nursing, Midwifery and Health Visiting (1992) *Code of Professional Conduct.* London: UKCC.

[UKCC] United Kingdom Central Council for Nursing, Midwifery and Health Visiting (1993) *Midwives Rules.* London: UKCC.

Von Neumann J & Morgenstern O (1947) *The Theory of Games and Economic Behaviour.* Princeton University Press.

Walt G (1994) *Health Policy: An Introduction to Process and Power,* ch. 6. London: Zed.

Weinstein MC & Fineberg HV, eds (1980) *Clinical Decision Analysis.* Philadelphia: WB Saunders.

Williams R (1976) *Keywords.* London: Fontana/Croom Helm.

Wilson B (1993) Why finders should be keepers. *MIDIRS* June 1994 **4**: 2.

Winterton N (1992) *Maternity Services,* vol. 1. Report of the House of Commons Health Committee. London: HMSO.

4

Willing handmaidens of science? The struggle over the new midwife in early twentieth-century England

Brooke V. Heagerty

The Midwives' Act of 1902 constituted a radical break with midwifery's past. At that time midwifery was unorganized, typically practised by working-class lay midwives, and was an integral part of the network of economic and social relationships which comprised working-class life and culture. The Act provided the legal power to reform the practice of midwifery, to alter the relationship between the midwife and the mother (and thereby the midwives' relationship to the working-class community), and to create and sustain a powerful apparatus of enforcement.

This break in the continuity of midwifery's past has been seen as the starting point of midwives' steady progress toward professional status and the social benefits derived from this accomplishment (Brierly, 1923b, 21; Harvey, 1951; Cowell and Wainwright, 1981; Rivers, 1981). Scholars have argued that midwives' failure to experience the same advances in autonomy and control of the work which other professions have achieved is largely the result of the rivalry and obstructionism of the male-dominated medical profession (Oakley, 1976; Donnison, 1977; Leavitt, 1986). These studies have provided much-needed knowledge about midwifery's legislative battles, the history of midwifery's leaders, the ideological constructs of women's behaviour that have passed for medical science, and the extent of the medical profession's power and control over the definition and delivery of obstetrical care.

Re-examination of midwifery's past, however, indicates that the conflicts rife within midwifery's development have not been fully explored. The middle-class and upper-class nurses and trained midwives of the Midwives' Institute who spearheaded the movement for midwifery reform shared the attitudes and biases of their class toward the working class. In matters pertaining to the working-class midwife and the women they attended, the Institute members expressed more kinship with those of their class – men and women, medical or lay – than with the women of the working class. In the first decades of the twentieth century midwifery reformers of both sexes and various professions battled with rank and file midwives over the scope of midwives' work, the nature of their relationship to the working-class women they attended and to the government officials to whom they were expected to answer under the provisions of the Act. Rank and file midwives' myriad forms of resistance to and participation in the redefinition of midwifery shaped its development as much as the strategies and actions of the Institute and its allies. The struggle between them, shaped and given texture as it was by conflicting class interests and ideologies and differential access to power, form the roots of twentieth-century midwifery and have marked its development ever since (Esland, 1980; Chamberlain, 1981; Brickman, 1983; Davies, 1983; Little, 1983; Maggs, 1983; Holmes, 1984; Taylor-Ladd, 1988; Heagerty, 1990; Leap and Hunter, 1993).

'A SELECT PART, NOT THE RANK AND FILE'

From that evening in 1881 when the wealthy philanthropist Louisa Hubbard brought together a group of well-placed trained nurses and hospital matrons, the Midwives' Institute combined the purpose of providing respectable employment for middle-class women with the broader agenda of late nineteenth- and early twentieth-century social reform. The Institute's early members earned their nursing and midwifery credentials in some of the country's most prestigious training schools, but few ever practised as midwives. Rather, they were the supervisors of obstetric wards, matrons of maternity institutions and managers of philanthropic organizations. The signatures on the original Articles of Association reveal some of the more prestigious names in the medical profession as well as three members of Parliament (Nursing Notes, 1933a, p. 114). The leadership of the Institute, the core of women who went on to control the policies and administration of the organization, were all well-educated upper-class and middle-class women who had risen to managerial positions in their chosen field of health work. Several of those who were nurses had graduated from the reformed nursing programmes of Florence Nightingale, and all of them held the certificate of the London Obstetrical Society, the highest certification of formal midwifery training prior to 1902 (Nursing Notes, 1933a, p. 113). At a time when the word 'midwife' was hardly spoken in polite society, women such as Jane Wilson who served as secretary to Louisa Twining's Work House Infirmary Association (Nursing Notes, 1933a, p. 113), Emma Brierly whose father was marine painter in the court of Queen Victoria (Nursing Notes, 1933b, p. 129), Amy Hughes who succeeded Rosalind Paget as superintendent of the Queen's Jubilee Institute for District Nursing (Nursing Notes, 1901) and Paget herself, the daughter of a wealthy barrister born into a Liverpool shipbuilding family, niece to William Rathbone MP and 'endowed with a restless social conscience', brought the cause of midwifery reform legitimacy and cemented its respectability (Cowell and Wainwright, 1981). As Paget testified in 1910, the Institute did not pretend to represent all the women practising midwifery, but rather the 'aristocracy... a select part, not the rank and file – very well' (UK Privy Council, 1909a, [512–513]). The Institute had been integral to the formulation and passage of the 1902 Midwives' Act and its strength and influence on the Central Midwives Board (CMB), the regulatory and policy-making body the Act created, allowed ample opportunity to protect the interests of those it represented (Heagerty, 1990, pp. 7–11).

ORDERING SOCIETY THROUGH SOCIAL REFORM

For the leadership of the Midwives' Institute, the struggle for the reform of midwifery was inseparable from the broader movement for social reform going on around them. Beginning in the 1880s, middle-class social reformers had grown increasingly concerned about the conditions under which large sections of the working class lived out their lives. In particular, the poorest of the cities' populations experienced shorter life expectancy rates than the middle and upper classes, greater morbidity rates, and despite an overall decline in the general mortality rate, an alarmingly high rate of infant and maternal mortality (Booth, 1892; Rowntree, 1901). Such a population – wracked by poverty and ill-health – was hardly adequate either to defend the Empire or to labour productively for the British economy. Since the most debilitated of the working class also appeared to be the most prolific, reformers were increasingly alarmed that the 'worst' of the population would soon outnumber the 'best', that is, their more socially stable and physically sound class superiors (Weeks, 1981, pp. 122–126; Searle, 1976, 1981). These years saw the rapid formation of charity organizations dedicated to the moral reform of the urban and rural poor and, in the early part of the twentieth century, a wave of social legislation (of which the Midwives' Act of 1902 was part) aimed at ameliorating the worst conditions (McCleary, 1935; Weeks, 1981, pp. 126–127; Lewis, 1980; Oakley, 1984).

Reformers were as concerned about the social consequences of poverty and ill-health as they were about the suffering of the poor. In the philanthropic and welfare literature of the late nineteenth and early twentieth century the poor were 'generally pictured as coarse, brutish, drunken and immoral; through years of neglect and complacency they had become threats to civilization ...'(Stedman-Jones, 1971, p. 285; Davin, 1978). This philosophy was especially evident in district nursing – the prototype for much of late nineteenth-century welfare work and the area with which the Institute leadership was most closely associated. Philanthropic organizations sought to supplement the efforts of the Poor Law not simply by outright relief, but through uprooting what reformers believed to be the source of the problem – individual failing. Although they usually provided some kind of material help, these organizations generally considered that their real work lay in teaching the poor to adopt the appropriate values. 'Building up of the character of the community,' wrote Mary Minit (a Midwives' Institute vice-president) relied 'upon building the character of each individual' – the most important of which were ' "self" qualities: "self-knowledge", "self-reverence", "self-control" to which let us add "self-help" and "self-reliance" ' (Minit, 1925, p. 2; Chin, 1995, pp. 114–121). Because this process of education could only be carried out by those who already lived by these values, services were to be dispensed by middle-class welfare workers (many of them women), who, because of their superior social background, were considered to be most capable of exercising the proper influence on the recipient in his or her journey to an orderly and independent life (Minit, 1925, p. 3; Nursing Notes, 1906a). 'If one sentence could explain our work,' wrote Reverend Samuel Augustus Barnett of his Charity Organization Society, 'it is that we aim at decreasing not suffering, but sin' (Stedman-Jones, 1971, p. 271).

Institute literature was permeated with the sense that the working class, particularly its poorest members, were beings who were fundamentally different from their social superiors. Although many writers contributed to creating this image in the pages of the Institute's monthly journal, *Nursing Notes*, probably no one writer was more responsible for consistently bringing substance to this notion than the prolific writer and district nursing reformer, Marjorie Loane. Drawing on her experience as a nurse for the Queen's Jubilee Institute for District Nursing, Loane's rather crude and starkly drawn descriptions of working-class life served as indispensable translations for health workers who, committed to reforming the poor for 'their own good', were often bewildered by the frequent cultural clash of these two different worlds. 'The familiar "honour bright" of better-class nurseries is unknown,' Loane wrote, warning her readers of the poor's natural evasiveness and deceit, particularly when confronted by their social betters (Loane, 1906). Even a respectful attitude could be just another dodge. 'Mr Atkins at home always refers to us as "Lady Nurses",' she wrote, 'but occasionally his voice floats in at my open window and the more picturesque expression used then is "them Jubilee tramps"' (Loane, 1905a).

Working-class mothers came in for particular scrutiny. Some contributors to *Nursing Notes* conceded that working-class women faced considerable obstacles to providing a stable and ordered existence for their families, not least of which was the 'double standard of morality' of which feminists complained (MD, 1910; Nursing Notes, 1908a, 1914a; Bland, 1986). More frequently, articles blamed the mother for her own plight and focused on reforming her behaviour rather than considering the need for any systemic changes (Nursing Notes, 1904a, 1906b; Loane, 1912a). For many, the ignorance of working-class women was matched only by their contempt for the efforts of those who sought to 'improve' them (Nursing Notes, 1907a; May, 1915). Loane graphically captured the haunting sense of danger when she described 'the slattern with one wretched infant in her unmotherly arms and five in their untimely graves, [who] listens with scarcely veiled contempt and mutters a coarse version of a coarse proverb as the baffled nurse turns away' (Loane, 1905a). If social stability and the future of the nation depended upon the ameliorative influence of middle-class health workers, what would be the consequences of their failure to influence such charges?

The attitudes expressed toward working-class women in *Nursing Notes* seem at odds with the leadership's commitment to the principles of feminism and the struggle for suffrage. The leadership was drawn to the cause for the same reason they were drawn to midwifery reform – a desire to make a change in society. The right to share in the same political and social rights granted to men of their class was no abstract precept for them. As Sandra Holton has shown, feminists did not 'seek merely an entry to a male-defined sphere', rather they wanted the 'opportunity to redefine that sphere' (Holton, 1986, p. 18). With many other feminists of their day, the leadership subscribed to what historians have called 'essentialism', the belief that women were bestowed by nature with a higher moral sensibility and natural altruism, qualities that ran counter to the immorality of men and their 'creed of brute force' (Nursing Notes, 1906c, 1907b; Wilson, 1915; Holton, 1986, pp. 9–28; Brown and Jordonova, 1986). They believed that by bringing 'a purer atmosphere into things political', women's involvement in 'the wide and beneficial ordering of the state' would end the social degeneration which men's immorality had caused (Nursing Notes, 1902b, 1907b,c, 1908a, 1909a; Loane, 1912b; Bristow, 1977; Soloway, 1982; Jeffries, 1985; Holton, 1986, p. 15; Kent, 1987; Heagerty, 1990, pp. 34–42). The vote was not a mere symbol of political equality, but a means to reconstruct society according to their moral sensibilities and social reform priorities.

The leadership's vision was not one of equality and democracy, however. They took for granted that the vote would be extended to women of property only and that most working-class women would continue to be excluded from political participation. They believed that social reform would best be served by the preservation of a strictly hierarchical class system in which the working class knew its place and adopted the behaviours and values their social superiors thought most appropriate for them. Training the working class to accept their place in society as the Empire's factory hands, labourers and childbearers was as important an aspect of the midwives' work as providing safe maternity attendance. The Institute promoted trained midwives, armed with their knowledge of antisepsis, as standard-bearers of science in the home. The inculcation of the values and morality of bourgeois society was an indispensable element of this 'science' and one which fused midwives' work to the preservation of the proper relations between the classes. 'As willing handmaidens of Science,' the nursing leader Albinia Broderick wrote and *Nursing Notes* approvingly quoted, nurses and midwives must 'inculcate always and everywhere the principle of self-control and self-discipline... to remove ignorance and dirt, in short, wherever [she] may find it' (Nursing Notes, 1913a). The working-class wife and mother was the crucial link in the chain of social order and her 'low ideals [and] inability to help' herself made intervention from above all the more urgent (Tonge, 1903; Nursing Notes, 1912a). Margaret French captured this sentiment when she wrote in *Nursing Notes*, 'We want to make these women ambitious. Ambitious, not to rise out of their own class, but to raise the standard of their own class to an altogether different plane' (French, 1915).

'ARRAYED ON THE SIDE OF MORALITY AND HEALTH'

At the time of the passage of the Midwives' Act and for almost two decades afterwards, the overwhelming majority of registered practising midwives continued to be working-class women who had no formal training (UKCMB, 1916, 1917). Since there were so few trained midwives in 1902, the Act had made specific provisions to allow lay midwives to continue in practice. If a midwife wanted to 'advertise as or call herself a midwife', she had until 1905 to register as 'bona fide' under the Act (Atkinson, 1907, p. 35). Lay midwives who did not register could still attend births, but they could not call themselves midwives and after 1910 they could no longer attend births 'habitually and for gain' without being under the immediate direction of a certified midwife or a physician. Stringent criminal and financial penalties accompanied these provisions.

That working-class lay midwives were allowed to practise in any capacity was a substantial blow to the Institute's class goals and professional aspirations. More galling, however, was that these women were allowed to register with the same status and on equal terms as the trained midwife. In commonly referring to lay midwives as 'illiterate, ignorant', 'faculties blunted from want of trained exercise' and 'superstitious and often of very low character', *Nursing Notes* correspondents and editorials alike left no question as to midwifery reformers' views (Nursing Notes, 1900; Brierly, 1923a). What status or prestige could there be for women of refinement and education to belong to a body of practitioners which included such women? Moreover, the Institute had fought for state licensing and regulation in order to remove the influence of working-class midwives from the working-class home. Instead, the Act had given legal credence to a class of practitioners who 'share their views and prejudices' (Wilson, 1904). For those who were 'arrayed on the side of morality and health', such a situation was intolerable (Dock, 1910).

It is a matter of debate whether lay midwives fitted reformers' descriptions of them, but more important for the moment is that this perception so common among midwifery reformers was verified and given substance in the form of a character not from life, but from fiction – Sairey Gamp the lay midwife in Charles Dickens' novel *Martin Chuzzlewit*. Sairey worked both as a midwife and a layer-out of the dead (making her an agent of infection), was fond of gin (thus throwing her personal morality into question) and refused to show the appropriate amount of deference to her social betters (thus making her a dangerous influence on her patients and a threat to the social order). This simple image of an old, drunken and wilful working-class woman served to crystallize the full range of middle-class attitudes toward the poor, their contempt for working-class life and culture, and their anxieties over the potential consequences of the failure to reshape and control working-class behaviour and values.

It was in contradistinction to this character that the new midwife was given shape and texture. Where Sairey flaunted her penchant for gin, the Institute championed temperance; where Sairey's personal morality was in question, the Institute supported every institutional and legal means possible to enforce dominant standards of personal and sexual morality on all registered midwives. Where Sairey was always on the lookout to turn a penny for herself, the Institute lauded service and self-sacrifice; and where Sairey confidently proclaimed her expertise and independence, the Institute insisted upon submission and humility before the medical profession and her social superiors. In the Institute's terms, Sairey was not even a woman, but a freak of nature. As Sairey's opposite and in step with the broader agenda of social reform, the new midwife would take her place as the primary attendant in normal midwifery.

'A midwife who knew when to send for the doctor' was the first goal of the regulations formulated by the Central Midwives Board (UK Privy Council, 1909a, [604]). The Board's approved training programmes prepared a midwife to perform the tasks that had been delegated to her by the Rules of Practice (the Board's regulations governing midwives' practice) – attendance on normal midwifery cases (strictly defined), the prevention of infection through the use of antiseptic techniques, and the summoning of medical aid in the event of complications. Pupils were taught the 'nature, causes and symptoms' of puerperal sepsis and the technical procedures to guarantee that the patient and the lying-in room were properly protected against infection. They were prepared through instruction in 'elementary anatomy of the pelvis and generative organs', the principal complications of pregnancy, and the 'symptoms, mechanism, course and management of natural labour' to manage those labours designated as normal under the Rules. In every other instance, except for the 'uncomplicated vertex or breech', a midwife was to send for a doctor. Under no circumstances was the midwife to make judgments as to condition or care (Nursing Notes, 1905; Atkinson, 1907, pp. 79–80). Dr Stanley Atkinson, the Institute's representative on the Board from 1907 to 1910, summarized this underlying premise of midwifery training when he approvingly quoted from comments made by Lord Balfour of Burleigh in a parliamentary debate on the question of licensing legislation: 'It is not the function of a Midwife to diagnose, but as with all "first- aid" practice, when in difficulty or in doubt to send at once for a doctor' (Atkinson, 1907, p. 72).

However, the new midwife was more than a technically proficient midwifery practitioner. Before she was allowed to sit for the certification examination or gain bona fide status, a midwife had to offer written proof from individuals acceptable to the Board that she was 'trustworthy, sober and of good moral character', and she was thereafter required to conduct her life and practice in accordance with those precepts (Atkinson, 1907, p. 60). Inevitably, midwifery reformers defined these qualities according to their own values and beliefs. Temperance, purity in sexual matters, a willingness to sacrifice and to serve others and the willing submission to the social hierarchy drew an immediate line between the new midwife and the Gamp.

Since alcohol made up a vital part of working-class culture for both men and women, it was predictable that it would gain the attention of middle-class reformers. Ellen Ross found that in the East End of London before the War, drinking and going to the pub were part of working-class women's social life. Midwives were often included in 'wetting the baby's head', the traditional toast celebrating the baby's birth. Although recent research has shown that working-class families made a distinct difference between having a drink and habitual drunkenness, middle-class reformers made no such distinction (UKCMB, 1911; Ross, 1983, pp. 10–11). 'The effect of alcohol,' wrote Institute Council member Agnes Duffield, 'is to undermine will power, destroy the intellect and take away moral responsibility' (Nursing Notes, 1915a). Midwives who drank or participated in working-class customs associated with alcohol not only helped to perpetuate dangerous and unhealthy behaviour, but reinforced the connection with working-class life that reformers fought to sever. So that midwives might remain above any association with alcohol or the iniquities of its effects, midwifery reformers advocated total abstinence and urged trained midwives to convince their patients to do the same (Nursing Notes, 1909b; Peart, 1910).

As an occupation of women, midwifery was inevitably judged by social proscriptions regarding women's sexuality. A woman was considered reputable if she kept her sexual life within the confines of a monogamous married life. Stepping outside these boundaries was cause for social stigmatization and shame. Reformers demanded that trained midwives stand as a living example, particularly to the working-class woman, of the proper conduct of sexual life. Her enquiries during the pregnancy, her attendance at the birth, her daily presence in the home for the 10 days postpartum that the Rules required meant that the midwife was, if even briefly, a part of a family's life. There were temptations and many possibilities for misunderstandings. A midwife who conducted herself properly would leave no room for question on either score and would thereby guarantee midwifery's privileged access to the patient's home (Nursing Notes, 1913d, 1916d; Nursing Notes, 1915b,c, 1916a; Heagerty, 1990).

The trained midwife was considered most 'womanly' in her anxious willingness to sacrifice her own needs in the service of others. The Institute argued that women's natural altruism, rooted in the capacity to reproduce and mother, was the missing element in social and political life. Trained midwives were mothers to their patients, the mother 'who loves, cherishes and admonishes all those who come under her care' (Nursing Notes, 1916b). In contrast to the almost aggressively arrogant Gamp who showed little interest for anyone's interests but her own, the new midwife displayed, in the words of Catherine Wood, a prominent nursing leader and a vice-president of the Midwives' Institute, 'the giving of one's best for another that is the highest of all woman's privileges' (Wood, 1901; Nursing Notes, 1914b; Mathieson, 1915).

Self-help, self-reliance and individual responsibility were considered as indispensable to the trained midwife as her elevated personal and sexual morality and her sense of service and willingness to sacrifice. Any actions midwives took, whether individually or collectively, had to reinforce those values that upheld the workings of the market. When midwives complained that physicians would not answer their call for medical aid until the family or the midwife guaranteed his fee (many families could not afford the fees of both midwife and doctor), the Institute recommended, and some took their advice, that midwives form insurance funds upon which they could draw the money to pay the fee themselves if necessary (Nursing Notes, 1913b,c). Similarly, at the urging of the Institute, some midwife groups formed defence funds to pay the legal expenses of their members who were called before a local tribunal or the Central Midwives Board for discipline (Nursing Notes, 1907f, 1911a). These kinds of solutions preserved the 'wholesome competition' between midwives so necessary to 'keep up efficiency', and prevented unseemly confrontations with the medical profession and local officials (Nursing Notes, 1917a).

Imbued with the proper values, the new midwife was to accept her place in the professional and social hierarchy, deferring to her natural superiors the medical profession, the officials of the Act and the elite leadership of the Midwives' Institute. The 'strict obedience to the physician's or surgeon's power and knowledge', as Florence Nightingale wrote (quoted by Gamarnikow, 1978), were for the leadership the first and lasting hallmarks of a good nurse and a good midwife (MIRC, 1912a). The leadership expected trained midwives to be treated with respect, but they never (except during a rare fit of pique) entertained the possibility that midwifery would extend its reach beyond the limited scope to which it had been assigned (Nursing Notes, 1907g). They considered midwifery to be 'the inferior branch of the healing profession', and medicine its 'natural leader and superior' (Nursing Notes, 1915d). Midwives' responsibilities did exceed those of the nurse, but her legal and technical authority was always, like the nurse, circumscribed by the physician.

Relations between midwives were to be the same as the relationship between the different classes of women. The elite would lead and the rank and file would follow. It was natural that rank and file trained midwives be placed in a subordinate position to women 'whose education, experience and position make them worthy to be leaders of that great army of women such as is represented by the Midwives Roll' (Nursing Notes, 1910a). Although unequal, both leaders and followers nevertheless had crucial roles to play. Women of status and education laboured on the 'truly thankless task of fighting the battle for their profession' and rank and file midwives made their most important contribution by upholding the Institute's vision of social order – deferring to the natural hierarchy, obeying the officials of the Act and abiding by the Rules, and conducting their lives and practice accordingly (Nursing Notes, 1907d).

There is little doubt that by defining the new midwife in this way the leadership sought to mollify those who were sceptical of educated women's entrance into paid employment or critical of midwifery's protected status under the Act. The history of any profession is the attempt to 'constitute and control a market for [its] expertise' and through this monopoly provide a living for its members (Friedman, 1965; Friedson, 1970; Johnson, 1972; Larson, 1976; Melosh, 1982; Tomes, 1983). Professions typically mask their protected status and the privilege derived from it through their claim of altruism and interest only in the public good. While self-serving, this vision was not simply opportunism. The leadership believed that these qualities were the building blocks of woman's essential nature. Society had said so already, but had hypocritically denied them their full scope. Service, sacrifice, and morality – these were not silly, empty sentiments, but the principles that guided them in their struggle to advance the interests of their class. With passionate devotion, the leadership disseminated these ideas in *Nursing Notes*, made every effort to publicize the activities of those who espoused them, and made the Institute itself into a place where the full range of social issues could be discussed and debated (Nursing Notes, 1908b,c,d, 1910k, 1911b,c, 1912b). 'It was in dear old Buckingham Street,' Emma Brierly recalled, 'that some of us began to realise for the first time we, as midwives, had glorious work to do, and that, please God, we would do that work faithfully' (Brierly, 1923b, p. 21).

ENFORCEMENT THROUGH DISCIPLINE

The majority of practising midwives during these years shared a common cultural background and life experience with the women they attended (Chinn, 1988, pp. 130–147; Ross, 1983, 1993; Heagerty, 1990, pp. 64–81). They too were wives and mothers overburdened by a life lived on slim resources and the responsibilities of keeping a household together and a family clean and fed. Many midwives lived and practised in the same neighbourhood for years, some in the neighbourhoods in which they were born (UKPRO cases 005, 015, 038, 067 – see Box 4.1). Over the years, these women attended hundreds of labours and knew the women they attended throughout their lives. The Institute vociferously denounced these practitioners, but evidence from various sources indicates that, as a general rule, these women provided a relatively safe and reliable service both prior to the Act and after (UKCMB, 1911, pp. 8–9; 1914, pp. 8–9; Nursing Notes, 1931; Chamberlain, 1981, pp. 112–114; Little, 1983, pp. 61–63).

Although not without their ups and downs, in general midwives' relationships with the women they attended were characterized by a natural familiarity which contrasted with the more distanced and formal ideal promulgated by the Institute and the medical profession. Elizabeth Roberts found that in some cases midwives could be as close as friends with the women they attended (Roberts, 1984, pp. 106–107). However, a woman did not have to befriend her midwife to share a deep and abiding bond with her. She faced real dangers during childbirth and as she endured the long and often anxious hours of labour nothing could replace the steady nerves and comforting hand of an experienced midwife. Midwives and the women they attended were known to protect and defend each other's interests and well-being against local authorities and social superiors. Trained and lay midwives alike covered up abortions gone wrong, or falsified official records to protect the family (Nursing Notes, 1910m, 1911h, 1914d, 1915g, 1916c, 1917d; UKPRO cases 047, 062, 063, 066, 072). When families pleaded with them to delay sending for the doctor whose fee they could not pay, midwives often abided by their wishes. In turn, if their midwife got into trouble with authorities, the women and their families would often write letters of support, collect signatures in the neighbourhood on her behalf or refuse to co-operate with local officials against her (Nursing Notes, 1909d, 1918; UKPRO cases 033, 038, 048, 057, 065).

If reformers were going to effect the necessary changes in working class behaviour, these 'close barriers [which] are firmly erected and closely guarded by the poor' had to be dismantled (Loane, 1905b). The midwife who considered herself accountable first to the woman and the standards of her community rather than to the legal power and authority of the Act and its officials was part of the foundation of this formidable bulwark against outside intrusion. Reversing this equation, and thereby establishing the proper relationship between midwife and patient, was the task of the Central Midwives Board.

The Central Midwives Board had been created by the Midwives' Act of 1902 and empowered with authority over all aspects of registered midwifery, but midwifery reformers believed that, as *Nursing Notes* asserted, 'the penal part of the Board's work is nearly, if not quite, the most important part of its duties' (Nursing Notes, 1904b, 1907e). The Board was composed of representatives from government bodies and various organizations, including the Midwives' Institute, which had a vested interest in midwife regulation. Of the nine representatives who sat on the Board, five (including the Institute's representative) were either members or supporters of the Institute, including the chairman, the obstetrician Sir Frances Champneys (Nursing Notes, 1902a, 1907d, 1908e). Rosalind Paget sat on the committee responsible for developing the Rules of Practice and, with a shifting cast of Institute members and supporters such as Jane Wilson, Sir Frances Champneys, Lady Mabelle Egerton and Mrs Latter, sat for years on the Board's disciplinary arm, the Penal Cases Committee (Nursing Notes, 1904c). The Board and the Local Supervisory Authorities (LSA), local bodies which oversaw the practice of midwives registered in their jurisdiction, were granted extensive powers under the Act to supervise and discipline registered midwives. In the name of controlling the bona fide midwives and making midwifery an instrument of social improvement, these powers provided the basis for the evolution of an extensive apparatus of control which operated throughout the country.

Because the Rules of Practice were at once so detailed regarding specific procedures and so encompassing as to cover the midwife's personal life as well as her practice, the powers which the Board bestowed upon the LSAs amounted to almost unrestrained authority over midwives' lives and work. Because the Rules required her to make her practice open to periodic inspection, the midwife had little choice but to submit to official investigations. Some Midwifery Inspectors recognized that the poverty and ill-health of the women whom midwives attended presented real difficulties for good practice and appreciated the resourcefulness with which the midwives answered these challenges and still provided a safe service (UKCMB, 1911, 1914; Davies, 1975, 1978; Pember Reeves, 1979). Others, however, were often patronizing, domineering and at times vindictive, their behaviour crossing the line from routine supervision to harassment (Nursing Notes, 1906e, 1911i, 1915h; UKPRO cases 022, 031, 041, 048, 070). If charged with a violation of the Rules, midwives defended themselves against the combined resources and expertise of the LSA and the Board. The Board and the LSA worked together on preparing the cases and the Board underwrote all the expenses from collecting depositions to paying travel and lodging for witnesses called to testify against the accused. Midwives were allowed to attend their hearings and to bring either counsel or a friend to represent them. They were also given the right to appeal against the Board's verdict in the High Court. Many, however, did not even have the resources to attend their own hearings, let alone pay to mount an appeal. With the Board given the legal power not only to charge and prosecute but also to stand in judgment, it is not surprising that guilty verdicts were rendered in the overwhelming majority of cases (Heagerty, 1990, pp. 284–285).

Hundreds of cases were brought before the Board on the LSA's recommendations in the first two decades of the twentieth century. A random sample of surviving files of cases heard between 1905 and 1919 gives an indication of the pattern of charges and verdicts. In the sample, charges were concentrated in those areas of the greatest concern to midwifery reformers – misconduct (particularly, alleged drunkenness and promiscuity), and failure to advise and send for a doctor. Almost 70% of all the midwives were charged with the failure to send for a physician in the event of complications. The Board rendered a verdict of guilty in 93% of these cases. Twenty per cent of the cases involved charges of misconduct (of which all but two involved midwives trained after the Act), and in almost 90% of these, the defendant was struck off. In the overall sample, training made little difference in the type of charge or the verdict. Trained and bona fide midwives were charged and received the severest penalties – cancellation of their certificates – in roughly the same percentages. In the sample, 58% of the bona fide midwives and 54% of the trained midwives were struck off the Roll. In the 'failure to advise and send' category the Board cancelled the certificates of 55% of the bona fide midwives and 53% of the trained midwives (Heagerty, 1990, pp. 284–290).

In its regular Central Midwives Board column, *Nursing Notes* consistently publicized the disciplinary work of the Board and the crimes of the women brought before it. While it reported on cases of trained midwives, the reporters reserved their most descriptive and sensational language for the transgressions of bona fide cases, the majority of cases printed in these columns. With name after name listed in dulling succession, the reporters gave witness to the continued dangerous and repulsive existence of Mrs Gamps throughout the country. The cases of Emma Jones who had to be 'picked up from a flower bed in the garden hopelessly drunk', or Sara Elizabeth Carford who 'had been sentenced to twelve months hard labour for supplying lead pills with intent to procure abortion', Mary Elizabeth Davey whose trade was 'cleaning the internal parts of pigs' carcasses in her own house' or Jane Tween who was charged with 'feeding the infant on oatmeal and gin' were guaranteed to sent shivers up the spine of the reader (Nursing Notes, 1906f,g, 1908h, 1913e). How could anyone deny the Board its extensive powers when such women were still out there practising?

The official correspondence, Inspectors' reports, and depositions and testimonials found in the Penal Committee's case files reveal that the type of publicity that *Nursing Notes* provided the Board did not always conform with the reality of the dynamics and the process of supervision and discipline. In some of the cases, the documents in the case files indicate a clear pattern of responsibility. In many cases, however, these sources reveal that the process of supervision and discipline was alarmingly arbitrary, local officials and Board members alike relying upon personal opinion and prejudice to guide them in their evaluations and judgments. Guilty verdicts were rendered on charges originating in the obvious vindictiveness of the local officials involved, on evidence that was collected by coercing witnesses and threatening the midwife, and on the sole and unsupported testimony of a local official or a self-interested doctor (UKPRO cases 002, 022, 038, 040, 043, 045, 048, 053, 060, 065; Nursing Times, 1912). Even *Nursing Notes* occasionally acknowledged the Board's apparent capriciousness, noting that in the cases of both Anna Hooper and Mary Ann Spate 'very little direct evidence' was given in the first and 'very conflicting evidence' in the other. Both were struck off (Nursing Notes, 1911i, 1911d). In the sample, 72% of the midwives who were found guilty of the very serious 'failure to advise and send for a physician' had not failed to comply with this Rule at all, yet nevertheless were held responsible by the Board for, among other things, families who refused to go for the doctor despite the midwife's urgings, and for poor outcomes that resulted from the malpractice of the physicians who answered their summons for assistance (UKPRO cases 005, 012, 025, 027, 041, 052, 062, 064; Heagerty, 1990, pp. 290–291). In making its decision, the Board generally extended greater sympathy to women who expressed deference to the Board's authority, who could draw on the good graces of their 'friends', and whose class background or social connections were similar to its members (Nursing Notes, 1910n, 1912d, 1912e). Treatment for those who did not defer ranged from verbal abuse (midwives who had been judged innocent of all charges were no exception) to the loss of a midwifes' living (Nursing Notes, 1914e; Champneys, 1915; Nursing Notes, 1916e).

'The reasons for this wholesale clearance are interesting in themselves', *Nursing Notes* observed in 1914. 'Health authorities who are determined to rid themselves of inefficient and dangerous practitioners will require, instead, well-trained, up-to-date midwives' (UK Privy Council, 1909b, [926–935]; Nursing Notes, 1914c). Such a midwife would no longer be in danger of misplaced allegiances and could be counted upon to uphold the goals and aspirations of midwifery as defined by the elite. She could be expected to turn a deaf ear to the pleas of a mother too poor to pay the doctor's fee and call the doctor without delay. She could be expected to neither participate in nor hide criminal behaviour, but report it immediately. She could be expected to join with other midwives to 'Black List patients who have not paid' and to use her influence to form 'maternity clubs along provident lines' (Nursing Notes, 1911a; MIRC, 1922), so that 'independence is maintained and pauperism discouraged' among working-class mothers and their families (Nursing Notes, 1917a; Paget, 1918). If she yielded to the temptation to either fall back or 'get slack', the extensive supervisory apparatus and the disciplinary powers of the Board would be freely exercised to control her practice and personal life.

'UPHOLDING THE DIGNITY OF OUR CALLING...'

Discontent was widespread among midwives during these years. Their frustration emerges in many places – in their letters and articles in the nursing and midwifery press, in depositions and appeals in the Penal Committee's case files, and in correspondence to the Institute itself. Many took the path charted for them by the Institute and attempted to adopt the values and perspectives of the leadership. Others refused to submit to the Act and resisted officials' attempts to make them comply. Still others, envisioning a different future for midwifery than the one offered by the Institute and the Midwives' Act, organized to put an end to the Institute's monopoly over midwives' affairs.

Probably nothing was more widely resented by midwives than the restrictions on the scope of their practice and the apparatus that enforced those limitations. Women who had been in practice prior to the Act had learned over the years that many of the kinds of births the Rules had defined as beyond their province did not require a doctor's intervention, but were in fact manageable and normal (even if some were difficult and not routine). To the Board, of course, this amounted to diagnosis; to the midwife, simply common sense. 'As long experience of nearly 40 years,' wrote Mrs R–, 'when I saw a patient *ill* I recognized it and sent for a doctor' (UKPRO cases 070). Others were frustrated at the 'laundry list' of limitations which seemed to have little purpose other than to trip them up and get them into trouble at every turn. They were offended by the attitudes of inspectors and disturbed by the apparent capriciousness of the disciplinary process. 'Even should the investigation prove her blameless,' one midwife complained, 'the inquiry is harmful to reputation' (Nursing Notes, 1906d, 1908f, 1907h).

Midwives' resistance was threaded throughout the process of supervision and discipline. They were as creative about dodging an inspector as they were resourceful in taking care of women who were too poor to provide a change of linen for the bed or mend a broken window in the dead of winter. Neighbours would be enlisted to give wrong directions to the midwife's whereabouts. Inspectors would be left at the front door while the midwife went out the back. Or, perhaps she'd respond like Fanny Emory who was called before the Board for being 'abusive and resentful to the Inspector' (Nursing Notes, 1913f). Others refused to give up the work even after the Board had cancelled their certificates (UKPRO cases 038, 055; Nursing Notes, 1911e,f). Similarly, handy-women continued to advertise their midwifery services and after 1910, despite the law's restrictions, continued to practise, as one Lancashire midwife allegedly declared, 'in spite of the committee, the inspector and the devil' (Nursing Notes, 1910b, 1911g, 1912c, 1915g). Women who continued to practise illegally were heavily fined and, in some instance, jailed.

While most resistance was individualized and spontaneous during these years, midwives also organized to defend their interests. Midwives had begun to form local associations from the time the Act had first been implemented, but it was not until 1909 that events offered these groups of rank and file midwives the opportunity to challenge the existing method of their representation in midwifery affairs and to confront the power of the supervisory apparatus. That year, the government appointed a Departmental Committee to investigate how the Act was working, to evaluate its operation and to make recommendations if they considered any revisions in the legislation were necessary. At the same time, as a 'wave of industrial unrest swept the country', working-class women in a variety of trades organized themselves into trades unions under the Women's Trade Union League (WTUL) and joined with their male counterparts to protest at poor conditions and insufficient wages (Drake, 1984, pp. 47–67; Liddington and Norris, 1984; Lewis, 1984, pp. 176). On the one hand, this series of events held out the opportunity that the Act, the operation of the Board and the means by which midwives were represented in midwifery affairs might be reformed, and on the other gave momentum to the efforts of two national organizations, the National Association of Midwives and the 1910 British Union of Midwives. Both organizations sought to improve registered midwives' working conditions and to gain greater control for midwives over the policies that determined their practice. Both focused on organizing the rank and file midwife regardless of training and, with their close affiliations to the trade union movement, provided an alternative vision to that of the Institute, the Central Midwives Board and the broader network of midwifery reformers. The demands and programmes of both organizations were given voice by the *Midwives Record and Maternity Nurse*, a journal founded in 1906 for practising midwives and maternity nurses. In order to pool their resources, the Union of Midwives and the National Association became affiliated in 1911, although they remained organizationally distinct (Midwives Record, 1911a).

Of the two, we know less about the origins of the National Association, but it appears to have been created around 1908 from an amalgamation of local midwife associations based in and around Manchester. It was closely affiliated with the trade union movement and it was not uncommon for trade union women and National Association representatives to share the podium at organizing meetings (Nursing Times, 1910a). Mrs Margaret Lawson, the president of the National Association, a practising midwife and a Guardian for West Manchester, was often reported touring the North recruiting midwives into the organization (Nursing Times, 1910b).

The British Union of Midwives was founded in 1910 by supporters and readers of the *Midwives Record* in direct opposition to the policies and programme of the Midwives' Institute. In its early years, the journal had been associated with the Institute through the Certified Midwives Total Abstinence League, a temperance organization in which journal supporters and Institute members participated and who reported on its activities in both the *Record* and *Nursing Notes*. This connection was first strained, however, by the journal's growing criticism of the Institute, the Central Midwives Board and the status quo of midwifery power relations, and then broken by its demand for direct representation on the Board and its assistance in the formation of a midwives' trade union – the 1910 British Union of Midwives. The choice of Mary McArthur, the secretary of the Women's Trade Union League, to chair the Union's founding meeting symbolized the organization's intention to take an alternative path. In her opening remarks McArthur declared the new organization 'a trade union, a democratic body, a registered society and organization' committed to protecting midwives' economic rights to good work conditions and a decent standard of living (Nursing Times, 1910a–c; Midwives Record, 1910a,b).

The difficulty of making a living from the work was a crucial issue among midwives who sought to support themselves or their families through their midwifery. Midwives' complaints made it clear that the poverty of the women they attended kept the fees low, while the Rules' requirements drained a sizeable amount of even the small fee they received (Nursing Notes, 1908f). Rank and file experience confirmed the impossibility of wringing 'money from our poorer sisters' (Nursing Notes, 1910l). In contrast to the self-help, individualist and reforming ideology of the Institute, the Union's programme sought to increase government's responsibility for the individual and by doing so, help to remove the stigma of poverty that many of the women midwives attended were forced to endure. State aid – a maternity service 'run on national lines' – would provide a living for midwives and guarantee attendance for women too poor to pay (Midwives Record, 1909a). 'If a great imperial state can spend millions and millions a year upon instruments of death and destruction,' asserted F. V. Fisher, the *Record's* general manager, it could surely provide the comparatively small amount of resources to fund a maternity service (Midwives Record, 1908a).

Neither organization had time for the hierarchical, exclusive and non-representative nature of the Institute and its ideology, the organization of the Central Midwives Board or the limitations it had placed on the midwives' work. Both organizations were 'open to all women on the register', no distinctions being made as to training or background (Midwives Record, 1908b; Nursing Notes, 1908g). Both agreed that there were too many restrictions on midwives' practice and, as one Union representative remarked, midwives 'ought not have to send for the doctor at the slightest abnormality' (Nursing Times, 1910a,c). With many others, the *Record* raised serious concerns about the process of discipline meted out by the CMB, likening its methods to those of 'Star Chamber', before which midwives were 'hauled without any of the guarantees which even in a public court are rarely sufficient to protect the poor or the inexperienced' (Editorial, 1911; Midwives Record, 1909b).

Both the Union and the National Association believed that better working conditions, greater scope to the work and just representation in all matters was obstructed by the power relations enshrined within the CMB. The sentiments and programme of the two organizations clearly delineated the differing interests of the elite represented on the CMB and the rank and file midwife who, since she had no say in the election of her representation, remained voiceless. Both organizations believed that the rank and file would never have 'the power of ventilating grievances and demanding justice' without the right to directly elect their representatives to the CMB 'by the popular vote' (Nursing Notes, 1908g, 1909e). Perhaps no issue was more controversial or more vociferously argued, or more clearly illustrated the political nature of their challenge. Without such representation, the *Midwives Record* asserted, midwifery would remain in 'the swaddling-clothes of semi-benevolent, semi-hostile interests; [it will be] cribbed and confined by those interests, and midwives individually and collectively will suffer accordingly' (Editorial, 1910; Midwives Record, 1908c).

The activities and positions of the two organizations were frequently publicized in the midwifery press and their representatives often spoke at public meetings and at nursing and midwifery conferences, debating the merits of a midwives' trade union and their direct representation on the CMB (Midwives Record, 1909c, 1911b). Throughout 1909 and 1910, the Union and the National Association held a series of public meetings to recruit midwives to their cause, and reports indicate that the meetings were well attended and well received (Nursing Times, 1910b,c). These midwives perhaps agreed with Annie Taylor who, in response to a charge in *Nursing Notes* that the Union was undermining the dignity of midwifery by advocating a trade union, wrote, 'Let us combine and insist upon receiving good pay for good service rendered and thus shall we "uphold the dignity of our calling"' (Taylor, 1910).

The general social unrest, the activity of these organizations and the relative isolation of the Institute from the vast majority of the rank and file was enough to prompt a serious response from the leadership. In several articles, *Nursing Notes* depicted both organiz-ations as ungrateful and rather unruly children who did not 'fully recognize that they owe their existence to the dauntless efforts' of the very Institute against which they were organizing (Nursing Notes, 1910c). Articles represented the Institute as the more experienced, more rational – 'hysterical shouting will do no good' – which 'far from being a private concern of a few Club members' was open to providing the necessary links between organizations around the country (Nursing Notes, 1909c). At the same time, the Institute initiated a recruitment campaign to extend its influence among the rank and file, albeit with those who would submit to the narrow representation and strict adherence to policy which the leadership demanded as a condition of affiliation. In 1909, the Institute counted 1140 members, '600 or 700' of whom were registered midwives, many drawn from the more prestigious midwifery institutions and prominent philanthropic organizations (UK Privy Council, 1909a, [514–515]). There were over 29 000 midwives who registered that year, of whom a little over 13 000 had notified their intention to practise (UKCMB, 1910). Elizabeth Glanville and her associate Miss Eaton worked tirelessly, visiting midwife associations up and down the country, lecturing and urging midwives to join the Institute (MIRC, 1912b; 1916). Although the Institute increased its membership during these years to include more rank and file midwives, the power remained firmly within the hands of the elite. As a 1917 study by the Fabian Society observed, 'Practicing midwives who are members of the Institute themselves take very little part in its government' (Nursing Times, 1917; Nursing Notes, 1910d, 1915e; MIRC, 1922).

The concept of a trade union for midwives violated every principle upon which the Institute's ideology and programme for the future of midwifery was based. While the Institute fought to distance midwifery from its working-class roots, a trade union only strengthened that connection. 'Midwifery,' *Nursing Notes* asserted, was 'not a trade, but a profession called into being by the needs and weaknesses of humanity' (Nursing Notes, 1910e). While the Institute promoted competition and the operation of the free market, a trade union was founded on the necessity to curb the operation of the market by limiting competition among the workers and enforcing their demands through the withholding of their labour. And finally, the outright appeal to 'the bread and butter side of the issue' threw into question the magnanimity of midwives' motives, the purity of which was essential for any profession to justify its privileged status (Nursing Notes, 1910l). If midwives allowed their 'commercial spirit to become paramount at the expense of altruism,' *Nursing Notes* warned, 'a retributive justice may be expected to make itself felt' (Nursing Notes, 1910e,f,g).

When it came to upholding the power of the supervisory and disciplinary apparatus, the Institute leadership was resolute. To suggest that flaws existed in the system of midwives' regulation and control was to attack the professional and class aspirations of the elite leadership and members of the Board, and to undermine the protection and privileges which had been bestowed upon that elite by the Act. They acknowledged that 'the powers given to the Local Supervisory Authority by these Rules may open the door for much vexatious interference' (Nursing Notes, 1903), and were particularly angered by the spectacle of trained midwives of a higher social standing being called before the Board under the same conditions as bona fide midwives (Nursing Notes, 1907e, 1910h,i, 1911d). They considered this to be a result of inexperienced and poorly trained individual inspectors, however, rather than any fundamental flaw in the system itself. Appointing officials with the proper attitude and knowledge would easily remedy the problem (Hall, 1914; Nursing Notes, 1915f, 1917b). The Institute firmly maintained that the Board and its Rules were, as Rosalind Paget told her audience of health workers, a 'protection to the good midwife', and for this reason midwives should remain loyal to its officers and their authority (Nursing Notes, 1917c). A midwife who did not conform to these prescriptions, regardless of the circumstances, failed to fit the criteria of a 'good midwife' and had to take responsibility for the consequences.

Direct representation transgressed the leadership's vision of a social order based on a natural hierarchy and threatened the Institute's and its constituents' ability to promote their views without challenge. Fighting to establish and maintain a system of control over the thousands of women who were registered and practising (trained or not) absorbed a considerable amount of the leadership's time and energy. They played a significant and pivotal role on the Central Midwives Board and in upholding and publicizing its decisions. They became involved in organizing midwives, but this was to tie them more closely to 'the central authorities, who are responsible for the direction and government of the profession' (Nursing Notes, 1909c). Their exclusive representation on the Board allowed them to advance the views and pursue the proposals that best served their real constituency. For the Institute, direct representation meant that the same rank and file the Institute sought to control would now be making the decisions. The midwifery electorate as a whole was composed of 'ignorant and illiterate' women (Nursing Notes,

1910j) whose votes, *Nursing Notes* warned, 'would swamp those of the trained ones' (Nursing Notes, 1908e). The trained rank and file, however, had little more to recommend them. The qualities needed by a representative (such as stating her 'opinions without stuttering or sputtering') were not 'commonly found among those who have spent years practising an all-absorbing profession that has given little time or opportunity for the cultivation of wider interests' (Nursing Notes, 1908e). Predictably, the Institute admonished those midwives who proposed to breach the established order and counselled them to accept the natural hierarchy led by women who had the 'means, leisure and the necessary technical knowledge' (Nursing Notes, 1907d; Glanville, 1908).

Appeals for midwives to submit to a natural social hierarchy did not sit well. Unlike the Institute, the leadership of both the British Union and the National Association believed that midwives had the right to a voice in the affairs of midwifery simply by virtue of their status as practitioners of the work. Neither organization recognized the Institute as a legitimate representative of the interests of the majority, but rather considered it an ally of those groups who were currently the source of midwives' problems, 'the "bossing" on the Central Midwives Board of doctors and non-registered nurses' (Midwives Record, 1910c). They welcomed the end to the Institute's privileged position as the exclusive representative of registered midwives (Nursing Mirror, 1910). An editorial in the *Midwives Record* clearly articulated the class and cultural divide which the struggle over representation revealed:

> At the recent meeting in the Cavendish Rooms one lady (who seemed to be associated with the Institute) objected to the principle of direct representation, on the feeble plea that working midwives could not find the time to sit on the Board. At the same meeting five smartly dressed women rose and rudely left the meeting, giggling hysterically like naughty schoolgirls, while Mrs Lawson, the respected president of the Association of Midwives, was speaking. These exhibitions of grandes dames *and the patronesses of midwives, 'dressed in a little brief authority' do not tend to inspire respect among working women. Serious-minded midwives, intent on the practice of a great science and on the elevation of their profession, do not need to be fussed over and patronized. They are tired of 'charity-mongers'; they are sick of being 'bossed'. Strange as it may seem to these outsiders, they have the audacity to believe that they know what they want better than their would-be patrons, and that they can get on very well without the help of the latter.* (Midwives Record, 1910c)

Although they did not take such a strident class position, others also questioned the Institute's opposition to direct representation. The *British Journal of Nursing* was quoted as considering such a position 'an inconceivable attitude in our mind' (Midwives Record, 1909d). Probably the most damaging defection was the Institute's own representative to the CMB, Dr Stanley Cullingworth, who argued as early as 1908 that to deny registered midwives direct representation 'constitutionally ... is wrong' and urged revision of the Act in this regard (Midwives Record, 1908d). As far as the *Midwives Record* was concerned, if the Institute refused to be brought 'into line with the great body of rank and file midwives. The sooner the Institute is smashed the better' (Midwives Record, 1910c).

FIGHT FOR OUR INTERESTS AND NOT AGAINST US

When the 1910 Departmental Committee decided to recommend only minor revisions in the Midwives' Act, the rank and file midwives' organized challenge to the legitimacy of the Midwives' Institute and the power of the supervisory apparatus eventually vanished from the national nursing and midwifery press. Yet the rank and file's dissatisfaction did not. Sources indicate that at least until 1914 the Union of Midwives and the National Association continued to promote direct representation and the creation of a state maternity service. In that year, these organizations lost an important advocate when the *Midwives Record* merged with the *Nurses' Own Magazine* and the proprietors gradually abandoned the *Record*'s passionate and militant defence of the rank and file midwife in favour of a generalized format aimed at a nursing audience. Rank and file midwives continued to use other journals such as the *Nursing Times, Nursing Mirror* and *Nursing Notes* to protest their treatment at the hands of the supervisory apparatus and demand, as one midwife wrote in 1919, that they 'should have more freedom of action and less rule and regulation. The chairman at a CMB meeting told a midwife to be more humble. The day for humility in England's workers (be they men or women) is gone by; it is buried in the graves of our soldiers' (Nursing Mirror, 1919a, 1925; Nursing Notes, 1927). Among some midwives, the Institute continued to be regarded as part of the problem. That Institute members sat on the Central Midwives Board, 'is no recommendation', one midwife wrote, 'rather it is a deterrent. They only administer the Rules' (Nursing Mirror, 1919b; Midwives' Institute Executive Club and Council, 1914). Neither did all the midwives who joined with the Institute agree with its policies, particularly those that required close collaboration between the associations – organizations meant to defend midwives' rights – and local officials – individuals who were part of the apparatus charged with supervising and disciplining midwives. Dissatisfied midwives argued these policies weakened their efforts to protect themselves. 'When we look to the Association for help and protection we find it helping those who oppress,' one Association member wrote to the Institute in 1927. 'We look to you to fight for us and not to put us off with platitudes about ideals when we need practical help ... [to] fight for our interests and not against us' (MIRC, 1923, 1926, 1927a,b).

CONCLUSION

Twentieth-century midwifery was born from a particular historical moment, one in which class relations were being renegotiated and social reform more extensively utilized as a method of mediating the inevitable conflict between the classes. The ideology promulgated by the Institute and its allies and the apparatus created and given force by the Midwives' Act of 1902 was part of the broader attempt to shape working-class life and culture to support and further capitalist relations. One way of thinking and behaving had to replace the other, reformers believed, if the essential thrust of social reform was to be realized.

For the leadership, discipline and division were necessary tactics to guarantee the rank and file did not interfere with their vision. The supervisory and disciplinary apparatus created by the Act supplied the power to control midwives' lives and practice on almost a daily basis. The Institute's strategy of exclusion supplied a clear image of an enemy that could be held responsible for all of society's ills and for all the problems trained midwives experienced. The Institute's upholding of capitalist social and economic relations, its monopoly of representation and its restrictions on participation within the organization

---

Box 4.1   Penal Committee cases

A random sample of 73 cases (brought against 74 midwives) was drawn from a list of surviving case files of midwives who had been charged by the Penal Committee of the Central Midwives Board between 1905 and 1919. The surviving penal files probably represent a little under half of the estimated 1500 cases against midwives during these years. The official correspondence, reports and testimony contained in each of the files provide insight into the dynamics of local supervision and the attitudes of the inspectors, the relationship between the midwife and the women she attended, and between the woman and local midwifery officials as well as the midwife's place in the community. For a discussion of this source, see Heagerty (1990) pp. 284–289. The individual case files are referred to by number rather than name for purposes of confidentiality, as required by the UK Central Council. The following list of cited case files includes the number assigned by the author, the training of the midwife (BF, bona fide; CMB, Central Midwives Board; LOS, London Obstetrical Society); and the year of the disciplinary hearing.

002 BF, 1906	038 BF, 1917	060 LOS, 1917
004 BF, 1908	040 BF, 1918	062 LOS, 1918
005 BF, 1909	041 BF, 1918	063 BF, 1918
011 CMB, 1911	043 BF, 1918	064 LOS, 1919
012 BF, 1912	045 BF, 1918	065 LOS, 1919
015 BF, 1912	047 BF, 1919	066 Salvation Army, 1908
022 CMB, 1915	048 BF, 1919	067 Manchester Maternity,
025 CMB, 1918	052 LOS, 1908	1909
027 CMB, 1916	053 LOS, 1911	070 Coombe Hospital, 1916
031 CMB, 1917	055 LOS, 1913	072 CMB, 1916
033 BF, 1918	057 LOS, 1915	

---

itself ensured that its ideology would become a powerful and defining force in the development of midwifery.

Some of the rank and file did adopt the views of the Institute and supported its exclusionism. Unfortunately, many midwives found that these tactics were no guarantee against their own expulsion. This was proved in the 'wholesale clearance' under the Midwives' Act of 1936, legislation formulated with the assistance of and promoted by the Midwives' Institute, which set the conditions for thousands of women trained as midwives to be replaced by a 'new' midwife – the preferably young, single midwife trained as a nurse (Heagerty, 1990).

The Institute assisted in building an apparatus of control over the rank and file midwife, but its strategies were not successful in achieving exclusive control over midwifery for the leadership itself. A firm class alliance underlay the principles of the Board and its composition, but there were inevitably conflicting professional interests among the members and the constituents they represented. No amount of ideology could mask the real power differential between the medical profession and midwifery. The leadership did not dare to fundamentally question this relationship, however, because the alternative – an alliance with the rank and file – was, for them, impossible.

Midwives' resistance to the Act represented an upholding of the new as much as it did a defence of the old. When midwives defied the Act outright they were struggling to preserve the relations of the past. The midwives of the British Union and the National Association, on the other hand, did not question the Act itself, but rather sought to reform its worst abuses. In this, they represented the embryonic beginnings of a new midwife created by the Act, if not the new midwife that the Institute had envisioned. They were unable to dislodge the Institute from its position, but their calls for greater democracy, an improved standard of living and increased government involvement in the provision of maternity care offered the rank and file an alternative vision to that of the hierarchical, individualist future proposed by the Institute leadership. In their defence of the mother and their refusal to turn the midwife away from her, these demands reveal the essential continuity even within the midst of change.

REFERENCES

Atkinson S (1907) *The Office of Midwife in England and Wales.* London: Baillière, Tindall & Cox.

Bland L (1986) Marriage laid bare: middle class women and marital sex, c. 1880–1914. In: Lewis J (ed.) *Labour and Love.* Oxford: Basil Blackwell.

Booth C (1892) *Life and Labour of the People in London.* London: William & Norgate.

Brickman JP (1983) Public health, midwives and nurses, 1880–1930. In: Lageman EC (ed.) *Nursing History: New Perspectives, New Possibilities.* New York: Teachers College Press.

Brierly E (1923a) In the beginning. *Nursing Notes* January: 9–10.

Brierly E (1923b) In the beginning. *Nursing Notes* February: 21–22.

Bristow R (1977) *Vice and Vigilance: Purity Movements in Britain since 1700.* London: Gill & Macmillan.

Brown P & Jordonova LJ (1986) Oppressive dichotomics: the nature/culture debate. In: Cambridge Women's Studies Group, *Women in Society: Interdisciplinary Essays.* London: Virago.

Chamberlain M (1981) *Old Wives Tales.* London: Virago.

Champneys F (1915) Address delivered to the Association of Inspectors of Midwives. *Nursing Notes* July, 169–170.

Chinn C (1988) *They Worked All Their Lives: Women of the Urban Poor in England, 1860–1939.* Manchester University Press.

Chinn C (1995) *Poverty Amidst Prosperity: the Urban Poor in England, 1834–1914.* London: St Martin's Press.

Cowell B & Wainwright D (1981) *Behind the Blue Door: The History of the Royal College of Midwives 1881–1981.* London: Baillière Tindall.

Davies ML, ed. (1975) *Life as We Have Known It* (originally published by the Hogarth Press, 1931). New York: WW Norton.

Davies ML, ed. (1978) *Maternity: Letters from Working Women* (originally published by Bell, 1915). New York: WW Norton.

Davies C (1983) Professionalizing strategies as time- and culture-bound: American and British nursing. In: Lageman EC (ed.) *Nursing History: New Perspectives, New Possibilities.* New York: Teachers College Press.

Davin A (1978) Imperialism and motherhood. *History Workshop Journal* 5: 66–95.

Dock L (1910) Book notes: review of hygiene and morality. *Nursing Notes* September: 222.

Donnison J (1977) *Midwives and Medical Men.* New York: Schocken.

Drake B (1984) *Women in the Trade Unions* (originally published by the Labour Research Department, 1920). London: Virago.

Editorial (1910) The Midwives' Bill. *Midwives Record and Maternity Nurse* December: 374–375.

Editorial (1911) The Penal Cases and the CMB. *Midwives Record and Maternity Nurse* May: 135–136.

Esland G (1980) Professions and Professionalism. In: Esland G, Salaman G (eds) *The Politics of Work and the Professions.* Milton Keynes: Open University Press.

French M (1915) The educative influence of the midwife. *Nursing Notes* October: 240.

Friedman L (1965) Freedom of contract and occupational licensing, 1890–1910. *California Law Review* **53**: 487–534.

Friedson E (1970) *The Profession of Medicine.* New York: Harper & Row.

Garmarnikow E (1978) Sexual division of labour: the case of nursing. In: Kuhn A, Wolpe AM (eds) *Feminism and Materialism.* London: Routledge & Kegan Paul.

Glanville NE (1908) Representation, or benevolent despotism. *Midwives Record and Maternity Nurse* July: 32.

Hall E (1914) Inspection from the midwives' point of view. *Nursing Notes* June: 173.

Harvey G (1951) *The Eternal Eve.* New York: Doubleday.

Heagerty BV (1990) *Class, Gender and Professionalization: The Struggle for English Midwifery, 1900–1936.* Unpublished PhD dissertation, Michigan State University.

Holmes L (1984) Alabama granny midwives. *Journal of the Medical Society of New Jersey* **81** (5): 389–391.

Holton SS (1986) *Feminism and Democracy: Women's Suffrage and Reform Politics in Britain, 1900–1918.* Cambridge University Press.

Jeffries S (1985) *The Spinster and her Enemies: Feminism and Sexuality 1880–1930.* London: Pandora.

Johnson T (1972) *Professions and Power.* London: Macmillan.

Kent SK (1987) *Sex and Suffrage in Britain, 1860–1914.* Princeton University Press.

Larson MS (1976) *The Rise of Professionalism.* Berkeley: University of California Press.

Leap N & Hunter B (1993) *The Midwives Tale.* London: Scarlet Press.

Leavitt JW (1986) *Brought to Bed: Childbearing in America, 1750–1950.* Oxford University Press.

Lewis J (1980) *The Politics of Motherhood: Child and Maternal Welfare in England, 1900–1939.* London: Croom Helm.

Lewis J (1984) *Women in England, 1870–1950.* Bloomington: Indiana University Press.

Liddington J & Norris J (1984) *One Hand Tied Behind Us.* London: Virago.

Little R (1983) *Go Seek Mrs Dawson. She'll Know What to Do – The Demise of the Working Class Nurse/Midwife in the Twentieth Century.* Unpublished thesis, University of Sussex.

Loane M (1905a) Notes added to 'The District Nurse as Health Missioner'. *Nursing Notes* September: 139.

Loane M (1905b) Book notes: review of the Queen's poor. *Nursing Notes* December: 179.

Loane M (1906) The ethics of the poor. *Nursing Notes* September: 137.

Loane M (1912a) Infant mortality. *Nursing Notes* February: 38–39, 93–94.

Loane M (1912b) Infant mortality. *Nursing Notes* May: 120–121.

MD (1910) Preventable disease. *Nursing Notes* December: 291–292.

Maggs C (1983) *The Origins of General Nursing.* London: Croom Helm.

Mathieson A (1915) The eternal in woman. *Nursing Notes* December: 271.

May E (1915) Teaching the mothers. *Nursing Notes* May: 112–113.

McCleary GF (1935) *The Maternity and Child Welfare Movement.* London: S. King.

Melosh B (1982) *The Physician's Hand: Work, Culture and Conflict in American Nursing.* Philadelphia: Temple University Press.

Midwives' Institute Executive Club and Council (1914) Minutes, July 3. Letter to Miss Goodlass, June 10. Royal College of Midwives Archives, London.

[MIRC] Midwives' Institute Representative Committee (1912a) Minutes, July 4. Royal College of Midwives Archives, London.

[MIRC] Midwives' Institute Representative Committee (1912b) Minutes, November 8. Royal College of Midwives Archives, London.

[MIRC] Midwives' Institute Representative Committee (1916) Letter to Miss Coleman, December 11. Royal College of Midwives Archives, London.

[MIRC] Midwives' Institute Representative Committee (1922) Minutes, March 17. Royal College of Midwives Archives, London.

[MIRC] Midwives' Institute Representative Committee (1923) Minutes, June 15. Royal College of Midwives Archives, London.

[MIRC] Midwives' Institute Representative Committee (1926) Letter to Mrs Mitchell, March 24. Royal College of Midwives Archives, London.

[MIRC] Midwives' Institute Representative Committee (1927a) Letter to 'Ladies', October 22. Royal College of Midwives Archives, London.

[MIRC] Midwives' Institute Representative Committee (1927b) Letter to Mrs K–, December 17. Royal College of Midwives Archives, London.

Midwives Record (1908a) The Midwives Record at home. *Midwives Record and Maternity Nurse* August: 12.

Midwives Record (1908b) The bona fide midwife. *Midwives Record and Maternity Nurse* February: 9.

Midwives Record (1908c) Representation, or 'benevolent despotism'. *Midwives Record and Maternity Nurse* July: 7–8.

Midwives Record (1908d) The direct representation of certified midwives on the CMB. *Midwives Record and Maternity Nurse* December: 18.

Midwives Record (1909a) The present and future remuneration of midwifery. *Midwives Record and Maternity Nurse* October: 345–346.

Midwives Record (1909b) Penal cases. *Midwives Record and Maternity Nurse* January: 22–23.

Midwives Record (1909c) The Nursing and Midwifery Conference and Exhibition: the direct representation of midwives. *Midwives Record and Maternity Nurse* May: 186–188.

Midwives Record (1909d) Enemies within camp. *Midwives Record and Maternity Nurse* July: 213.

Midwives Record (1910a) The 1910 Union of Midwives. *Midwives Record and Maternity Nurse* March: 71–73.

Midwives Record (1910b) The 1910 Union of Midwives. *Midwives Record and Maternity Nurse* February (supplement).

Midwives Record (1910c) Treasons, stratagems and spoils. *Midwives Record and Maternity Nurse* May: 138.

Midwives Record (1911a) National Association and the Union of Midwives. *Midwives Record and Maternity Nurse* November: 37.

Midwives Record (1911b) The Nursing and Midwifery Conference. *Midwives Record and Maternity Nurse* May: 145–152.

Minit M (1925) *District Nursing in Towns*. Bishop's Stortford: Mardon Bros Observer. (Reprinted by Queen's Institute, London).

Nursing Mirror (1910) The Nursing and Midwifery Conference. *Nursing Mirror* 7 May: 385.

Nursing Mirror (1919a) Everybody's opinion: midwives of today. *Nursing Mirror* 25 January: 257.

Nursing Mirror (1919b) Everybody's opinion. *Nursing Mirror* 11 January: 225.

Nursing Mirror (1925) Midwifery under present conditions. *Nursing Mirror* 23 October: 81.

Nursing Notes (1900) Rural midwives. *Nursing Notes* November: 162.

Nursing Notes (1901) Miss Amy Hughes. *Nursing Notes* September: 118.

Nursing Notes (1902a) The Central Midwives Board. *Nursing Notes* December: 153–154.

Nursing Notes (1902b) The midwives question and women's suffrage. *Nursing Notes* April: 44–45.

Nursing Notes (1903) The Rules of the Central Midwives Board. *Nursing Notes* October: 135.

Nursing Notes (1904a) Nurses in Council. *Nursing Notes* April: 63.

Nursing Notes (1904b) The CMB and its proceedings. *Nursing Notes* July: 105.

Nursing Notes (1904c) District nursing notes. *Nursing Notes* May: 73.

Nursing Notes (1905) Practical notes for practising midwives. *Nursing Notes* August: 119.

Nursing Notes (1906a) National Health Society. *Nursing Notes* January: 7.

Nursing Notes (1906b) Notes on mothers and factory work. *Nursing Notes* April: 53.

Nursing Notes (1906c) The nurse and the midwife as citizens. *Nursing Notes* December: 173–174.

Nursing Notes (1906d) ? *Nursing Notes* July: 102.
Nursing Notes (1906e) Penal Cases (Elizabeth Patillo). *Nursing Notes* June: 85.
Nursing Notes (1906f) Penal Cases (Emma Jones). *Nursing Notes* June: 85.
Nursing Notes (1906g) Penal Cases (Jane Tween). *Nursing Notes* March: 36.
Nursing Notes (1907a) The working mother. *Nursing Notes* June: 90–92.
Nursing Notes (1907b) Notes: the Spectator on women's suffrage. *Nursing Notes* April: 52.
Nursing Notes (1907c) National vigilance. *Nursing Notes* September: 136–137.
Nursing Notes (1907d) Midwives' representation. *Nursing Notes* July: 103.
Nursing Notes (1907e) The Penal Cases. *Nursing Notes* June: 87.
Nursing Notes (1907f) Midwives' defence association. *Nursing Notes* August: 124.
Nursing Notes (1907g) Central Midwives Board. *Nursing Notes* November: 175.
Nursing Notes (1907h) Central Midwives Board. *Nursing Notes* December: 196.
Nursing Notes (1908a) Mothers and the state. *Nursing Notes* May: 93.
Nursing Notes (1908b) Votes for women. *Nursing Notes* July: 138.
Nursing Notes (1908c) The suffrage. *Nursing Notes* June: 130.
Nursing Notes (1908d) Members in Council. *Nursing Notes* August: 107.
Nursing Notes (1908e) Direct representation. *Nursing Notes* October: 201–202.
Nursing Notes (1908f) Midwifery as a profession for gentlewomen. *Nursing Notes* May: 108.
Nursing Notes (1908g) Northern midwives meeting. *Nursing Notes* September: 181.
Nursing Notes (1908h) Central Midwives Board (Sara Elizabeth Carford). *Nursing Notes* January: 11.
Nursing Notes (1909a) Eugenics. *Nursing Notes* July: 144, 166.
Nursing Notes (1909b) Midwives' notes: midwives and temperance. *Nursing Notes* June: 94.
Nursing Notes (1909c) Linking up. *Nursing Notes* December.
Nursing Notes (1909d) Central Midwives Board (Mrs Pittman). *Nursing Notes* July: 140.
Nursing Notes (1909e) Central Midwives Board. *Nursing Notes* December: 242.
Nursing Notes (1910a) The 1910 Union of Midwives. *Nursing Notes* February: 28.
Nursing Notes (1910b) Defiant midwife. *Nursing Notes* October: 254.
Nursing Notes (1910c) Union is strength. *Nursing Notes* April: 81.
Nursing Notes (1910d) The practising midwife. *Nursing Notes*, November: 272.
Nursing Notes (1910e) Midwives and trades unions. *Nursing Notes* February: 31.
Nursing Notes (1910f) Strikes for midwives. *Nursing Notes* July: 170.
Nursing Notes (1910g) Midwives and trade unionism. *Nursing Notes* October: 245.
Nursing Notes (1910h) CMB. *Nursing Notes* February: 35.
Nursing Notes (1910i) The Monmouthshire training home. *Nursing Notes* August: 194.
Nursing Notes (1910j) The representation of midwives. *Nursing Notes* June: 134.
Nursing Notes (1910k) Preventible disease. *Nursing Notes* December: 291.
Nursing Notes (1910l) Midwives and trade unionism. *Nursing Notes* November: 276.
Nursing Notes (1910m) Central Midwives Board (Maria Penfold). *Nursing Notes* January: 16.
Nursing Notes (1910n) Penal Cases (Mary Jane Barrett). *Nursing Notes* August: 198.
Nursing Notes (1911a) Committee of Representatives. *Nursing Notes* February: 48.
Nursing Notes (1911b) Midwives and the vote. *Nursing Notes* January: 8.
Nursing Notes (1911c) Nurses in the suffrage procession. *Nursing Notes* July: 173.
Nursing Notes (1911d) The protection of the midwife. *Nursing Notes* December: 295.
Nursing Notes (1911e) Still practising though removed from the Roll. *Nursing Notes* May: 128.
Nursing Notes (1911f) Gloucester. *Nursing Notes* February: 40.
Nursing Notes (1911g) From far and near. *Nursing Notes* February: 40.
Nursing Notes (1911h) Central Midwives Board (Sarah Dean). *Nursing Notes* January: 16.
Nursing Notes (1911i) Penal Cases (Anna Hooper; Mary Ann Spate; Ellen Leatherland). *Nursing Notes* July: 178.
Nursing Notes (1912a) Practising midwife: the influence of the midwife. *Nursing Notes* January: 12.

Nursing Notes (1912b) Notes on a debate at the Midwives' Institute and Trained Nurses Club. *Nursing Notes* December: 334.

Nursing Notes (1912c) Correspondence. *Nursing Notes* October: 182.

Nursing Notes (1912d) Central Midwives Board (Mary Ann Preece; Mary Ann Southern). *Nursing Notes* July: 196.

Nursing Notes (1912e) Penal Proceedings *Nursing Notes* March: 74.

Nursing Notes (1913a) Letting in the light. *Nursing Notes* September: 243.

Nursing Notes (1913b) Ipswich and Suffolk Association of Midwives. *Nursing Notes* March: 82.

Nursing Notes (1913c) Doctor's fee. *Nursing Notes* March: 78.

Nursing Notes (1913d) Penal Board (Sophia Alice Brockway Cook). *Nursing Notes* December: 346.

Nursing Notes (1913e) Penal Board (Mary Elizabeth Davey). *Nursing Notes* August: 226.

Nursing Notes (1913f) Penal Session *Nursing Notes* January: 12.

Nursing Notes (1914a) The care of the mother. *Nursing Notes* May: 136.

Nursing Notes (1914b) What am I doing for England? *Nursing Notes* December: 323.

Nursing Notes (1914c) Vacancies for certified midwives. *Nursing Notes* July: 206.

Nursing Notes (1914d) Central Midwives Board (Jane Harvey). *Nursing Notes* January: 16.

Nursing Notes (1914e) Penal Cases (Emilie Victoria Pocock). *Nursing Notes* January: 16, 18.

Nursing Notes (1915a) Midwives' total abstinence war league. *Nursing Notes* September: 218.

Nursing Notes (1915b) Stock vs Central Midwives Board. *Nursing Notes* June.

Nursing Notes (1915c) Midwives and moral character. *Nursing Notes* August.

Nursing Notes (1915d) The higher training of midwives. *Nursing Notes* April: 182.

Nursing Notes (1915e) Representatives of the midwives' associations affiliated to the Midwives' Institute. *Nursing Notes* February: 46–47.

Nursing Notes (1915f) Why was the Midwives' Act passed? *Nursing Notes* March.

Nursing Notes (1915g) Central Midwives Board (Charlotte Elizabeth Downscll). *Nursing Notes* July: 176.

Nursing Notes (1915h) Penal Session (Catherine Seabury). *Nursing Notes* March: 70.

Nursing Notes (1916a) Supplement: Annual General Meeting. *Nursing Notes* February: ii–iv.

Nursing Notes (1916b) The Local Supervisory Authority. *Nursing Notes* October: 209.

Nursing Notes (1916c) Central Midwives Board (Ethel Irwin). *Nursing Notes* July: 160.

Nursing Notes (1916d) Penal Board (Elizabeth Morgans). *Nursing Notes* September: 200.

Nursing Notes (1916e) Penal Board (Agnes Sarah Quinton). *Nursing Notes* April: 92.

Nursing Notes (1917a) Municipal midwives. *Nursing Notes* June.

Nursing Notes (1917b) The delegation of the inspection of midwives. *Nursing Notes* March: 45–46.

Nursing Notes (1917c) Co-operation meeting at Whitechapel. *Nursing Notes* February: 35.

Nursing Notes (1917d) Central Midwives Board (Alice Louise Roadnight, CMB certified). *Nursing Notes* July: 120.

Nursing Notes (1918) Central Midwives Board (Charlotte Risebrook) *Nursing Notes* February: 30.

Nursing Notes (1927) Why will not – or, at any rate does not – the well-educated woman who must earn her living practise as a midwife? *Nursing Notes* August: 108.

Nursing Notes (1931) The toll of motherhood. *Nursing Notes* March: 36.

Nursing Notes (1933a) A short history of the Institute. *Nursing Notes* August: 112–115.

Nursing Notes (1933b) Nursing notes and midwives chronicle. *Nursing Notes* September: 129–132.

Nursing Times (1910a) National Association of Midwives. *Nursing Times* 3 September: 740.

Nursing Times (1910b) Midwifery: the National Association of Midwives. *Nursing Times* 22 January.

Nursing Times (1910c) The 1910 British Trade Union of Midwives. *Nursing Times* 26 February: 180.

Nursing Times (1912) Injustice to a midwife. *Nursing Times* 25 May: 574.

Nursing Times (1917) Organization of midwives. *Nursing Times* 28 April: 467.

Oakley A (1976) Wisewoman and medical man: changes in the management of childbirth. In: Mitchell J, Oakley A (eds) *The Rights and Wrongs of Woman*. Harmondsworth: Penguin.

Oakley A (1984) *The Captured Womb*. London: Basil Blackwell.

Paget R (1918) Midwives, are you awake! *Nursing Notes* May: 66.

Peart IF (1910) Midwifery and alcohol. *Nursing Notes* September: 215–216.

Pember Reeves M (1979) *Round About a Pound a Week* (originally published by Bell, 1913). London: Virago.

Rivers J (1981) *Dame Rosalind Paget. A Short Account of her Life and Work.* London: Midwives Chronicle.

Roberts E (1984) *A Woman's Place.* Oxford: Basil Blackwell.

Ross E (1983) Survival networks: women's neighborhood sharing in London before World War I. *History Workshop Journal* **15**: 4–27.

Ross E (1993) *Love and Toil: Motherhood in Outcast London, 1870–1918.* Oxford University Press.

Rowntree BS (1901) *Poverty: A Study of Town Life.* London.

Searle GR (1976) *Eugenics and Politics in Britain 1900–1914.* Leyden: Noordhoff.

Searle GR (1981) Eugenics and class. In: Webster C (ed.) *Biology, Medicine and Society 1840–1940*, pp. 217–242. Cambridge University Press.

Soloway RA (1982) *Birth Control and the Population Question in England, 1877–1930.* Chapel Hill: University of North Carolina Press.

Stedman-Jones G (1971) *Outcast London.* Oxford University Press.

Taylor A (1910) Midwives and Trade Unionism. *Nursing Notes* November: 276.

Taylor-Ladd M (1988) Grannies and spinsters: midwife education under the Sheppard–Towner Act. *Journal of Social History* **22**: 255–276.

Tomes N (1983) The silent battle: nurse registration in New York State, 1903–1920. In: Lageman EC (ed.) *Nursing History: New Perspectives, New Possibilities*, pp. 107–132. New York: Teachers College Press.

Tonge G (1903) How to instruct the working mother on the care of infants. *Nursing Notes* April: 57–58.

[UKCMB] UK Central Midwives Board (1910) *Report of the Work of the Board for the Year Ending March, 1910.* Royal College of Midwives Archives, London.

[UKCMB] UK Central Midwives Board (1911) *Report of the Work of the Board for the Year Ending March, 1911.* Royal College of Midwives Archives, London.

[UKCMB] UK Central Midwives Board (1914) *Report of the Work of the Board for the Year Ending March, 1914.* Royal College of Midwives Archives, London.

[UKCMB] UK Central Midwives Board (1915) *Report of the Work of the Board for the Year Ending March, 1915.* Royal College of Midwives Archives, London.

[UKCMB] UK Central Midwives Board (1916) *Report of the Work of the Board for the Year Ending March, 1916.* Royal College of Midwives Archives, London.

[UKCMB] UK Central Midwives Board (1917) *Report of the Work of the Board for the Year Ending March, 1917.* Royal College of Midwives Archives, London.

UK Privy Council (1909a) Departmental Committee to Enquire into the Working of the Midwives' Act, 1902. Minutes of Evidence, February 4, 1909, [508–844]. Courtesy of Miss Ann Bent.

UK Privy Council (1909b) Departmental Committee to Enquire into the Working of the Midwives' Act, 1902. Minutes of Evidence, February 17, 1909, [845–1068]. Courtesy of Miss Ann Bent.

[UKPRO] UK Public Records Office. Central Midwives Board 1905–1919. Penal Cases Committee.

Weeks J (1981) *Sex, Politics and Society.* London: Longman.

Wilson J (1904) *The Training of Midwives and the Organization of their Work in Rural Districts*, pp. 12–13. Royal College of Midwives Archives, London.

Wilson J (1915) War and women's work. *Nursing Notes* September: 207–208.

Wood CJ (1901) A retrospect and a forecast. *Nursing Notes* October: 132.

FURTHER READING

Brickman JP (1983) Public health, midwives and nurses, 1880–1930. In: Lageman EC (eds) *Nursing History: New Perspectives, New Possibilities.* New York: Teachers College Press. Examines the development of midwifery in the USA within the context of the struggle of the medical profession to establish a therapeutic basis for its monopoly over the market for obstetrical services and to implement a fee-for-service system of payment for those services.

Heagerty BV (1990) *Class, Gender and Professionalization: The Struggle for English Midwifery, 1900–1936.* Unpublished PhD dissertation, Michigan State University. Examines the development of English midwifery within the context of the class and professional goals of the elite of midwifery and medicine, the conflicts engendered with the rank and file over changing work and attitudes to the mother, and its impact on the development of maternity care and midwives' work between 1900 and 1936.

Leap N & Hunter B (1993) *The Midwives Tale.* London: Scarlet Press. Using oral interviews, provides a picture of the attitudes of midwives' practicing in the 1920s and 1930s toward their work, reproductive health, and the women they attended.

Little R (1983) *Go Seek Mrs Dawson. She'll Know What to Do – The Demise of the Working Class Nurse/ Midwife in the Twentieth Century.* Unpublished Thesis, University of Sussex. A detailed picture of the life, social networks and experiences of handywomen within the context of the class relations of the first decades of the century.

Roberts E (1984) *A Woman's Place.* Oxford: Basil Blackwell. An oral history of working-class women's lives between 1890 and 1945. Particularly relevant for midwifery history are the chapters 'Marriage' (including sexual relationships, birth control, childbirth and infant mortality) and 'Families and Neighbours' (including relationships between the women and their midwives).

Ross E (1993) *Love and Toil: Motherhood in Outcast London, 1870–1918.* Oxford University Press. Examines the meaning of motherhood for working-class women during these years, their attitudes toward their children and their childrearing practices, their knowledge of reproduction and their interaction with the increasing intervention by state health workers attempting to change their values and behaviours.

Taylor-Ladd M (1988) Grannies and spinsters: midwife education under the Sheppard–Towner Act. *Journal of Social History* **22**: 255–276. Examines the conflicts between US public health workers working under the Sheppard–Towner Act in the 1920s and the lay Black, Hispanic and immigrant working-class midwives that came under its influence.

5

Support and control in labour: doulas and midwives

Diane Walters
Mavis J. Kirkham

HISTORICAL BACKGROUND

Throughout most of history, and in much of the world today, women in labour are supported by women they already know well. Those whom we may call midwives care for childbearing neighbours as part of the fabric of their domestic life, and birth takes place in a domestic setting, supported and witnessed by women friends and kin. As midwives became more skilled this support has continued (e.g. Allison, 1996).

In 1944 Grantly Dick-Read observed:

> *One of the most gratifying features of a normal labour is the personal interest and undivided attention given by the attendant of the parturient woman. This applies particularly to primaparae. However great the confidence and courage, the knowledge that someone competent to understand is nearby affords a comforting sense of security.* (Dick-Read, 1944)

In the second half of the twentieth century the centralization of medical expertise in hospitals led to the institutionalization of birth, a transition that was seen as increasing medical control in the event of unpredictable complications and which gave working-class women a brief respite from unrelenting domestic toil. Within the institution, however, the woman laboured on the professionals' territory, which was organized to render their work efficient, and the professionals' aims were primarily concerned with physical monitoring and care. When the woman entered hospital, therefore, the emotional support provided by women of her family and community was left behind. She was then in the presence of attendants skilled in understanding physiology and its adjustment rather than in understanding her experience.

With the move of birth into ever larger institutions came a separation of physical care and emotional support for labouring women. The growth of technology around birth and ever more complex forms of monitoring produced a great increase in physical tasks for the attendant to perform. Failure to perform these tasks became a serious and visible omission, whereas failure to give support is much less visible. Another aspect of the growth in technology was the availability of information on the condition of mother and fetus which was gathered by technical means rather than from the mother in conversation. Information flow is a crucial component of support, and rendering the mother largely redundant as a source of information affected the balance of power in relationships with carers. The source of vital information has to be cared for and maintained, and much of this maintenance work in labour turned towards machines rather than the relationship between the mother and the midwife. The feedback of information to mothers was in the control of professionals, many of whom saw this information as concerning them more than the woman from whom it was technologically derived.

The use of more effective forms of analgesia and anaesthesia in labour also greatly affected the relationship between the woman and her carer. With increasing medical powers of control over pain and progress in labour, enhancing the mother's ability to cope with her labour was no longer the key midwifery skill. There was a growing sense in which medicine rather than the mother was doing the physical coping. The close link between emotional and physical coping was also seen as open to medical solution as in obstetricians' recommendation of epidural anaesthesia to very young or very frightened women in labour because 'we don't want to make trouble for ourselves' (Kirkham, 1987). With complex technology came a need for control over the woman to whom the equipment was attached. The technology also offered the means for control of behaviour which was welcomed by many women as well as by doctors and midwives.

At the same time, the organization of the workforce in hospitals meant that care was fragmented and a woman was very unlikely to have previously met her carer during labour or to see her again. This, together with changes in carer during labour, made it much more difficult to provide emotional support. A relationship of trust, which must precede effective support, had therefore to be built anew in each episode of care. The low priority given to support by medical powerholders, and the fact that a woman well supported may make choices inconvenient to the smooth running of a labour ward (Kirkham, 1987), led to support becoming a neglected art in large maternity hospitals in the 1970s and 1980s. There were, however, always notable exceptions, which were possibly more likely to be found in the community or in very small units where the relative absence of modern technology meant that the midwife must still cherish the mother in order to gain her co-operation and enhance her ability to cope with labour.

A situation was reached where: 'Childbirth is now lonelier and more psychologically stressful. For some mothers left to labour largely on their own, birth becomes a "solitary confinement".' (Klaus et al, 1993). An awareness that all was not well was probably part of the move for partners to be present during labour in the 1970s and moves towards both privacy and professional support for women in labour.

RESEARCH

Much research has been done on the effect of support on the outcomes of labour. This is summed up on the cover of a recent research-based leaflet on the subject:

The constant presence of a supportive birth companion is one of the most effective forms of care in childbirth introduced in the last 25 years.   *(MIDIRS, 1996)*

Ten randomized, controlled trials, including 3336 women, were carried out between 1980 and 1993 to examine the effect of the continuous presence of a support person on women in labour. In each study the supporters had received brief training and did not know the women they were supporting before labour. The results are remarkably consistent (Hodnett, 1995), showing increased physical benefits, a reduction in complications and considerable emotional benefits for the mother.

Outcomes of support in labour

The original studies of this series took place in Guatemala. Sosa et al (1980) randomly assigned 20 primiparous women to a control or experimental group. The experimental group were supported by lay women who remained with them from admission until delivery. It is significant that 103 women had to be admitted to the control group in order to obtain 20 uncomplicated deliveries, whereas the experimental group achieved this with 33 women. Women in the experimental group had average labours of 8 hours compared with 19 hours for the control group. The supported mothers smiled at, talked to and stroked their babies more than the control group and suffered significantly fewer perinatal problems. The study was repeated in the same hospital 6 years later (Klaus et al, 1986) with similar, statistically significant findings. The supported women had shorter labours, fewer caesarean sections and less use of oxytocin to augment labour.

Kennell repeated the study in a US hospital (Kennell et al, 1991) where 412 women were enrolled into three groups: control, supported and 'inconspicuously observed'. The latter category of mothers had outcomes slightly better than those of the control group. The caesarean section and forceps delivery rate for the experimental group was significantly lower and postnatal outcomes were improved.

These early studies concentrated on clinically measurable outcomes around the time of birth. This is hardly surprising, as Oakley (1988) explained, 'since maternity care policy-makers tend to be more impressed by evidence of clinical effects, it is these effects that (from this point of view) need to be highlighted as outcome measures'. Longer-term emotional outcomes are also of significance. A study in Johannesburg (Hofmeyr et al, 1991) reported that companionship had no measurable effect on the progress of labour; this was perhaps because the women were labouring in a 'familiar community hospital' where epidural anaesthesia was not available. In the supported group, 'diastolic blood pressure and the use of analgesia were modestly but significantly reduced'. The most important results were that 'the psychological responses and perceptions of the group were strikingly different ... Companionship ... had a striking effect on the way that the participants reported experiencing labour'. The supported group were more likely to report that they felt that they had coped well during labour, their reported labour pain was less and their state anxiety scores were lower than in the control group. Their breast-feeding outcomes were markedly better. This latter finding, together with other studies, led the authors to conclude that 'conventional hospital care may interfere with the confidence needed to breast-feed'. Overall, they concluded that 'if feelings of competence initiated during labour, a time of intense emotional impressionability, are important to a woman's ongoing sense of competence as a mother and ability to breast-feed successfully, then this finding is of considerable importance'. This fits with the findings of a large English survey of women's expectations of experiences around birth (Green et al, 1988), which found that women's sense of control in their birth experience was linked with positive emotional outcomes postnatally. As childbearing remains a vivid and integral part of a woman's personal story and self-image for many years (Simkin, 1991), probably for the rest of her life, 'conventional hospital care' may interfere with confidence in many long-term senses.

A later study by the same Johannesburg research team (Wolman et al, 1993) followed up the two groups of women and found the supported mothers' self-esteem rising in the 6 weeks after delivery, while the self-esteem of the control group fell; depression scores were also significantly higher in the control group.

It is perhaps obvious, though highly unusual in trials of interventions in labour, that no negative outcomes have been associated with support in labour (Hodnett, 1995).

The nature of support

With such striking – though not entirely consistent – results from studies of support in labour, it is important to look at the nature of that support. Women in labour have been described as having a profound need for companionship, empathy and help (Simkin, 1992). Support in labour has been described as having four dimensions (Hodnett and Osborn, 1989):

- emotional support: encouragement, praise, reassurance, continuous physical presence
- informational support: explanations and advice
- physical support: comfort measures such as massage
- advocacy: interpreting the woman's wishes to hospital staff, acting on her behalf

While the mere presence of another person may slightly affect outcome, and I (M.K.) have had the chastening experience of being thanked for 'being there' while in the role of unobtrusive observer of a labour, it cannot be assumed that those who are meant to be there are actually giving support. McNiven et al (1992) piloted a work sampling technique to determine the amount of time intrapartum nurses at a Toronto teaching hospital spent in support activities as defined above. Their finding was 9.9%. They concluded that 'the technologic tasks associated with medical intervention tend to be more highly valued and occupy more of nurses' time than supportive care' and identified very different philosophies to explain this:

> *Medical intervention and obstetric technology embody a conceptual system that emphasizes fragmentation and separation, whereas support and empathy derive from a perspective that emphasizes connection between individuals.* *(McNiven et al, 1992)*

These nurses are there to be with the medical system, not with the women.

Those who are present during labours, not surprisingly, differ in the support they give. Radin et al (1993) looked at the influence of nurses' care during labour and delivery on the caesarean rate for healthy, nulliparous women in a US hospital. Nurses were selected because of their presence at either low or high numbers of caesarean births during the previous year. This was a carefully designed, statistically sophisticated study which controlled for a large number of variables. 'Large differences' were found in the caesarean rates of the women cared for by the two groups of nurses. The women in the care of the 'low caesarean' nurses also had fewer forceps and vacuum extractions and shorter labours. There was no difference in fetal distress or Apgar scores between the two groups. Analysis of the actual differences in care awaits further studies.

An examination of Hodnett and Osborn's four dimensions of support (see above) can be useful in determining who can give support effectively. All four categories require the carer to focus on the labouring woman in order to give support that is appropriate. This is clearly difficult if they have other priorities such as monitoring and attending to information collection, or being responsible for another woman in labour at the same time. Conflict of loyalties can also occur at a philosophical as well as a physical level. Oakley (1992) sees two different tasks and philosophies in 'supporting women rather than medicalizing them'.

The information dimension of support may at first sight appear straightforward. This is clearly important to women. Fleissig (1993) found, 'Women who felt staff had given them enough information during labour and delivery were more likely to say that labour and delivery were managed as they liked than those who wanted more explanation'. Staff and clients may not have the same perceptions of information given. In a study by McKay and Smith (1993), 'caregivers' perceptions of the quality of their information giving is more positive than mothers' perceptions'. Considerable skill is required in giving appropriate information to individual mothers: women are reluctant to ask questions of carers whom they perceive as 'busy' or not welcoming questions (Kirkham, 1987), and 'unvoiced fears' (McKay and Smith, 1993) loom large. The hierarchical organization of hospitals creates further barriers to information flow (Kirkham, 1987). It is difficult to praise within a medical system where the active role is the medical role and not the maternal role. Indeed, it is difficult to praise where the value system pervades the language, and the woman's performance in labour may bear a label including the word 'failure' or one of her key obstetric organs may be described as 'incompetent'. It is interesting that in the study by Hofmeyr et al (1991) support was 'not informative except to the extent of simple advice derived from personal experience, as the companions had no medical, nursing nor traditional midwifery experience, but all had children of their own'. Perhaps the supporters changed the emotional atmosphere to the extent that professional carers gave more information to these women. There is no way of knowing that, but it is often observed in midwifery that support is infectious, as is lack of support.

Hofmeyr et al (1991) identified the factors that they thought were important in support:

• The companions were not part of the hospital hierarchy, and may therefore have been seen as an ally without a vested interest in the hospital establishment.
• They were drawn from the same community as the women in their care and were therefore 'able to communicate easily with and share common values with the participants'.
• They were not known personally to the participants and therefore did not have to meet expectations or keep up appearances.
• The specific elements which the companions were repeatedly told to concentrate on were comfort, reassurance and praise.
• The emotional support seemed to be genuine. The companions worked as volunteers with small payment for expenses only. Yet they 'showed a remarkable ability to maintain a commitment to their vocation'.

- 'The fact that someone with no other functions whatsoever was allocated on a full-time basis to be with the women in labour may have conveyed a message of concern for and value of them as individuals.'

If these are key factors, they clearly limit the extent to which professionals or family members can take on the role of supporter.

ORIGINS AND DEVELOPMENT OF THE DOULA MOVEMENT

Doula (pronounced 'doola') is a Greek word literally translated as 'in service of'. The term 'doula' was first used for women with a broad knowledge of breast-feeding who helped new mothers nurse their babies (Raphael, 1976), and is also the name given to women who provide support for the mother at home after the baby is born (postpartum doulas).

Definition:

> In the context of childbirth, a doula is a non-medical professional experienced in birth who provides continuous emotional, physical and informational support to both the mother and her partner throughout labour and delivery.

The doula movement and doula training programmes have been developed in the USA to accommodate the needs of pregnant women who have a belief in natural childbirth. This was in a situation where the continuing campaign to restrict or eliminate midwives meant that most women gave birth in hospital with a physician who only appeared when birth was imminent. Women felt isolated and, though cared for by nurses, were often left on their own during labour and heavily sedated, sometimes not even knowing that they had given birth until hours afterwards. Practices are now changing, but feelings of loneliness and isolation are still often reported.

To make birth more humane and to help women have more positive experiences, the 'labour coach' emerged, who told women when and how to breathe and when to push, usually involving very structured breathing patterns. Subsequently the role of the labour coach evolved to one of providing support and listening to the needs of the women who wish to give birth in an instinctive and natural way. This has been supported by various studies clearly showing the benefits of doula support. There are now numerous doula associations and training programmes in the USA, the oldest being the National Association of Childbirth Assistants. Local training programmes have evolved in various regions of the country, including the Pacific Area Labour Support, organized and led by Penny Simkin in Washington, and Birth and Bonding in California, who initiated an international training programme in the UK in 1991.

THE DOULA

If midwife is the first word pregnant women should be well acquainted with, doula is the second.
(Arms, 1994)

The doula's primary function is to ease the birth experience, making it a more positive one by helping to reduce the levels of anxiety and fear experienced by the couple. This is achieved in part by her assurance that she will be with the couple continuously throughout the entire labour until the birth of their baby – they will not be left alone at any time. This assurance gives the couple a profound sense of being cared for and supported and it is in this nurturing space that the woman is able to freely give herself up to giving birth.

> *Feeling completely safe with another human being creates a kind of freedom that enables a woman to begin to test the limits of her own capacities possibly not recognized before – or perhaps recognized but not risked. This freedom to be one's true self produces feelings of empowerment and creativity.*
> *(Klaus et al, 1993)*

The presence of the doula is valuable not only for first-time mothers but also for subsequent births. As one experienced mother reported to her doula after her third child's water birth at home:

> *I was able to be so focused on what was happening to my body because I knew you were there for me taking care of everything. It gave me the freedom to concentrate on the birth and what I had to do. It was brilliant!*   *[mother's feedback to her doula]*

It is a woman-led philosophy – the doula is guided by the woman's own individual needs during labour and she is sensitive to the way those needs will change as labour progresses, i.e. what felt right during one contraction might not feel right during the next, so she must be prepared to be adaptable. Sometimes she will be active, sometimes not, depending on the couple's needs, but at all times they know she is 'there' for them. She is never critical or judgmental – her role is to inspire confidence in the woman's ability to give birth and to reduce the fear of the unknown. Her presence is always positive.

The doula will 'listen' both to what is said and what is not said, i.e. will be instinctive and intuitive in order to care for the woman in ways that are right for her. In this way she is able to help the woman find her own strengths and abilities. She will help the woman work with her labour rather than against it, guiding her on how to stay as relaxed and comfortable as possible using various support measures if appropriate, e.g. stroking, verbal encouragement, eye contact and visualization. She will sense when a woman needs the reassurance of touch or at other times the need for encouraging words, or sometimes just her undivided attention will be enough to let the women know she is cared for.

> *By listening, establishing a sense of rapport and responding to the woman's changing needs the support person becomes a valuable resource.*   *(MIDIRS, 1996)*

The doula explains what is happening as labour progresses, helping to ease the anxiety that comes with unfamiliarity. She keeps the couple informed of progress, knowing that they need to be reassured that the sights and sounds of labour are normal. When they know what is happening and have constant affirmation that they are doing well, they have a more positive feeling of being able to succeed. Without the right kind of support and encouragement it is easy to lose confidence in your body. If the course of labour changes and other decisions have to be made, the doula is able to assist and support the couple in making other choices.

As Nancy Weiner Cohen said:

When a woman is begging for medication during labour, we believe she is really asking for support. She wants information that what is happening to her is okay. She wants reassurance that the pain she's feeling is normal... that she's not alone. She wants a loving touch... and eye contact. She wants someone to remind her that she's strong and healthy and there's a baby coming.   *(Cohen, 1983)*

What a woman in labour needs most of all is positive emotional and verbal reassurance from all those attending her and it is for this reason that the doula, if she has given birth herself, needs to have cleared her own birth experiences so as not to carry over any of her own unresolved anxieties to the women under her care. Ina May Gaskin (1977) talked about the quality of the energy of people attending births having a significant effect on the course of the labour. As she observed, 'anyone whose presence is not an actual help is requiring the emotional support that should be going to the mother'. For this reason the doula needs to have created a support network for herself in order to talk through or debrief after each birth she attends, so that she can approach the next birth with clarity.

Doula support during pregnancy and birth

Ideally the doula meets the couple some months before the baby is due. They have several meetings to discuss the couple's expectations about the birth, what their hopes and fears are, and what is important to them. Discussing their choices and options with the doula in advance helps them to define their objectives. These meetings also provide an opportunity for a relationship to develop, for a sense of familiarity and trust to emerge.

The experienced doula will also know local hospital protocols and will be able to advise first-time parents of hospital policies. During these meetings the doula can encourage the couple to practise positions for labour together and suggest support and relaxation techniques. It is also an opportunity for the woman to let the doula know what comfort measures she enjoys that might be helpful during labour.

The couple have the assurance that the doula will be available for them when they feel the need for her support: this could be in early labour or later, whatever feels right for them. Having the doula with them lessens their initial anxiety and the couple will often remain at home longer than if they were on their own. At this stage the doula needs to be sensitive to the couple's relationship and allow them to find their own rhythms together, helping and encouraging when necessary, but allowing them to share this early phase together. This is also the time for the couple and doula to talk through any anxieties they may have, and also to build a rapport with one another if they have not met often.

As labour progresses and becomes more intense, the doula becomes more involved in touching, hugging, stroking and reassuring, always letting the woman and her partner know what is happening. It is at this point that the partner may feel overwhelmed by the change of intensity in the labour and can become alarmed and unsure, and also be in need of support and reassurance. The doula will recognize this, and her ability to verbalize what is happening helps to ease their anxieties. She will also, at this time, encourage the partner to support the woman in ways that are right for him and up to the level that he is able so that he does not feel solely responsible for her care. She is 'there' for them both – her focus is their emotional well-being.

When the birth becomes imminent the midwives or doctors are in charge but the doula still remains close to the woman, encouraging and supporting. She does not interfere with the decisions of the medical staff but will remain a constant source of emotional and physical support to the woman and her partner, helping them both to a more positive experience. Following the birth of the baby, she will help to ensure that the couple's wishes for the moments after the birth are respected and fulfilled. If labour does not proceed as planned, the doula still plays an important role in helping the parents to understand what is happening by verbal explanation. Her continuing positive support and calming presence will be deeply reassuring for them at this time, as will her assurance that she will not leave them.

A few days following the birth, the doula will meet again with the family to talk through the birth. This debriefing is an essential part of their shared experience – she is able to fill in information about what happened or things that were said that the mother (and father) may have forgotten. It is an opportunity to reaffirm how well the woman coped with her labour – how strong she was and what courage she showed, as well as to talk through any difficult situations that might have occurred. This positive feedback serves to increase her feelings of self-confidence and self-esteem. (This is her 'birth story' – see Chapter 9.) The woman and her partner also express their feelings – sometimes negative ones in relation to the way they feel they coped; from the doula's feedback they can gain a new perspective on the experience and their part in it. If there were complications the doula will encourage the couple to talk about feelings of disappointment or distress, and will help them integrate the experience.

> *I found [the doula] to be a wonderful source of support from the time I met her during pregnancy through to the birth of my son and then afterwards in discussion. After a caesarean section I was keen to experience a normal, natural vaginal delivery. I believe that working with [her] enabled me to achieve my aim … On every occasion that we met she gave freely of her time. We worked through both my anxieties and my hopes as thoroughly as was necessary and at all times she gave her support unconditionally and without judgment. She was also a great source of information and advice and this enabled me to secure the care of my preferred medical officer at the hospital … I felt secure with her and her confidence in my ability to birth my baby helped me prepare emotionally for a normal labour and birth. Not only did I achieve my desire but I did so being able to enjoy pregnancy, labour and the birth itself. I consider it to have been a marvellously healing experience; one that has empowered me and given me back my belief in my body and my abilities as a mother. I sincerely thank my doula with all my heart.*   *[Doula-supported vaginal birth after previous caesarean section, 1994]*

The doula and the father

> *A father is rarely able, moment to moment, to appreciate what is happening with the mother and whether each change is a normal part of the actual events of labour. An easier role for him is to give emotional support to the mother while the doula is there to support them both during labour.*   *(Klaus et al, 1993)*

A father's presence at the birth of his child has undergone major changes since the 1950s. Then it would have been considered radical behaviour to have a father in the labour ward – they were left to pace hospital corridors and to celebrate the eventual birth with a drink in the pub with their male associates. By the 1970s it was commonplace for fathers to be in attendance, and by the 1980s it was expected behaviour.

Most women want their partners to be with them; they need to know they are there for them in a loving and supportive way – but although partners may have attended childbirth classes and be sensitive to the woman's needs, their experience in labour is limited and their close emotional tie to the woman makes it difficult for them to remain objective while also dealing with their own intense feelings. As one father observed:

> *With our first baby I was so overcome emotionally that I couldn't make any rational observation about what was happening and I truly believed there was imminent danger at every stage of labour.*
>
> *(Klaus et al, 1993)*

Berry (1988) concluded that it was unrealistic to expect fathers to be highly supportive during labour as they were 'concerned about their abilities to help while wrestling with. . . and trying to hide their own feelings'. Considering the level of the partners' emotional involvement, it is scarcely surprising that Bertsch et al (1990) found that labour support from fathers was not associated with the improved outcomes linked with labour support from lay women. Chapman (1992) found that the role most commonly adopted by fathers during labour was that of witness.

A doula is not a replacement for the father – her role is to free him from feeling totally responsible for his partner's well-being and to allow him to participate during labour as and when he feels able. She is there to support them both and her presence equally benefits them, providing the father with the same emotional freedom as the mother. The mother is able to get on with giving birth feeling supported, and the father is able to participate knowing that he too is supported.

As Michel Odent says in *Birth Reborn*:

> *Men sometimes find it hard to observe, accept and understand a woman's instinctive behaviour during childbirth. Instead they often try to keep her from slipping out of a rational, self controlled state... it is not mere coincidence that in all traditional societies women in labour are assisted not by men but by other women who have had children themselves.* *(Odent, 1994)*

For most first-time fathers, the experience of birth can be overwhelming. They are often confused and uncertain of their role given the demands and emotions of intense labour, but with the doula gently encouraging and suggesting ways in which they can be of positive help to the woman, they are able to find their own level of involvement, at the same time feeling that they are a useful participant and an integral part of the process. The doula also serves as a role model on which they can base their own form of support and behaviour. As one doula reported:

> *I congratulated a new father on the wonderful support he'd given to his wife during an anxious labour and his instant reply was that he'd had a great teacher and all he'd done was copy what he'd seen me doing.* *[Personal communication from a doula]*

Sometimes the couple may be concerned that an outside person will take over and intrude on their birth experience, but the doula is there primarily to enhance that experience by her quiet reassurance and her sensitivity to both their needs. Conversely, many fathers welcome her presence, not only as a support person for their partners, but also so that they too will have one face in the labour room that is familiar to them – someone they feel they can relate to who will be with them throughout the entire labour.

> *A father may, for the most legitimate reasons, have difficulty in providing his labouring partner with the same undivided attention that a doula is able to give. For him, as much as for the mother, the birth of his child represents a rite of passage, involving a major emotional readjustment. He has to cope with fears for*

his partner's safety and his baby's, as well as dealing with his own emotions, the intensity of which may surprise him.

(Nolan, 1995)

It is relevant that the study by Breart et al (1992) found 'fewer unsatisfactory relationships between midwife and father' to be one of the positive results of the continuous presence of a supportive female companion in labour.

Doulas in the UK

There are a growing number of trained doulas in the UK as a result of the US-based Birth and Bonding international training programme initiated in 1991. The training takes place yearly and is currently evolving into a more British-based experience taking into account the differences in medical care between Britain and the USA. The training explores the physiological, psychological and emotional aspects of pregnancy, labour and birth through discussion, videos, lectures and experimental exercises. The course includes fetal development, anatomy, birth physiology, clinical terminology and hospital procedures, as well as focusing on the emotional and psychological aspects of giving birth and its significance in women's lives. Emphasis is also placed on enhancement of the parent–infant bond both prenatally and after the birth.

After completing the training, new doulas attend regular meetings and weekend workshops for further learning and the sharing of experiences and skills. These meetings serve to create an invaluable support group. Initially they will attend a certain number of births on a volunteer basis, but when sufficiently experienced will be employed privately by couples. Many doulas offer childbirth preparation classes and birth workshops, as well as being involved in home birth and vaginal birth after caesarean (VBAC) support groups.

Birth and Bonding in Oakland, California, currently have a volunteer doula team at their local hospital and their East Bay Doula Service, which works specifically with low-income women, is applying for government grants as a result of their non-profit status, in order that doulas can receive a fee for each birth attended. One of the largest and most prestigious teaching hospitals on the West Coast, University College of San Francisco, has now requested the services of a team of doulas, so Birth and Bonding are now initiating the San Francisco doula team. Doulas are also employed on a private basis by couples who wish to secure their services. Perhaps such schemes could emerge in Britain as the role of the midwifery support worker receives increasing attention.

The roles of doula and midwife

With regard to breast-feeding, Raphael (1981) states that, 'any supportive person including the midwife can fulfil the role of doula'. In labour the situation is more complex, largely because of the institutional setting of most labours in Britain. This is clear in the context of Hofmeyr's six points (see above). Doulas are identified as being 'on the mother's side', while the midwife is part of the hospital hierarchy and is usually employed by the hospital. There are, however, a few hospitals in the world that employ doulas in a clearly identified role (Klaus et al, 1993). The midwife's role is wider and she has other concerns besides 'comfort, reassurance and praise'. How far these concerns undermine her ability to give support is the crucial issue here.

Where institutional controls over women in labour are strongest, their need for support is likely to be great. It is significant that a doula service is now being developed for childbearing women prisoners (S. Kitzinger, 1996, personal communication). For prisoners choice and control are scarcely issues, and guards are ever-present during labour. In this context the presence of a 'birth companion' whose only role is support is likely to have a profound effect.

Where institutional controls over midwives are strongest, they are least likely to be able to meet their clients' needs for individual support. Where midwives are allied with the institution's controlling forces (medical, institutional or managerial) and they are employees, there are two possible effects on the support midwives can give to clients. The support for clients is usually lessened because of the strength of other pressures upon the midwife's time and sense of priorities. It is also possible that support can become institutionalized. This is prescribed by O'Driscoll et al (1993) as part of a medically controlled '*Active Management of Labour*' which, while effective, is very different from the support given by doulas.

Over recent decades midwives have come to fit the description by Freire (1972) of an oppressed group, who have taken on the technological and organizational values of the dominant group (medicine and later to some extent management) and experienced the suppression of their own original values of nurturing. There can then be seen the 'submissive aggression' where members of the oppressed group turn their frustration upon their own group. In such a situation it is hardly surprising that midwives often react with unease or hostility to the presence of an unknown lay person with a specific nurturing role during labour. Doulas are very aware of this. I (D.W.) do not use the word 'doula' when working with midwives, partly to avoid appearing threatening and partly because the word is not known. The woman is my advocate in this sense either in formulating her birth-plan, in explaining my role to her midwife, or when introducing me to her in the labour ward.

The midwife faces further dilemmas with regard to her relationship with her profession and her immediate colleagues or team. Professionalism is also an issue, which can be seen as ensuring that the midwife's primary loyalty is to her profession rather than to individuals in her care (Kirkham, 1996). It is ironic that with all these affiliations midwives so often lack a support network and the opportunities for debriefing which doulas see as essential. Midwives are working, as never before, to develop new ways of being 'with women', and there is evidence that changes towards continuity of care move midwives' primary allegiances towards their clients rather than towards their profession or employer (Brodie, 1996). Yet midwifery still bears the marks of its medicalized and institutionalized recent past.

A central issue here is that of defence reactions. The midwife has to cope with the pressures of institutionalized work and its attendant anxieties alongside the human need of those in her care. As Menzies-Lyth (1988) so tellingly described, there is a tendency to create routines in order to insulate oneself from the emotional stress provoked by conflicting human and institutional demands upon carers. This must have been a factor in care becoming fragmented originally. Yet defensive practice allows our human skills to atrophy. Years of defensive practice have tended to erode our trust in ourselves as practitioners, our colleagues and our clients. Trust, however, is vital in maternity care. Jessica James sees her role as a birth attendant as helping the labouring woman to have trust in herself:

I stay in constant contact, attempting to be in touch with what the labouring woman needs… I aim to help her to feel safe and to let go… shielding the labouring woman from the outside world and facilitating her capacity to trust her instincts and move into an inner state.   (James, 1990)

This sounds very much like being 'with women', the origin of the word 'midwife' long before that word was linked with descriptions such as 'oppressed group' and 'defence reactions'. It is perhaps not surprising that James (1990) goes on to describe midwives giving instructions rather than support: 'instructing women to breathe rather than doing it with them', and suggesting women move, but not helping them to get off the bed; and questions 'how much some midwives really want to get involved'.

As George Eliot's character in *Middlemarch* so tellingly observed, 'We do not expect people to be deeply moved by what is not unusual. Tragedy in frequency – our frames could hardly bear it' (Eliot, 1871). Yet the doula and midwife frequently deal with life's most moving experiences. It is difficult to deal, on a frequent basis, with what Taylor (1996) sees as 'real dangers in all midwives' practice … death, sex, madness and love'. Providing real support involves close contact with these dangers and women's perceptions of them; all this in an institutional context which also requires them to control uncertainty and manage risk. She concludes that 'midwives therefore have good reasons to have developed psychological and institutional defence mechanisms against these dangers. But if they are to implement *Changing Childbirth* [DoH, 1993] they cannot use these defences'. In the context of 'this necessary dismantling of the psychological and institutional defences' midwives need, at the very least, the support networks which doulas see as essential. This is difficult as we have also developed an ethos of battling on with what we have, even if the structures we have were built for a different era and purpose.

James (1990) sees the midwife as primarily concerned with 'progress or the baby's heartbeat', and without these concerns she is 'able to make a good relationship and possibly a closer one than the midwife's'. It is important to examine how far the several aims of monitoring and support may be in conflict. It is true that midwives seem to be elsewhere just at those points in labour when women most need support: when they are clearing up after procedures, summoning medical assistance, preparing equipment or liaising with other services. But these are institutional arrangements, not integral parts of the midwife's role. With appropriate technical and personnel support for the midwife, she need never leave a woman in labour at these crucial times. It is because midwives in hospitals are seen as being in a support role to medicine that they run errands and leave their clients with inadequate support. Furthermore, because they are so efficient in moving swiftly from task to task, they are often required to care for two women in labour at once, thus giving continuous support to neither. If midwives were seen as key professionals who themselves needed technical support, the midwife could remain with woman.

It may be claimed that the doula's role is highly specialized and the midwife's highly technical. Indeed James claims that 'midwives cannot stay in constant contact [with the client] unless there are two of them – one for each role'. Such division of labour, at a time of economic constraints, would be likely to lead to less midwifery time spent with each client and thereby a 'dilution' in the skilled clinical observation which a woman receives from a midwife as she receives support (Cronk, 1996, personal communication). A midwife's clinical skill is one part, though far from the whole, of what equips her to give support, for her continued support assures the mother that all is clinically normal, or the diagnosed problem is being treated.

As a mother holds her growing child (Winnicott, 1992), midwifery support can hold the situation in which the woman labours. The midwife's clinical knowledge assures the mother that all is well and as is to be expected and thereby provides her with a safe and cherished space in which to cope (Main, 1989). Such holding increases the space within which the mother can act; it does not restrain her. The midwife thus holds open a safe space in which the mother is the main actor. It is a delicate task to hold in such an empowering manner, for very often the clinician's technical expertise holds clients in a grip that constricts their freedom of action and inhibits their instinctive responses. Thus the midwife has a tremendous potential for giving support, but is less likely than the doula to succeed in doing so.

Prioritizing technical tasks may leave the carers' supportive skills to atrophy, which is why midwives feel that women receiving obstetric care also need the care of a midwife. By this same logic it could be said that a woman receiving midwifery care should also receive the care of a doula. Yet the further this division of labour is carried, the more potential there is for misunderstanding and the more impoverished the role of the midwife may become. It is ironic that it is the medical innovators of '*The Active Management of Labour*' who stress, as part of their medically controlled management of labour, that:

> *The nurse [sic] must appreciate that her primary duty to the mother is to provide the emotional support so badly needed at this critical time and not simply to record vital signs in a detached manner.*
>
> *(O'Driscoll et al, 1993)*

It must also be said that O'Driscoll's unit requires medical students to stay with labouring women and provide support. It is professionally ironic that a book much used in the training of doulas in Britain (Klaus et al, 1993) contains a chapter on 'The Dublin Experience' by O'Driscoll and Meagher.

There is also the wider issue of who is best placed to give support in labour. This is a time of heightened emotions, the prelude to the forging of new relationships with the newborn. In a real sense, therefore, the key actor is the mother and the key supporters are those who love her and the baby. In Nicky Leap's view:

> *Much has been written in recent years about the concept of 'empowerment' through birth. Speaking from a midwifery perspective, the process of empowering women means making sure that the people the woman has chosen do all the tender supporting during labour, not us. It means we take a step back and ensure that we disturb the process as little as possible, providing a 'safety net' presence, sometimes encouragement and little else. Putting into practice the theory that 'the less we do the more we give'....*
> *Our job as midwives is to watch, listen and respond with all our senses, including our intuition, so that we know when to inform, suggest, act and most importantly when to remove ourselves.*   *(Leap, 1992)*

Before we can even start upon this we need to abandon all the ways in which midwives' actions may inhibit or limit women by suggesting an expected way in which they should be good patients. The exercise of such intuition may then lead a midwife to take a doula role, to facilitate other supporters or to protect a woman using her own inner resources. The variety of women's reactions and the reactions of any one woman during her labour is infinitely richer than the prescribed support and 'the need to keep every woman in labour on a tight emotional rein' laid down by O'Driscoll et al (1993). Institutionalization prevents intuition being developed and used as Leap describes. This, in itself, must be a reason for birth ceasing to be institutionalized and becoming personalized, wherever it happens, through close relationships between client and carer built up over a pregnancy. Doulas are skilled in supporting women in an alienating setting, but the setting needs to be changed. This does not mean that women will cease to need support or doulas. Relationships also need to be changed. The addition of a new set of relationships, with the doula, runs the risk of simply bypassing the problems inherent in the existing relationships between parents, midwives and obstetricians. If there is a need for advocacy and clarification between mother and midwife then that relationship really needs to be readdressed. If the labouring woman feels lonely and isolated then staffing levels need to be reassessed. Present relationships are too powerful to be bypassed. If mothers, doulas and midwives can work together to recreate maternity care in terms of its organization, relationships and values, then there is a massive task on which it is worthwhile for us all to work together. The use of doulas to fill the gaps in an alienating and underresourced maternity service sounds tragic. In the meantime, as midwives and doulas, we must do our best for those women in labour now, as well as building for the future.

DOULAS AND MIDWIVES: IMPLICATIONS FOR PRACTICE

- In their relationships with clients, midwives and obstetricians exercise considerable power including the power to structure and define the woman's experience of labour. The institutional pressures on midwives and obstetricians mean that they are not continuously present with women in labour and this literally leaves space for another role of supporter. Yet, without a reassessment of these power relationships, support which mediates within structures that are alienating can only be partial. The structures within which care is given need to change and much work is now being done with that intention. The existence of doulas serves to remind midwives that change must occur in relationships as well as in structures. It is chastening to remember that doulas came from a setting without midwives, yet they are greatly appreciated here by women who are also attended by a midwife.
- Midwives can also learn from the non-hierarchical, supportive way in which doula care is provided and doulas themselves are supported. There is need for a real awareness of the parallel processes between the way we care for women and the way we are cared for as workers (Eckstein and Wallenstein, 1958), the way we are managed and the way we manage labour, and the way we are supervised and the way we in our turn supervise others. Such awareness can only be developed in a supportive culture. Without such an awareness there is always the danger that we will act out of defensiveness or aggressive oppression rather than a true desire to give support. We therefore need to radically rethink the culture within which we work as midwives. We are in an era of change, and the structures and responses of an era of hierarchical control are highly inappropriate to an era of choice and control for the women in our care. Doulas offer midwives an example of non-hierarchical ways of approaching issues of support for ourselves and for clients, together with fresh insights into issues such as debriefing and supervision. We need particularly to examine our defences against the anxiety generated by the uncertainties of practice and by constant organizational change.

Defences are never there for nothing. The bigger the defence, the more sure one may be of the need for it.
(*Main, 1989*)

Just as the doula needs help to clear her own birth experiences so as not to carry over any of her own unresolved anxieties to the women under her care, so midwives need facilitation to protect women cared for in the present from the effects of past institutionalization and medicalization.

- In and after such rethinking there is much that midwives and doulas can learn from each other as well as from the women in our care. Doulas can teach midwives much about being aware of their own needs and seeking and taking as well as giving support.
- Some student midwives have already gained much from training as doulas in the UK and arrangements are now in place for amended training and course fees for midwives and student midwives. Maybe one day doulas could receive similar recognition in midwifery training.
- To be 'with woman' or to be 'mothering the mother' we need to reflect on the role of that woman as mother. Motherhood is a universal symbol of support and caring; it is a highly active role, but in the sense of facilitation not of control. This role for which we prepare our clients is concerned with fostering growth, not with control which fosters powerlessness. To be a doula, a midwife or a mother we need fundamentally similar skills, for our roles run parallel. In the immense task of changing childbirth so that it is woman-centred there must be room for all of us to learn from each other.
- Together we could learn much, for there is much to learn, about coping, support and empowerment for ourselves and for women in our care.

The contact address for doulas in the UK is:

c/o 22 Tavistock Drive
Mapperley Park
Nottingham
NG3 5DW

REFERENCES

Allison J (1996) *Delivered at Home.* London: Chapman & Hall.

Arms S (1994) *Immaculate Deception II.* Berkeley: Celestial Arts.

Berry L (1988) Realistic expectations of the labour coach. *Journal of Obstetric and Gynaecological Nursing* 17: 354–355.

Bertsch TD, Nagashim-Whalen L, Dykeman S et al (1990) Labour support by first time fathers: direct observation with a comparison to experienced doulas. *Journal of Psychosomatic Obstetrics and Gynaecology* 11: 251–260.

Breart G, Mika-Cabane N, Kaminski M et al (1992) Evaluation of different policies for the management of labour. *Early Human Development* 29: 309–312.

Brodie P (1996) *Australian Team Midwives in Transition.* Paper given at International Confederation of Midwives. 24th Triannual Conference, Oslo.

Chapman J (1992) Expectant fathers' roles during labour and birth. *Journal of Obstetric, Gynaecological and Neonatal Nursing* 21: 114–119.

Cohen NW (1983) *Silent Knife.* New York: Bergin & Garvey.

[DoH] Department of Health (1993) *Changing Childbirth*. Report of the Expert Maternity Group. London: HMSO.

Dick-Read G (1944) *Childbirth Without Fear*. New York: Harper.

Eckstein R & Wallenstein RS (1958) *The Teaching and Learning of Psychotherapy*. New York: Basic Books.

Eliot G (1871) *Middlemarch*. Harmondsworth: Penguin (republished 1980).

Fleissig A (1993) Are women given enough information by staff during labour and delivery? *Midwifery* **9**: 70–75.

Freire P (1972) *Pedagogy of the Oppressed*. Harmondsworth: Penguin.

Gaskin IM (1977) *Spiritual Midwifery*. Summertown, TN: Book Publishing Co.

Green J, Coupland VA & Kitzinger JV (1988) *Great Expectations*. Child Care and Development Group, University of Cambridge.

Hodnett ED (1995) Support from caregivers during childbirth. In: Enkin MW, Keirse MJMC, Renfrew MJ, Neilson JP (eds) *Pregnancy and Childbirth*; Module of the Cochrane Database of Systematic Reviews. London: BMJ Publishing.

Hodnett ED & Osborn RW (1989) Effects of continuous intrapartum professional support on childbirth outcomes. *Research in Nursing and Health* **12**: 289–297.

Hofmeyr GJ, Nikodem VC, Wolman W et al (1991) Companionship to modify the clinical birth environment: effects on progress and perceptions of labour, and breastfeeding. *British Journal of Obstetrics and Gynaecology* **98**: 756–764.

James J (1990) On being a birth attendant. *New Generation* June: 22–25.

Kennell J, Klaus MH, McGrath S et al (1991) Continuous emotional support during labour in a US hospital. *Journal of the American Medical Association* **265**: 2197–2201.

Kirkham MJ (1987) *Basic Supportive Care in Labour: Interaction with and around Labouring Women*. Unpublished PhD thesis, University of Manchester.

Kirkham MJ (1996) Professionalisation past and present: with women or with the powers that be? In: Kroll D (ed.) *Midwifery Care for the Future*. London: Baillière Tindall.

Klaus MH, Kennell JH, Robertson SS & Sosa R (1986) Effects of social support during parturition on maternal and infant morbidity. *British Medical Journal* **293**: 585–587.

Klaus MH, Kennell JH & Klaus PH (1993) *Mothering the Mother: How a Doula Can Help You Have a Shorter, Easier and Healthier Birth*. New York: Addison-Wesley.

Leap N (1992) Our heritage: midwifery tales of the unexpected. *Proceedings of the Second International Homebirth Conference*, University of Sydney, Australia.

Main T (1989) *The Ailment and Other Psychoanalytic Essays*. London: Free Association.

McKay S & Smith SY (1993) 'What are they talking about? Is something wrong?' Information sharing during the second stage of labor. *Birth* **20**(3): 142–147.

McNiven P, Hodnett E & O'Brian Pallas LL (1992) Supporting women in labour: a work sampling study of the activities of labour and delivery nurses. *Birth* **19**(1): 3–7.

Menzies-Lyth I (1988) *Containing Anxiety in Institutions*. London: Free Association.

[MIDIRS] MIDIRS and the NHS Centre for Reviews and Dissemination (1996) *Support in Labour*. Bristol: MIDIRS.

Nolan M (1995) Support in labour: the doula's role. *Modern Midwife* March: 12–15.

Oakley A (1988) Is social support good for the health of mothers and babies? *Journal of Reproductive and Infant Psychology* **6**: 3–21.

Oakley A (1992) Commentary: the best research is that which breeds more. *Birth* **19**(1): 8–9.

Odent M (1994) *Birth Reborn*. London: Souvenir Press.

O'Driscoll K, Meagher & Boylan P (1993) *Active Management of Labour*, 3rd edn. London: Mosby.

Radin TG, Harmon JS & Hanson DA (1993) Nurses' care during labour: its effect on the caesarian birth rate of healthy, nulliparous women. *Birth* **21**(1): 14–21.

Raphael D (1976) *The Tender Gift: Breastfeeding*. New York: Schocken Books.

Raphael D (1981) The midwife as doula: a guide to mothering the mother. *Journal of Nurse-Midwifery* **26**(6): 13–15.

Simkin P (1991) Just another day in a woman's life? Women's long-term perceptions of their first birth experience. *Birth* **18**(4): 203–210.

Simkin P (1992) The labor support person: latest addition to the maternity care team. *International Journal of Childbirth Education* **7**(1): 19–24.

Sosa R, Kennall J, Klaus M et al (1980) The effect of a supportive companion on perinatal problems, length of labour and mother–infant interaction. *New England Journal of Medicine* **303**: 585–587.

Taylor M (1996) An ex-midwife's reflections on supervision from a psychotherapeutic viewpoint. In: Kirkham MJ (ed.) *The Supervision of Midwives.* Hale: Books for Midwives Press.

Winnicott DW (1992) *Babies and Their Mothers.* Merloyd Lawrence Classics in Child Development Series. New York: Addison-Wesley.

Wolman WL, Chalmers B, Hofmeyr GJ & Nikodem VC (1993) Postpartum depression and companionship in the clinical birth environment: a randomised controlled trial. *American Journal of Obstetrics and Gynaecology* **168**(5): 1388–1393.

6

Control for Black and ethnic minority women: a meaningless pursuit

Euranis Neile

The woman must be the focus of maternity care. She should be able to feel that she is in control of what is happening to her and able to make decisions about her care based on her needs, having discussed matters fully with the professionals involved.   *(DoH, 1993, p. 8)*

CARE, CHOICE AND POLICY

This chapter examines the concepts of choice, continuity and control for Black women in the context of the report, *Changing Childbirth* (DoH, 1993). The available evidence is used to explore whether midwives can provide planned individualized, holistic care for Black and minority ethnic women. The multicultural knowledge of midwives is questioned through the results of the research which investigates it. The research findings are used as an opportunity to discuss positive action for the future.

Some of the terms used in this chapter are defined in Box 6.1.

Planned individualized care

Midwifery puts great emphasis on the claim that it offers planned individualized care. However, the medicalization of childbirth and growth in technology means that 98.7% of births take place in hospitals (Campbell and Macfarlane, 1994; Tew, 1995). The trend towards hospital births has led to greater segmentation of care, and an increase in interventions and instrumental deliveries, with little regard for individual needs and preferences. Innovations such as birth plans, where the woman is encouraged to plan and write down her wishes for the conduct and her care in labour, have brought about limited improvements, but only for some sectors of society. The Black report (Townsend and Davidson, 1982) and *The Health Divide* (Whitehead, 1987), amongst other contributions to the inequalities debate, established that middle-class educated people have the power and ability to assert their right to good services from all institutions, while people in the lower social classes have not. These reports failed to debate the position of Black and

---

Box 6.1   Definitions used in this chapter

The term 'Black' is used in the political sense of the word. It refers to anyone who is not white and is likely to experience racism as a result of colour.

'Racism' is prejudice combined with power.

The term 'race' can be used as one of convenience but not as a true definition. It is a term that socially describes a group of people who look alike because of their physical appearance and superficial features such as skin tone, hair texture and stature. The term is biologically irrelevant.

'Cultural dominance' is the ability of the white majority to determine what will be the available choices.

---

minority ethnic people within the health services in the UK. Where issues of race and health were mentioned in the most recent of the reports (Benzeval et al, 1995) they were mainly marginalized by being given only a token mention. Black women often fall outside this powerful group of middle-class educated people, and for them a problem is created by racism, class differences and poverty (Neile, 1995a).

Planned individualized care should result in continuity of care. However, the majority of a woman's care in pregnancy, labour and the postpartum period is concentrated in the hospital where she may be seen by more than 30 professionals in the course of just one pregnancy (Flint and Poulengeris, 1987). The emphasis will be on monitoring and treatment, much of which – for those who do not need it – is a waste of time and money. These resources could be concentrated on those who really need them. At the same time many social and psychological needs of women will be left unmet.

What are the choices?

In the 1980s women worked through the consumer movement for choices in childbirth. Theoretically a woman is able to choose from a wide range of options for maternity care. She has a statutory right to midwifery care, and can choose between hospital consultant care, general practitioner care, and care solely by a midwife in a variety of settings including in her own home. She is able to choose between a wide range of drugs, medical procedures and natural childbirth. In reality, a woman will find it extremely difficult to arrange a natural birth without any medical interference or the use of routine technology (Lawrence Beech, 1991).

The majority of Black and minority ethnic women originated from cultures where birth is a family event, taking place mainly at home. The hospital was reserved for abnormal births, sometimes from choice and sometimes because the hospitals were not available. With the exception of those Black and minority ethnic women who have been strongly influenced by the process of colonialization, or feel largely culturally British, the majority of Black and minority ethnic women would possibly choose to give birth either at home, or at the home of their parents or in-laws. Many middle-class Black and minority ethnic women have been educated under the British system. They have learnt to abandon many of the natural practices which were prevalent in their countries of birth. A proportion of those colonial educated women who have immigrated to Britain, and even some who have remained in the ex-colonies, still aspire towards Western ideals. Clearly this is a paradox, where educated White British women are seeking the type of natural childbirth which some educated Black and minority ethnic women have learnt to abandon. British-born Black and minority ethnic women would find it easier to make decisions regarding the choices between technological and natural childbirth practices if they knew the facts regarding safety and the place of birth. They are already advantaged because natural birth is part of the life experience of their foreparents, which many will have learnt from them. Many Black and minority ethnic women have hospital 'high technology' births because these have been chosen for them by the dominant culture.

Lack of choice

During the 1980s many initiatives and reports suggested that the maternity services were not meeting the needs or wishes of women, especially those of Black and minority ethnic groups (Ahmed and Pearson, 1985). The Association of Radical Midwives, in *The Vision* (ARM, 1986), recognized that Britain was a multicultural society and that women have diverse cultures with different needs. Publication of *The Vision* was followed swiftly by the Royal College of Midwives (RCM) booklet *Towards a Healthy Nation* which included the following statement:

> *Regional variation and the multi-ethnic nature of our society will give rise to a range of social, cultural and religious needs. A standard pattern of service is not likely to meet all these needs and a range of options will be required for different individuals and communities.*   *(RCM, 1987, p. 3)*

Despite these initiatives and pressures to develop a more considerate and sensitive maternity service, the inequalities in care persist. Statements were written but not translated into action. *The Vision* (ARM, 1986) reached a relatively small number of midwives, but the RCM has the largest membership of midwives in the UK, and therefore represents the majority of them. A copy of *Towards a Healthy Nation* was delivered to every midwife who was a member of the RCM at the time of publication; yet it does not appear to have changed midwifery practice and education. In 1991 every household received a copy of the short version of *Health of the Nation* (DoH, 1991). It gave the impression that the needs of Black people were being officially recognized and fostered the hope that many Black midwives had felt when the RCM booklet was published in 1987. Black people have, however, grown used to empty rhetoric. The evidence to date does not suggest that the hope that each new pronouncement brings, will be made concrete in policy and practice (Henley, 1979, 1980; Clarke and Clayton, 1983; McNaught, 1987; NAHA, 1988; Phoenix, 1990; Ahmad, 1993; Neile, 1995a).

Reports and policy for changing childbirth

The House of Commons Health Committee second report on the maternity services (Winterton, 1992) stated that many voices have been saying that all is not well in the maternity services and that women have needs that are not being met. The committee highlighted the dilemma that unsatisfactory care can exist despite reductions in perinatal mortality. The reduction of perinatal mortality rate remains a primary measure of excellence in maternity services and measures to reduce it paramount (Macfarlane and

Mugford, 1984; DoH, 1991; NHS, 1991). Yet figures from OPCS *Monitor* show that although perinatal mortality rates have halved in recent years, they remain unacceptably high in areas of low socioeconomic status and with large Black populations, such as Bradford. The perinatal mortality rate in England was 8.9 per thousand births, while in Bradford, perinatal mortality was 13.5 per thousand births (OPCS, 1991). More recent reports have shown overall improvements, but differentials still exist between geographic areas with large and small minority ethnic populations. When the perinatal mortality rates are compared on the basis of the mother's country of birth, vast differences can be seen (OPCS, 1995).

All three reports mentioned here have in common the fact that they recognized the association between poverty, ill-health and perinatal mortality. Although the Winterton report (Winterton, 1992) expressed concerns about families living in poverty and recommended increases in benefits to alleviate poverty, the following 3 years have witnessed decreases in benefits when measured in real economic terms. The expectations of the Short report (Short, 1980) were that increased maternity care in a hospital-based, technological environment would compensate for poverty. There was no evidence to support this expectation. Attempts to evaluate the effectiveness of more hospital-based and technological care have suggested that an increase in maternal satisfaction and a reduction in perinatal mortality and morbidity are associated with midwife-led care, in a community and non-technological environment (Campbell and Macfarlane, 1994; Tew, 1995). *Changing Childbirth* (DoH, 1993), recognized the value of greater commitment to women from midwives through better services offering more choice, continuity and control, but midwives cannot compensate for poverty and inequality. If government policy is to make an impact upon the health and welfare of Black and minority ethnic women, then the policy must be supported by adequate and long-term financial commitment.

The reports of the 1980s highlighted many areas of deficit in care and provision for Black and minority ethnic women. These have been reiterated in both the Winterton report (Winterton, 1992) and in *Changing Childbirth* (DoH, 1993). To achieve positive and lasting effects, structural and political changes are necessary through policies and positive action initiated by the state and implemented by its institutions. These changes should be directly aimed at promoting equality of opportunity and outcome for all clients. Examples are given throughout this chapter to demonstrate how the policy recommendations of *Changing Childbirth* have been weakened through inadequate resources.

THE EXPERIENCE OF BLACK AND MINORITY ETHNIC CLIENTS

Black women and women from the ethnic minorities in the UK experience inequality of access to the maternity services, with limited communication. They are unlikely to be offered the same range of choices as educated White women. Many services are inappropriate for their perceived needs, and there are no provisions for specific cultural needs that deviate from the British norm. They are often treated insensitively, and many have to cope with racism. Women from a variety of ethnic backgrounds are given little information about options for pregnancy and labour and may be prescribed medication without being given any information about effects and side-effects (Durward, 1990; Parkside CHC, 1992; Neile, 1993a, 1995b).

Some women have said that the institution (including doctors and midwives) takes control of their pregnancy and denies them choice, particularly during labour (Kitzenger, 1983; Flint and Poulengeris, 1987; Lawrence Beech, 1991). These women say that health professionals often neglect to inform them of their rights and choices, especially if the woman's expectations are culturally different.

Inequality of access

Black women are distinctive by their colour and make visible targets for racial discrimination in the maternity services. Equality of opportunity in the maternity services can only be realized when all women have equal access to services that are appropriate and adequate to meet their varying individual needs. Part of the ethos of the Health Service since its establishment in 1948 is equality of access, meaning the same services for everyone, everywhere, but the established 'usual policies' and 'normal' practices assume that the population is English-speaking and White, and may be totally inappropriate for most Black and minority ethnic women. At the same time midwifery claims to offer planned individualized care. This poses a dilemma for most midwives who are entrenched in the medical model of care, because they cannot treat everyone alike and at the same time differently to satisfy individualized needs. Black women do not use the maternity services as early and as much as White women because of their experiences of insensitivity, stereotyping, discrimination and racism within the NHS (Larbie, 1985; NAHA, 1988; Phoenix, 1990; Clarke and Clayton, 1983; Parsons et al, 1993; CRE, 1994; Barj, 1995).

The uptake of services is influenced by many factors such as convenience, social relevance, acceptability and previous experience. These criteria, though laudable, are defined by the same middle-class senior professionals who designed and deliver the maternity services, and not from the norms and expectations of minority ethnic groups.

Accessibility in geographic terms will have different meanings to a woman who is well-off with her own means of transport, or easy access to public transport. It will have a different meaning to any poor woman, or to a minority ethnic woman who wears traditional dress and is likely to be singled out on her journey to the maternity clinic for ridicule and abuse. She may very well face further abuse on arrival at the maternity clinic.

A middle-class White woman with her own mode of transport will not be inconvenienced by having to travel a few miles to the nearest antenatal clinic for her maternity care. A lower social class woman on benefits will find it difficult, but for an unemployed Black woman who is unaware of her right to claim benefits it may be impossible to attend. A service is only socially relevant if it caters for the perceived needs of the population that is using it. A minority ethnic woman may not attend an antenatal clinic if she has learnt that the information and advice will conflict with her cultural norms. A service will be unacceptable to a woman whose previous experience was negative. As Weller, speaking of the NHS, said:

> *This service remains essentially geared to the attitudes, priorities and expectations of the majority population, which is considered White, middle class and nominally Christian.*   (Weller, 1991)

Access is meaningless where communication is poor, as it is only by having clear information about what is available that women can try to seek access. Women who speak English as a first language are often poorly informed about the availability of – and their rights to – the full range of maternity services. The problem is worse for those whose English is poor or non-existent. They are even more greatly disadvantaged; to them choice is meaningless, unless the language barrier is broken down. It is not the inability of a woman to speak English that denies her information, but the attitudes and behaviour of midwives, policy-makers and others who have a responsibility to deliver an equitable service. Bhaat and Dickinson (1992) showed that many maternity units are lagging behind in the provision of information in appropriate languages, and that as a result many minority ethnic women who qualify for benefits continue in poverty as they are unaware of their eligibility. The use of advocates or interpreters would ideally give these women access to information, but this facility is as yet not widely available. Although not all minority ethnic women are literate in their first language, where an interpreter is not provided, the availability of leaflets in a range of languages would at least enable access to those women who are literate.

For the majority of women, the general practitioner will be the first point of contact in pregnancy, as many women will see the doctor for confirmation of pregnancy. However, many Black women experience difficulties registering with a GP (Balarajan et al, 1989). They are often told that the GP's list is full, without being given any suggestion of the alternatives that are available. They could be given the list of GPs showing who is qualified to give obstetric care, or be advised to seek the help of the community health council (CHC). A study in Leicester showed that more Asian women were likely to be registered with GPs who were not on the approved obstetric list, which demonstrates that they have the requisite training and qualifications to give obstetric care in general practice. Access to competent professionals will to a great extent influence the quality of care that women receive. Lumb et al (1981) showed that 64% of Asian mothers in Bradford had less than 4 months of antenatal care compared with 20% of non-Asian mothers. In Leicester only 64% of Asian women had over 5 months supervised antenatal care, compared with 80% of British-born non-Asian mothers (Clarke and Clayton, 1983). Women who are dissatisfied with the maternity services often vote with their feet.

Efforts are being made to improve access by some UK maternity services. Bradford, for example, has responded specifically to the needs of its diverse community by setting up a mobile maternity service to increase access to Asian and other isolated communities. This has so far been a great success. However, this initiative was funded by a Department of Health *Changing Childbirth* grant. This grant of £12 000 had to be won through competition, and while it provided for setting up and launching the service, its maintenance in the long term will be dependent upon the support of the health-care trust. The grant was insufficient to buy a bus, which would have been ideal for the project. The midwives managed to hire a share in an old multiuse bus from the Community Trust. Women who would traditionally default antenatal care would arrive at the bus for services including booking, parenting education, and antenatal and postnatal support. Not only did the women use the bus for maternity care, but the communities used it for health education and advice. Jan Eubank, one of the midwives involved with the scheme, expressed the disappointment of the midwives in having to tell the women that they could no longer provide the service, as the bus was unexpectedly withdrawn towards the end of 1995 (J. Eubank, 1996, personal communication). The midwives had put a lot of 'time, effort and hard work' into setting up the scheme, it was 'running well then it was taken away. We are trying hard to find new funding' to continue a service from which midwives gained a high level of job satisfaction and from which Black women had greatly benefited.

This situation should not occur, given the rhetoric of *Changing Childbirth.*

Stereotyping

The definition of stereotyping, derived from Allport (1954), is that of making inaccurate judgments about each individual in a whole group based upon the supposed character-istics of that group. Many ideas abound about the characteristics of Black women. These perceptions are held by individuals, and more disturbingly, are institutionalized into the structures of organizations and systems. Black women in the health services are generally labelled as 'at risk' and problematic. They give birth effortlessly, yet are demanding, thick, smelly, and when things go wrong they do so because Black women are unco-operative. None of these accusations is substantiated by evidence (Clarke and Clayton, 1983; Larbie, 1985; Bowler, 1993; Neile, 1993a).

It has become fashionable in the UK for women to have their partners present at the birth, but some Black and minority ethnic women are averse to having men present when they give birth. In many of their cultures childbirth is traditionally the women's affair. Both the women and their husbands have often felt pressured into having the husband present at the birth. Alibhai (1988) interviewed a young Turkish woman who took her sister to support her through birth, and was alarmed at the assumptions which were made about her husband. Midwives further generalized about other Turkish men. Unfortu-nately, midwives remain ignorant to the subsequent detrimental effects (such as marital difficulties) of their behaviour upon the marriages and lives of many clients. Michel Odent (1985) was one of the early pioneers to encourage husbands to support and share the experience of birth with their partners. He has more recently come to the conclusion that men are a hindrance to labouring women. They often try to impose their will upon the woman and sometimes slow down the progress of labour by increasing the woman's level of stress. For this reason Odent (1991) now suggests that men should be kept away from the birth. What many labouring women need is a 'good midwife'. Many European men have themselves complained of this modern pressure and have expressed their feelings of guilt and helplessness at watching their wives in pain. Some have reported periods of impotence following the birth owing to their fear of putting their wives through further gruelling birthing experiences.

Black women at risk?

The risk scoring system used by obstetricians and midwives to assess the likelihood of a woman developing an obstetric problem with the need for consultant care often includes 'race' (usually meaning Black), as a criterion. This social construction of Black women as being at risk can be associated with an oversimplification of perinatal and maternal mortality in the British Black populations (Radical Statistics Health Group, 1987; Phoenix, 1990; Parsons et al, 1993). Macfarlane (1986) demonstrated the higher mortality rates amongst women from the 'New Commonwealth' published in successive reports in the Confidential Enquiries into Maternal Deaths in the 1970s. Further, and more comprehensive, studies of mortality amongst Black women in the 1980s showed that maternal mortality was lower for women of the Indian subcontinent than for women from Africa and the New Commonwealth (Marmot et al, 1984). Although there is a narrowing of the gap between mortality rates amongst women who were born in the 'New Commonwealth' and those born in the UK, the likelihood of childbirth-related death is still greater for women from Africa and the Caribbean (Radical Statistics Health Group, 1987; OPCS, 1995).

Once labelled 'at risk', women are likely to be exposed to more obstetric intervention, not because clinicians have found anything wrong in their pregnancies, but 'just in case'. This label will effectively deny them the rights and choices that are available to other women and will take away any control they might have had over the events and outcomes of their pregnancies. It is by now well established that more antenatal care does not necessarily mean better care, and that more care for women who do not need it is at best a waste of time, and more dangerously can lead to more intervention (Clement et al, 1996). More intervention for Black women can mean a greater likelihood of death.

Black women are at greater risk of being anaesthetized because of their increased exposure to obstetric interventions. Under anaesthesia the risk increases, as many midwives cannot differentiate between Black women's normal colouring and their colouring when they are cyanosed or pale. Removing the 'at risk' label should reduce the rate of interventions to Black women. Greater vigilance in observing those who of necessity are anaesthetized should help to reduce mortality and morbidity. An increase in the availability of Black medical and midwifery staff in areas of high Black populations should also help, as they should be more likely to recognize cyanosis and pallor in other Black people. An increase in Black staff could also help to increase the acuity of White colleagues, who as they work alongside healthy Black people, if they have an interest in doing so, may become more likely to recognize deviations from the norm.

It has been established that there is a relationship between low birthweights and perinatal morbidity. Black women tend to have smaller babies than white women; however, it is incorrect to conclude that babies born to Black women are more likely to suffer greater rates of perinatal morbidity because of their lower birthweights. The evidence suggests that lower birthweight babies born to Black women may have better survival rates than babies of equivalent weights born to White women (Institute of Medicine, 1985).

The usual response to high mortality and morbidity rates is to provide more of the same care that has previously failed, then blame the victims for poor uptake. What Black women need is more sensitive care, and the knowledge that they will be made to feel welcomed by midwives and clinicians, to increase their trust and reduce the fear of having to confront racism in their maternity care.

Chinese women

The Chinese are the third largest minority ethnic group in the UK, after those from the West Indies and the Indian subcontinent. The Chinese population in the UK was assessed at 157 000 in the 1991 census (OPCS, 1993). This population is expected to increase owing to large-scale immigration from Hong Kong into Britain, as a result of the transfer to Chinese rule.

There is so little written about the needs of Chinese women that they may be the forgotten minority in the maternity services. There are very few studies that focus on their general health needs (Fong and Watt, 1994). The following statement summarizes their position:

> *We are not a vocal community... we have not made demands on scarce resources therefore we are not looked upon as a problem. But there are problems and our problems are no different from anyone else's; it is just because we are from a different cultural group and we have a certain cultural identity, they must be recognized within this.*   (*House of Commons Home Affairs Committee, 1985*)

A study of Chinese mothers in Hull (Neile, 1995b) showed that they face similar problems to other minority ethnic groups: difficulties with communication, poor access, lack of choice, and assumptions made by others about their needs and expectations. In the absence of clear communication, many procedures are carried out without informed consent.

Less than 15% of the Chinese population in Hull were estimated to be proficient in English. Chinese men achieve greater proficiency in English than women but they would not traditionally participate in maternity activities nor attend the birth. Relatives and close female friends would traditionally fulfil this role. It is also necessary for midwives to be flexible in their expectations regarding who supports the woman in labour rather than to expect her to adapt to what is considered normal by the dominant culture. Where a named midwife is caring for a Chinese woman, she will need to assess their ability to communicate and make arrangements to enhance communication prior to and during labour.

Many Chinese women tend to adhere to the principles of traditional Chinese medicine (humoral medicine), the basis of which is the maintenance of physical and psychological harmony and balance. Good health is dependent upon the accumulation of energy or vital life force called *qi* as well as the balance of 'cold' (*yin*) and 'hot' (*yang*), which are polar elements in the body (Koo, 1984; Reid, 1987; Tham, 1994). Food is categorized by its 'cold' or 'hot' properties and balance is maintained by eating the right foods (Anderson, 1987; Reid, 1987; Tham, 1994). The foods are categorized according to their physical properties and the environment in which they are grown, so that ice water is 'cold', and foods grown in ponds or damp soil are cold. 'Hot' foods are spicy hot, cooked by high temperatures and are usually high in energy content.

The system generally works well, with two exceptions, one of which is during pregnancy (Anderson, 1987). Pregnancy is defined as a 'hot' state, and many nutritious foods which are 'hot' such as red meats, eggs and fish are withheld to prevent the fetus from 'overheating' and growing too big, leading to a difficult delivery. There is no typical Chinese diet, as people tend to eat what is available in the provinces from which they derived. Many food taboos surround pregnancy and childbirth, and some Chinese women will not eat cold or uncooked foods after they have given birth and will only have hot drinks including water. Where communication is difficult, it may be necessary to use an advocate or interpreter who shares her language and cultural understanding to aid the midwife to enquire about what the Chinese woman is eating, and to work out an acceptable and balanced diet with her, if necessary (Neile, 1995b).

It may be best to avoid using the woman's husband as an interpreter, as research suggests that Chinese women are uncertain whether their husbands interpret everything that is said by the midwife. The results of a continuing study at the University of Hull should provide an evidence base for the future planning and development of policy and services to this community. However, in the meantime it is necessary to address the

---

Box 6.2   UK legislation affecting travellers

Section 80 of the Criminal Justice and Public Order Act 1994 repealed the Caravan Sites Act 1968, and local authorities no longer have a duty to provide sites for gypsies, and no longer receive central grants to cover the cost of acquisition and site construction. Sections 77–79 confer powers on local authorities to make directions to remove unauthorized campers from the land.

---

maternity needs of Chinese women by improving communication, giving them more information to allow greater access to services. Midwives need to be non-judgmental and non-discriminatory in their approach when dealing with Chinese mothers.

Travellers

Travelling women are routinely evicted from unofficial caravan sites during pregnancy, childbirth and the early postnatal period (Box 6.2). Eviction exacerbates the already segmented maternity care which they receive, owing to the inadequate provision of suitable official caravan sites (Neile, 1993b).

The 'Safe Childbirth for Travellers' campaign demonstrated that prior to the Criminal Justice and Public Order Act 1994, traveller mothers experienced great difficulty in achieving equity in maternity services and care. The Criminal Justice and Public Order Act 1994 is likely to increase the number of situations where traveller families are moved on while mothers are in the middle of their maternity care, and where babies are left behind in special and intensive care units. Even dedicated midwives who strive to provide an equitable service for travellers are facing a greater challenge to provide just adequate care for families who have no security of stability in encampment. Furthermore, it is likely that many midwives are totally ignorant of the plight of travellers and are likely to share the views of those who see them as a strain on the system rather than as women with equal rights to satisfactory maternity services and care. The case of the travellers demonstrates the subtle yet powerful differences between government policy and legislation. These conflicts suggest that traveller women and their families will be deprived of choice, continuity and control in childbirth.

THE WAY FORWARD

This chapter has so far established that practising midwives lack the knowledge and willingness to fulfil the needs of clients. Midwifery needs a dynamic programme of education to begin to address the deficit in knowledge of issues of race and culture which exists in the profession. It cannot be assumed that students entering midwifery education will bring with them any multicultural knowledge from their previous education.

Research on the present position

No evidence of a multicultural curriculum content in midwifery education in 1991–1993 was found by a survey (Neile, 1993a) investigating how much midwifery education in

England had been permeated by issues of race and culture. A 10% sample of the midwifery education population was randomly selected for the research. Six semistructured interviews were carried out, and 126 questionnaires were sent to midwife teachers with a return rate of 77% (97). A further 318 questionnaires were sent to student midwives and midwives who had qualified within the previous year, with a return rate of 77% (245). Many midwifery education institutions were merging with nursing schools, swiftly followed by further mergers with universities, at the time of the research. These mergers led to the closure of some schools of midwifery which had agreed to participate in the study. Questionnaires sent to institutions that had closed were returned uncompleted. Again due to the mergers, a few questionnaires were completed by nurse teachers and maternity care nurses, and those were not used in the analysis. In the end 62 questionnaires from midwife teachers (49% of those issued) were suitable for analysis, and 150 from students and newly qualified midwives (47% of those issued).

The research questions were as follows:

1. How much preparation had midwife teachers themselves had to enable them to teach about issues of race and culture?
2. What curricular provision is made for the teaching of issues of race and culture in institutions providing midwifery education?
3. What learning do midwife teachers facilitate about race and culture?
4. What multicultural knowledge have student midwives learnt during their programmes of education?
5. What do student midwives think that they should learn about race and culture?

The knowledge of midwife teachers

Approved midwife teachers were chosen as interview subjects as they were traditionally the heads of midwifery education, and powerfully influenced the curriculum development and implementation process. Four of the six interviewed had not learnt anything about race and culture in their own initial teacher training and education. Midwife teachers were similarly lacking; typical answers to questions regarding how much they had learnt were 'not at all' and 'hardly at all'.

The majority (approximately 60%) of midwife teachers had not acquired any multicultural knowledge over the last 10 years. Only 22.6% (14) of the remaining 40% of teachers had currency of knowledge, that is knowledge gained in the last year.

A small minority who had been initiated through people of vision, or because they had lived abroad, had studied issues of race and culture to postgraduate levels. These few teachers demonstrated that they were continuously learning and teaching.

Midwife teachers experienced difficulties persuading their managers to second them to courses on multiculturalism, therefore not surprisingly those teachers who acquired any knowledge explained, as it was expressed by one, that it was 'progressive, self-taught and sought'. Seven per cent had spent more than a day, 24.2% (15) less than a day and the remaining 67.7% had not spent any time on updating their multicultural knowledge over the last 10 years.

Issues of race and culture in the curriculum

The midwifery curriculum does not reflect the multiracial nature of British society. The comparative study showed that teachers were more likely than students to be optimistic

Table 6.1 Investigation of multicultural curricula.

Content	Structure	Assessment	Resources
Equal opportunity	Content explicit	Assessed/	Books
Race Relations Act	Theme	not assessed	Videos
Food	Module	How assessed	Slides and tapes
Customs	Unit	Formative	Films
Religion	Day	Summative	
Challenging racism			

about the amount of multicultural curriculum content and to say that it was explicit, but the majority of subjects (both teachers and students) stated that it was sadly lacking. Sixty-three per cent of teachers said that the multicultural curriculum content was explicit, but only 43% of the students agreed.

Students and teachers were asked about the content and structure of the multicultural curriculum, assessment and the resources that were available for teaching and learning. Some of the aspects covered by the survey are listed in Table 6.1.

Student midwives bemoaned the lack of multiculturalism in their curricula, just as their teachers had done about their initial teacher training and education curricula. The research showed that students were more likely to be taught subjects that were pathological and of a sensational nature, than those outlined. The majority of teachers who commented on what they have taught or information that they have given to colleagues, gave examples of pathological conditions such as:

> *Touched on in relation to the topic under discussion, e.g. appropriate insulins for diabetics with specific beliefs.*

> *Organized a study day for the students next month for the Sickle Cell Association.*

It is absolutely necessary and good practice to teach these pathological subjects, but it is only the tip of the iceberg. Midwives need a broad understanding of both the cultural and political issues relating to race and culture. Looking at pathological issues in isolation may reinforce stereotypes or diminish the importance of the subject. It would appear that even the multicultural subjects that are covered are either not taught in sufficient depth or not assimilated by students. This was confirmed by Dyson et al (1995) who examined midwives' knowledge of haemoglobinopathies and found that it was very limited.

Where does midwifery education go from here?

It will be necessary to plan a programme of education which is implemented from both 'bottom up' and 'top down' to meet the needs of students, managers and staff. The broad aims should be to enable midwives to:

- acquire a credible knowledge in issues of race and culture
- to promote an awareness of the covert and overt racism which exists within midwifery and society
- to develop strategies to challenge and combat racism

It will be necessary for midwives to learn about the subtle ways in which people are socialized by institutional racism, thus developing negative stereotypical and racist attitudes. The programme needs to be intensive to compensate for the many years that both general and professional education have neglected to include multiculturalism in the curriculum.

In reality, not everything that is worthwhile can be covered in 18 months or even in a 3–4 year midwifery programme, but the environment can be created that establishes the importance of the subject. The individual can then be motivated to continue to learn beyond what is directly covered in the supervised portion of their learning outcomes. Educators should aim to enable students to take responsibility for their continuing professional education and development, which is part of the accountability that every qualified midwife must accept (UKCC, 1992). If this is achieved, and coupled with the realization that issues of race and culture are as important as the rest of the curriculum, then the learning process should continue.

Qualified and managerial staff will need to attain the same minimum level of knowledge, albeit through different avenues to those open to students. Without a good knowledge base they cannot plan a good service.

An effective midwifery programme of education should enable midwives to acquire:

- knowledge of the different biological, social and psychological needs of minority ethnic women in maternity care
- knowledge of racism and its effects
- knowledge of migration
- thorough understanding of equal opportunity legislation, clients' rights and staff responsibilities under the law
- awareness of their own attitudes and prejudices and how these may affect their interactions with Black and minority ethnic clients
- insight into cultural and religious rights, foods and customs
- the ability to recognize when to use the knowledge and skills of Black and minority ethnic people as client advocates and as a resource for teaching and learning

The important aspects of all curricula feature prominently as themes, modules or units and are revisited throughout the course. There are two schools of thought regarding multiculturalism: one is that it should be identifiable as a distinct module or unit in the curriculum; the other is that it should be integrated throughout the course, with special options as well (DES, 1989; Shah, 1989).

As a specific module or unit of the course, the subject will be identifiable and will be less open to selective dismissal by those who do not appreciate its importance to good midwifery practice. There are also disadvantages; the students may apply themselves to the module then put aside the knowledge, forgetting that effectiveness in practice is the whole essence of professional education. Schon (1987) would agree that unless practitioners are able to apply theory to practice then theoretical knowledge is not achieving its primary objective. Therefore a strategy should be applied which both allows the student to focus on the subject but also to revisit it constantly. Such a programme would also allow qualified midwives to take up the module or share learning in the same programme where it is appropriate.

Who should teach and learn about race and culture?

The research showed that issues of race and culture were currently being taught mainly by midwife teachers, despite their general lack of preparation. Students, mentors, mothers/clients, social scientists and link workers contributed to teaching it in different parts of the country.

Teachers

Midwife teachers carry the responsibility for the delivery of the curriculum. It is they who thread the themes which run through the curriculum. Unless they have a good understanding of the subjects that impinge upon health and race, as well as of the politics of how the race of clients will affect their life chances and their health, issues of race and culture will not be explicit in the midwifery curriculum but will be, as one said:

> ... 'mentioned' when thought appropriate by the teacher. It is not explicit, but rather ad hoc.

Since midwife teachers are doing most of the teaching, it is essential for them to gain a sound knowledge base to enable them to teach these issues credibly.

Students

Seeing a deficit in their education, some students chose to do seminars and special projects on race. Some of these students were themselves of minority ethnic backgrounds (e.g. Jewish), or had worked or studied abroad, or were finding it challenging to deal with the minority ethnic population in the clinical area where they were working. Some students were learning from their mistakes, but this should not happen as it could be damaging both to the students and the clients. The statement quoted below typifies many similar comments made by students:

> I knew nothing about what young Black or Asian women's lives were like when I did a community placement at ... and this information was sorely missed.

Qualified staff

Mentors are teaching students about race and culture but the students did not express great confidence in their knowledge. The following quote, including her learning outcome, from one of the students discussing her end of placement assessment, suggests that it is with good reason:

> '1. The student should be able to discuss ethical issues relating to midwifery practice.'
> My mentor insisted that 'ethical' has the same meaning as 'ethnic' and because I cared for an Indian lady I was capable of achieving this outcome!

In November 1995, I questioned 54 midwives from all over the UK, who were on a Royal College of Midwives refresher course, about their equal opportunity policies. All 54 knew that their NHS trusts had policies, but only five had read them. Equal opportunity policies are worthless unless staff have read them and have been given training on the meaning and implementation of equality of opportunity. Staff who recognize that there is a deficit in their knowledge should also take the responsibility to ask for education and training.

Managers

The recently published results of the Policy Studies Institute (PSI, 1995) survey of 14 000 midwives and nurses in the NHS confirm previous findings that not only were managers not taking responsibility for implementing equal opportunity policies but that they were condoning the negative behaviour of staff and were themselves joining in. The report reiterated that racial harassment by patients, colleagues and managers was widespread. Managers were not doing enough about these problems; racial harassment was 'accepted' as part of the job (PSI, 1995).

Antiracist education and equal opportunity training are essential for managers and teachers as it is they who have the power to hire and fire, and have a moral and statutory responsibility for the behaviour of employees under the Race Relations Act 1976:

> *An employer is liable for any discriminatory act done by an employee in the course of his or her employment even if the act was done without the employer's knowledge or consent, unless the employer took all reasonable and practicable steps to prevent discrimination.*
>
> *(Section 32, Race Relations Act 1976)*

Midwifery has inherited the hierarchical structure of the NHS, therefore it seems unlikely that managers and teachers would be willing to share learning with students in their own institutions. In large institutions there would be scope for setting up specialist workshops in an accredited study programme on equality of opportunity, health and race. The programme could be planned to permit incremental learning, allowing managers and teachers to confront issues such as challenging racism in self and others in workshops, while having time for reading, writing, reflection and presentations, between workshops. Smaller institutions could send their staff on credible courses and study days.

Making the most of people

Staff in all sectors of midwifery need to learn to look around their own environment to see who is available and how these people could benefit their institutions. Many teachers may be surprised to find that even if they live in areas with very small minority ethnic populations, there will be organizations and support networks with which they could forge mutually beneficial links.

Firstly, there are the teachers and students who are already in the system but have never been asked to contribute. Some of these will be Black, but many will be White. Students often recognize the need for such education, and some may be making the only multicultural contribution to the curriculum. Students pointed out that Black teachers were more likely to mention other cultural practices than many White ones. Some teachers and students pointed out that they had family connections, and many had lived and worked abroad. Not all of these people will necessarily be interested in, or qualified to share their knowledge and experience but there is one way of finding out; ask them:

- if they have an interest in issues of race and culture
- about their background and knowledge base
- if they are willing to share their knowledge
- if they need any help and support with preparation

It cannot be assumed that Black and minority ethnic teachers will want to teach issues of race and culture. Although a multicultural staff can make very positive contributions to changing attitudes in an institution, and are invaluable as role models for minority ethnic students (DES, 1989), they cannot replace members of the community. If Black teachers are working in an oppressive environment they can sometimes find it easier to keep quiet for fear of marginalization, or even collude with the negative attitudes of the establishment. They may also become institutionalized and lose touch with the reality of what the Black and minority ethnic community really want from midwifery.

Teachers and students were asked if they had forged links with:

- community relations councils, now called race equality councils
- race relations forums
- local authority race relations advisors
- consultative groups with Black and minority ethnic representation
- any projects funded by the equal opportunities unit in their institutions

Many of those questioned had never heard of most of the above. Less than 18% (11) of the teachers and only 4% of students had made any links. They all explained that their involvement was as a result of personal interest, and while midwifery benefited from them, were not made as a result of any initiative from their institutions.

Using and valuing people

It is not possible to provide holistic midwifery care without any consultation with the people for whom we are providing the service. Yet even today, the majority of NHS board memberships, curriculum planning teams and community health councils have no minority ethnic representation. If we are to modify cultural dominance then it is essential that Black and minority ethnic people should be involved in the planning of services, as well as in the delivery.

How to make contact with black and minority ethnic people in your area
The more specialized the topic, the more important it becomes to bring in or buy in expertise. Topics such as the Race Relations Act, equal opportunities and immigration are examples of those that demand specialist delivery. Financial remuneration is important. Establishments often take the attitude that individuals from the community will give their services free of charge, while at the same time paying exorbitant sums for practitioners who are already salaried by the NHS, to give lectures which could be done equally well by midwife teachers. Furthermore, Black and minority ethnic people's contributions are unique and should be valued as such.

Telephone your local library and ask if there is a Race Equality Council (REC) in your area. The REC will know people in the different minority ethnic communities. Get in touch with them and negotiate times and fees.

It is most useful for your institution to join the REC, and any individual association of minority ethnic people that is willing to have you. Institutions should send a representative who is both interested and non-judgmental. This provides an opportunity to be in constant dialogue with the communities, thus enhancing the learning opportunities.

Although some teachers relied greatly on the input of the few students who were from Black and minority ethnic groups, the students did not always feel good about it. At times these students are made to feel that:

- They should be experts in everything to do with all minority groups.
- They are somehow personally responsible for the misdeeds of everybody in their own racial groups.
- They have come from or belong to a strange, exotic group and are expected to fulfil all the stereotypes associated with that group. British-born minority members often feel that they have to apologise for not meeting these expectations, and sometimes for not having the knowledge of their perceived cultural background.
- It is not recognized that they may be experiencing the effects of racism within the group and or institution, therefore this issue is not dealt with. As a result, rather than feeling valued for their contribution, they may feel undervalued and their confidence may be undermined.

The following quote from one of the students suggests developing awareness. There is recognition of the loneliness and isolation experienced by some minority ethnic students and gives expression and insight into how they may feel:

> *It's been suggested to me that as a group the black students are not involved in the group by other members, and tend to form a group of their own, and that their contributions to discussions, etc., are less valued by teachers than that of others, despite on the first day a great stress on supporting each other which was included in class negotiated ground rules and the need to value ourselves, etc. I haven't noticed this ... I probably don't notice subtle racism all the time either.*

Multiracial students often have the multilingual skills which many of the students indicated were missing, and for which they suggested the use of interpreters and link workers. Black and minority ethnic students also have a vital role to play in building up the confidence of minority ethnic women who use the maternity services. As midwives they could be visual symbols of a commitment to provide equality of care through staff who can understand, culturally, linguistically, and through their shared experience of belonging to a minority in the community.

Employing and promoting Black staff

Equality of opportunity can be a visible process, that is in situations where it is practised and not just preached. If the employees in each organization recruited the same percentage of Black and minority ethnic people as were living in their vicinities to meet equal opportunity targets, then equality would be reflected. The present reality is that they are more likely to be employed in situations where it is difficult to recruit staff or in menial roles, and not on the unbiased basis of the best person for the job.

Current attitudes and recruitment practices are negatively biased against minority ethnic staff. They appear to have to surmount a series of hurdles, firstly in gaining entry and qualifications, and also after qualifying. The PSI (1995) findings support the assertions that:

- there is unfairness in the allocation of training and promotion opportunities for minority ethnic groups
- minority ethnic midwives and nurses have not advanced very far up the grading structure

There has been a steady fall in the number of Black and minority ethnic NHS nurses and midwives since the 1960s and 1970s when they comprised over 50% of the workforce. The PSI (1995) estimated that they comprised 8% in the 1990s. The last population census showed that the White majority is an ageing population while the Black and minority ethnic population is youthful. Midwifery is therefore likely to miss out if recruitment attitudes are not changed. Almost half the minority ethnic population were born in Britain and nearly three-quarters are British citizens (OPCS, 1993). It is often said that young British Black people are reluctant to apply for entry to the NHS. It is only half of the truth. On the one hand, when they look at their parents who are already working in the NHS, they are not encouraged by seeing them at the bottom of the scale. They were born in Britain with the same expectations as their White peer group, and are not prepared to put up with the racism that their parents experience. On the other hand, the evidence from the CRE (1983) research suggests that Black applicants are less than half as likely to gain entry to jobs as Whites, even in areas where there are large minority ethnic populations.

IMPLICATIONS FOR PRACTICE

Midwifery has a long way to go before it can begin to claim that Black women have control over their maternity care. This chapter suggests that for the majority of Black and minority ethnic women the promises of *Changing Childbirth* are largely meaningless. Midwives cannot give to women what they do not have themselves, i.e. power, for they are themselves disempowered by a medicalized and technological midwifery service. Furthermore, the majority of midwives do not have the specific skills which are required to empower Black and minority ethnic women.

Providing continuity of care could help midwives to begin to take control of their profession. Where the money is available, recent innovations such as caseloads and team midwifery help midwives to provide continuity of care in situations where they are freed from the constraints of a medicalized and technological environment, such as in women's homes and in midwife-led centres. In these situations midwives must take full responsibility, and operate as true practitioners; therefore they must seek to increase their knowledge and skills to meet the needs of women.

There are specific areas of knowledge and skills that are particularly relevant to fulfilling the needs of Black and minority ethnic women. Good communication is essential, and it is impossible to achieve where midwives have negative attitudes towards Black and minority ethnic clients, as the attitudes will prevent them from trying. When a woman does not speak English, communication may be enhanced by:

- use of interpreters
- use of advocates or link workers who share the woman's language
- learning a few useful phrases to help her to feel welcomed and respected
- employing more minority ethnic and midwives who are multilingual

Women cannot gain access without information and it is through good communication that this is achievable. Give women information and they are given the power to take control. They can begin to ask the right questions, of the right people, and gain access to areas from which they have previously been excluded. Clearly, midwives cannot do this alone, and much of the responsibility needs to be taken at board and managerial levels, and should be reflected in policy, funding and practice. NHS trusts need to provide secondment for equal opportunity and race-related education, and training to allow midwives to learn, reflect and implement better practice. Only individuals can change their own attitudes, through a process of education and self-examination.

REFERENCES

Adorno TW, Frenkel-Brunswick E, Levinson DJ & Sansford RN (1950) *The Authoritarian Personality.* New York: Harper & Row.

Ahmad, WIU (1993) *Race and Health in Contemporary Britain.* Buckingham: Open University Press.

Ahmed A & Pearson M (1985) *Multiracial Initiatives in Maternity Care.* London: Maternity Alliance.

Alibhai Y (1988) Maternity care: black women speak out. *New Society* April: 2–3.

Allport GW (1954) *The Nature of Prejudice.* Wokingham: Addison-Wesley.

Anderson EN (1987) Why is humoral medicine so popular? *Social Science and Medicine* **25**(4): 331–337.

[ARM] Association of Radical Midwives (1986) *The Vision.* Lancs: ARM.

Balarajan R, Raleigh VS & Yuen P (1989) Ethnic differences in general practitioner consultations. *British Medical Journal* **299**: 953–957.

Barj K (1995) Providing midwifery care in a multicultural society. *Midwifery* **3**(5): pp. 271–276.

Benzeval M, Judge K & Whitehead M (1995) *Tackling Inequalities in Health.* Kings Fund.

Bhaat A & Dickinson R (1992) Analysis of health education materials for minority communities by cultural and linguistic groups. *Health Education Journal* **51**(2): 72–77.

Bowler I (1993) 'They are not the same as us': midwives' stereotypes of South Asian descent maternity patients. *Sociology of Health and Illness* **15** (2): 156–177.

Campbell R & Macfarlane A (1994) *Where to be Born: The Debate and The Evidence.* Oxford: National Perinatal Epidemiology Unit.

Caravan Sites Act (1968) London: HMSO.

Clarke M & Clayton D (1983) Quality of maternity care provided for Asian immigrants in Leicestershire. *British Medical Journal* **286**: 621–623.

Clement S, Sikorski J, Wilson J, Das S & Smeeton N (1996) Women's satisfaction with traditional and reduced antenatal visit schedules. *Midwifery* **12**: 120–128.

Coombs G & Schondveld A (1992) *Life will Never be the Same Again.* London: Health Education Authority.

CRE (1983) *Ethnic Minority Hospital Staff.* London: CRE.

CRE (1987) *Ethnic Origins of Nurses Applying for and in Training – a Survey.* London: CRE.

CRE (1994) *A Code of Practice in Maternity Services.* London: CRE.

CRE (1996) *Roots of the Future.* London: CRE.

Criminal Justice and Public Order Act (1994) London: HMSO.

DES (1989) *Responses to Ethnic Diversity in Teacher Training.* Report by HMI. London: HMSO.

DoE (1992) *New Proposals to Curb Illegal Camping by Gypsies and Travellers.* London: DoE.

[DoH] Department of Health (1991) *The Health of the Nation.* London: DoH.

DoH Expert Maternity Group (1993) *Changing Childbirth.* London: HMSO.

Durward L (1990) *Traveller Mothers and their Babies: Who Cares for their Health?* London: Maternity Alliance.

Dyson S, Fielder A & Kirkham M (1995) *Midwives' Knowledge of Haemoglobinopathies.* Leicester: De Montfort University.

Flint C & Poulengeris P (1987) *The Know your Midwife Report.* London: Heinemann.

Fong CL & Watt IS (1994) Chinese health behaviour: breaking the barriers to better understanding. *Health Trends* **26**(1): 14–15.

Henley A (1979) *Asian Patients in Hospital and at Home.* London: Pitman Medical.

Henley A (1980) Asians in Britain: *Asian Names and Records.* London: DHSS/Kings Fund.

House of Commons Home Affairs Committee (1985) *Chinese Community in Britain.* Second report, Session 1984–1985. London: HMSO.

Institute of Medicine (1985) *Preventing Low Birth Weight.* Washington: National Academy.

Kitzinger S (1983) *The New Good Birth Guide.* Harmondsworth: Penguin.

Koo LC (1984) The use of food to treat and prevent disease in Chinese culture. *Social Science and Medicine* 18(9): 757–766.

Kwhali J (1991) Assessment Checklist for DIPSW External Assessors. In: CCTSW, *One Small Step Towards Racial Justice.* Farnborough: Midas Press.

Larbie J (1985) *Black Women and the Maternity Services.* London: Training in Health and Race.

Lawrence Beech B (1991) *Who is Having your Baby: A Health Rights Handbook.* London: Maternity Alliance.

Lawton D (1983) *Curriculum Studies and Educational Planning.* London: Hodder & Stoughton.

Lumb KM, Congdom PJ & Lealman GT (1981) A comparative review of Asian and British-born maternity patients in Bradford, 1974–78. *Journal of Epidemiology and Community Health* 35: 106–109.

Macfarlane AJ (1986) Anaesthetics – The risk for Black women. *Maternity Action* 26: 6.

Macfarlane AJ & Mugford M (1984) *Birth Counts: Statistics of Pregnancy and Childbirth,* 2 vols. London: HMSO.

Marmot MG, Adelstein AM & Bulusu L (1984) *Immigrant Mortality in England and Wales 1970–1978.* Studies on Medical and Population Subjects no. 47. London: HMSO.

McNaught A (1987) *Health Action and Ethnic Minorities.* London: National Community Health Resource and Bedford Square Press.

[NAHA] National Association of Health Authorities (1988) *Action not Words: A Strategy to Improve Health Services for Black and Minority Ethnic Groups.* Birmingham, NAHAT.

[NAHAT] National Association of Health Authorities and Trusts (1990) *Words About Action – Review of Services for Black and Minority Ethnic people.* Birmingham: NAHAT.

[NHS] National Health Service Management Executive (1991) *Priorities and Planning Guidance for the NHS for 1992/93.* Executive letter EL(91) 103. London: DoH.

Neile EE (1993a) *Investigating Midwifery Education in a Multiracial and Multicultural Society.* Thesis, University of Hull.

Neile EE (1993b) Safe childbirth for travellers: sick birth caravans. *Nursing Standards* 7(33): 49.

Neile EE (1995a) Racism: a challenge for the RCM. *Midwives* 108(1): 284.

Neile EE (1995b) The maternity needs of the Chinese community. *Nursing Times* 91(1): 34–35.

Nixon J (1985) *A Teachers' Guide to Multicultural Education.* Oxford: Blackwell.

Odent M (1985) *Entering the World.* Harmondsworth: Penguin.

Odent M (1991) *Childbirth Need – Dreams and Realities.* Guest speaker, Grimsby branch of the RCM Study Day.

OPCS (1991) *OPCS Monitor* DH3 91/2. London: HMSO.

OPCS (1993) *Social Trends.* London: HMSO.

OPCS (1995) *OPCS Monitor: Infant and Perinatal Mortality – Social and Biological Factors 1994,* DH3 95/3. London: HMSO.

Parkside CHC (1992) *Women Speak Out.* London: Parkside CHC.

Parsons L, Macfarlane J & Golding (1993) Pregnancy, birth and maternity care. In: Ahmad WIU (ed.) *'Race' and Health in Contemporary Britain.* Buckingham: Open University Press.

Phoenix HG (1990) Black women and the maternity services. In: Garcian J, Kilpatrick R, Richards M (eds) *The Politics of Maternity Care.* Oxford: Clarendon Press.

[PSI] Policy Studies Institute (1995) *Nursing in a Multiethnic NHS.* London: Policy Studies Institute.

Race Relations Act (1976) London: HMSO.

Radical Statistics Health Group (1987) *Facing the Figures: What Really is Happening to the National Health Service.* London: Radical Statistics Health Group.

Reid D (1987) *Chinese Herbal Medicine.* Hong Kong: CWF.

[RCM] Royal College of Midwives (1987) *Towards a Healthy Nation.* London: RCM.

[RCM] Royal College of Midwives (1992) *Midwifery Philosophy.* London: RCM.

Schon D (1987) *Educating the Reflective Practitioner: Toward a New Design for Teaching and Learning in the Professions.* London: Jossey Bass.

Shah S (1989) Effective permeation of gender and race issues in teacher education courses. *Gender Education* 1(3): 221–236.

Short R (1980) *Perinatal and Neonatal Mortality.* Report of the House of Commons Social Services Committee. London: HMSO.

Tew M (1995) *Safer Childbirth? A Critical History of Maternity Care.* London: Chapman & Hall.

Tham G (1994) Child bearing practices of Chinese women. In: Rice LP (ed.) *Asian Mothers, Australian Birth.* Asumed.

Townsend HER & Davidson N (1982) *Inequalities in Health.* The Black Report. Harmondsworth: Penguin.

[UKCC] United Kingdom Central Council for Nursing, Midwifery and Health Visiting (1992) *Exercising Accountability.* London: UKCC.

Weller B (1991) Nursing in a multicultural world. *Nursing Standards* 5(30): 31–32.

Winterton N (1992) *Maternity Services.* Second report of the House of Commons Health Committee. London: HMSO.

7

Midwives and debriefing

Pauleene L. Hammett

There is a growing acceptance that, to be successful, labour and delivery should not only result in a physically healthy mother and baby, but should also be as positive a psychological experience as possible. *Changing Childbirth* (DoH, 1993) identified that the woman should be the focus of maternity care, able to feel in control of what is happening to her and enabled to make informed decisions about her care, having discussed matters fully with the professionals involved. This move towards a more consumer-led type of care may provide difficulties for midwives and women during labour. Women's increased expectations of the labour experience may not be fulfilled, which can lead to psychological difficulties (Green et al, 1988). Good psychological care thus becomes even more important. Midwives do not need to be psychologists in order to provide this care; Niven wrote:

> *Good basic psychological care involves respect, compassion, reassurance, the giving of information, the provision of choice, the acknowledgement of concerns, the sharing of joys and sorrows.*
>
> *(Niven, 1992, p. 3)*

Midwives are well aware of the psychological interventions that they apply to extraordinary situations such as stillbirth or neonatal death, but may not have considered psychological interventions which could be applied to all women giving birth, for example labour debriefing. This chapter aims to increase midwives' knowledge of women's reactions to birth experiences, and to consider the subject of labour debriefing, focusing particularly on what debriefing all women may mean for midwives.

What determines whether a woman has a joyful, fulfilling experience or a frightening, disappointing one appears to depend on many variables (Crowe and von Baeyer, 1989; Kitzinger, 1992), not least of which appears to be the care given during labour by the woman's attendants, i.e. midwives, doctors and birth supporters (Oakley and Houd, 1990; Kitzinger, 1992). Women who undergo what they perceive to be traumatic birth experiences appear to be at increased risk of developing psychological stress, yet understanding why one woman is deeply troubled by her birthing experience while another is not, can be complex and difficult (Kendall-Tackett and Kaufman Kantor, 1993). If midwives were to offer a labour debriefing session to all women in their care, the feedback they receive could help to increase their knowledge of trauma-producing incidents and thus inform their practice (Hammett, 1994). Ralph and Alexander (1994) feel that by incorporating this intervention into postnatal care, psychological disorders in women occurring as a result of childbirth may be reduced. Raphael-Leff (1991) believes that it is vital for a woman to discuss the birth:

> *In order to assume her new emotional liberty, a woman feels the need to establish a bridge between her pregnant self and the mother she is becoming by talking over the labour, working through the traumatic aspects of her birth, imposing meaning on the confusion of her current maternal experiences and integrating these extraordinary happenings into her ongoing life. ... Midwives have a focal role in debriefing after the birth.*
> *(Raphael-Leff, 1991, p. 336)*

These concepts need exploration: what is 'debriefing' and do midwives feel they have a focal role in debriefing after birth? Should all women receive this intervention? How could it be achieved and what skills, knowledge and attitudes does a midwife need to undertake such a task?

DEBRIEFING

The term 'debriefing' is common military parlance, and can be defined as the 'procedure of extracting facts, comments or recommendations concerning a previous assignment or experience' (Samter et al, 1993).

Military debriefing is used in combat psychiatry as a therapeutic intervention in the treatment of soldiers traumatized by battle (Samter et al, 1993). It refers to the process of recalling events and clarifying the details of traumatic combat experiences; recalling trauma in a factual way counteracts a tendency to suppress unpleasant events, reviewing details assists the process of integration and diminishes emotional reactivity (Samter et al, 1993). The objective of this debriefing is to reduce unnecessary psychological after-effects and it is known to be an effective intervention in preventing adverse reactions which may follow traumatic events (Samter et al, 1993).

Parkinson gives a simpler definition:

> *Debriefing provides a structured method of talking through the experiences and feelings of those involved.*
> *(Parkinson, 1993, p. 141)*

The normal structure used during a debriefing interview is as follows:

- introduction and rules
- facts
- thoughts and impressions
- emotional reactions
- normalization/symptom phase
- future planning and coping/teaching
- disengagement – summing up and follow-up resources (Dyregrov, 1989)

Parkinson (1993) felt that this model should not be medical or psychiatric, but that personnel from many disciplines can be trained to use it effectively. He believes that professionals can provide great assistance by not retreating behind their roles and erecting barriers to keep people and their problems at a distance, but by:

- being there and showing that they care

- using their own professional skills and knowledge
- understanding how trauma affects people, including themselves
- developing skills of listening and responding
- being aware of the debriefing process
- having the ability to debrief themselves (Parkinson, 1993)

In relation to postnatal debriefing it is important to consider the current knowledge concerning trauma-producing events around labour.

BIRTH EXPERIENCES

Rubin (1961) described three main phases of adjustment to motherhood: the dependent phase, the dependent-independent phase and interdependent behaviour. Rubin (1961) considered the first two postnatal days to be the dependent or 'taking-in' phase, when the mother looks to others to fulfil her own needs for comfort, rest, nourishment and closeness, indicating her need for protection and nurturing – 'mothering' – so that she is herself able to 'mother'. This phase is generally a time of great excitement and most women are keen to verbalize their experience of childbirth. Focusing on the labour, analysing it and accepting the experience helps the mother to move on to the dependent-independent phase. This is usually reached 3 days after delivery when, if the mother has received adequate nurturing and protection in the dependent phase, she feels ready to reassert her independence again: the 'taking hold' phase, which lasts for several weeks as the mother cares for her baby but seeks nurturence and support for herself. The interdependent or 'letting go' phase starts as integration of the baby into the altered family is achieved. The family moves forward as a unit with interacting members, and the relationship of the parents, although changed by the advent of the child, resumes many of its previous characteristics (Rubin, 1961).

Every labour is a unique event and may differ considerably from the experience the mother expected, or from the joyful event often portrayed by the media. These divergences may lead to unanswered questions in the mother's mind; if these questions are not addressed they could adversely influence the mother's psychological adaptation to motherhood (Affonso, 1977). By devoting time to discussing the woman's experience of labour, the midwife concerned may act as one of the bridges between pregnancy and motherhood in supplying answers which help to integrate the birth experience. This will assist the mother to progress to the 'taking hold' phase and thus promote psychological well-being (Konrad, 1987).

Poor birth experiences

It is not easy to define what constitutes a poor birthing experience. A search of the literature reveals many points for consideration.

Stewart (1985) ascribed an increase in postnatal psychiatric referrals to the establishment of antenatal classes which were highly committed to natural childbirth. She found that in the first 8 years of providing a psychiatric care service for women and their families within 6 months of delivery, only 0.6% of women referred attributed their psychiatric symptoms to the birthing experience. This contrasted greatly with 14% of women referred in the 2 years following the establishment of the antenatal classes, who attributed their symptoms to their birthing experience; all had attended the classes and felt themselves failures because they had required analgesia or intervention during labour.

Great Expectations is the title of a report of a prospective study of women's expectations and experiences of childbirth. Green et al (1988) studied the emotional well-being of 825 women by using questionnaires at 30 and 36 weeks of pregnancy and about 6 weeks after delivery. Overall, they concluded that women with low expectations of childbirth had worse psychological outcomes than women with high expectations. Low emotional well-being was associated with caesarean section, inadequate information, lack of control over staff or over own body, and dissatisfaction with what happened regarding interventions. Interestingly, obstetric interventions *per se* were not related to emotional well-being, nor whether the intervention was major or minor. What mattered to the woman was that she herself perceived the intervention to be necessary – 'the right thing was done'.

Thus women may feel that they 'failed' during labour, or that the experience was not what they expected, both of which result in negative reactions. Others may describe aspects of their experiences in very strong terms, feeling 'mutilated' or 'violated'; this is the language of rape, rather than of the supposedly happy event of birth (Kitzinger, 1992).

It is known that people experience depression after major surgery, yet Levy (1987) found that health professionals did not consider this would relate to caesarean section. Indeed, the very use of the term 'section' rather than 'hysterotomy' could imply that health professionals do not always consider the operation to be 'real' abdominal surgery. The terminology may also increase women's feelings of fragmentation after delivery. Martin (1987) quoted a mother's remark:

> Somehow being referred to as a 'section' after a caesarean does not help you feel a whole person.
>
> *(Martin, 1987, p. 82)*

It is also expected that women should feel happy after a caesarean delivery because their babies are safe, and of course the vast majority of women are. What is not always acknowledged is the anger and disappointment they may feel as a result of the delivery. Focusing on the product of labour, the baby, ignores the woman's concerns about her birth experiences. The results of studies examining possible links between negative birth experiences and postnatal depression are contradictory. Oakley (1983) found that obstetric intervention was related to depression, whereas Chalmers and Chalmers (1986) did not. O'Hara et al (1984) found obstetric complications linked to postnatal depression, whereas Whiffen (1988) and O'Hara (1986) did not. Kendall-Tackett and Kaufman Kantor (1993) suggested that this diversity of findings is related to the fact that these studies focused on objective birth events rather than the woman's subjective reactions to them. They also suggest that the objective focus was used because no conceptual model of aspects of birth that create traumatic experiences exists. Kendall-Tackett and Kaufman Kantor (1993) have devised such a model to aid understanding of women's experience, based on Finkelhor's traumagenics model (Finkelhor, 1987), which was initially developed to describe reactions to child sexual abuse and has been adapted to describe birth experience. The traumagenics model is based on the standard model of post-traumatic stress disorder (PTSD), expanded to include factors of an interpersonal nature such as the relationship between the woman and the doctor or midwife, which have an importance if reactions to birth are to be fully considered.

Post-traumatic stress disorder and labour

Post traumatic stress disorder is defined as occurring when a person has experienced an event outside the range of usual human experience and one that would be markedly distressing to anyone, for example serious threat to life or physical integrity or serious threat to one's child.

(Ralph and Alexander, 1994)

The idea that extreme situations provoke extreme reactions has been described for centuries. In Shakespeare's *Henry IV* Part II, Hotspur's wife described symptoms in her husband indicative of PTSD (Scott and Stradling, 1992). The two World Wars produced terms such as 'shell-shock', 'combat exhaustion' and 'war neurosis', all synonyms for traumatic stress. However, Scott and Stradling (1992), citing studies on non-combat populations such as survivors of fire, flood and concentration camps, showed these survivors to be experiencing similar symptoms. This has led to the idea that there is a single post-trauma syndrome which can be the result of various types of severe stressors. It has been related to patients who have endured traumatic illnesses or procedures in hospitals (Williams et al, 1994), particularly where intolerable pain has been experienced (Fisch and Tadmore, 1989). It may also follow events such as rape, accidents and natural disasters. Compton (1996) suggested that if the trauma was caused by human behaviour rather than natural catastrophe, the after-effects may be more severe. Williams et al (1994) described the criteria for PTSD established by the American Psychiatric Association (Box 7.1).

Ralph and Alexander (1994) postulated that PTSD can follow childbirth. They cited Moleman et al (1992), who recognized all the symptoms of PTSD in two women following difficult labours, yet felt that the diagnosis of PTSD could not stand because the researchers did not consider childbirth to be an event outside the range of normal human experience. Ralph and Alexander (1994) disagreed, believing that even 'normal' labour may be an 'unusual' experience to some women. It can be momentous, unbearably painful and uncontrollable, and women may be in real fear for their own or their baby's life.

Niven (1992) wrote that when she had the opportunity 3–4 years later to follow up women who had participated in her research in 1986 on 'factors affecting labour pain':

I found that most of these subjects recalled their childbirth accurately and with equanimity but that 5 out of 33 respondents reported that their recall caused them anxiety and distress. Four of these five subjects were reluctant to give birth again; three had experienced nightmares or, as one put it, 'daymares' – waking ones as well as sleeping ones; and one spontaneously reported postnatal problems in sexual adjustment. These results would suggest that there are a considerable number of women who suffer from a mild form of PTSD associated with childbirth. *(Niven, 1992, p. 133)*

Tylden (1990) described PTSD in relation to six women experiencing stillbirth or early neonatal death. Symptoms included anxiety and depression with disturbed sleep and horrifying nightmares. All women ruminated about the traumatic events, and acute anxiety attacks could be provoked by simply mentioning the names of the hospital, doctor or midwife, or clinical condition experienced. Some could not stay at home alone or return to work, and their children and partners suffered from the effects of the woman's depression and emotional lability. More recently, Ballard et al (1995) discussed

---

Box 7.1   American Psychiatric Association criteria for post-traumatic stress disorder

A. The event is persistently re-experienced in at least one of the following ways:
1. Recurrent and intrusive recollections
2. Recurrent distressing dreams
3. Sudden sense of reliving the experience
4. Intense distress at exposure to events that symbolize or resemble the event

B. Persistent avoidance of stimuli linked with the trauma or numbing of responsiveness (not present before trauma), as indicated by at least three of the following:
1. Efforts to avoid thoughts or feelings associated with the trauma
2. Efforts to avoid activities or situations that arouse recollections of the trauma
3. Inability to recall an important aspect of the trauma (psychogenic amnesia)
4. Markedly diminished interest in significant activities
5. Feeling of detachment or estrangement from others
6. Restricted range of feelings
7. Sense of a foreshortened future

C. Persistent symptoms of increased arousal (not present before trauma), as indicated by at least two of the following:
1. Difficulty falling or staying asleep
2. Irritability or outbursts of anger
3. Difficulty concentrating
4. Hypervigilance
5. Exaggerated startle response
6. Physiologic reactivity upon exposure to symbols of traumatic event

D. Duration of symptoms of at least 1 month

---

the prevalence of PTSD associated with childbirth and considered the possibility that many women may live with the condition undiagnosed (Beech and Robinson, 1985).

Parkinson defined post-traumatic stress as 'the normal reactions of normal people to events which, for them, are unusual or abnormal' (Parkinson, 1993, p. 24) – an abnormal event being one that is life-threatening or extremely disturbing. The reactions he described are very similar to those indicative of PTSD: he considered that the trauma disturbs our normal life beliefs, creating confusion, disbelief, vulnerability, a loss of meaning and purpose in life, and changes in self-image or self-esteem. Parkinson (1993) believed that post-traumatic stress could be managed by a sensitive debriefing after the traumatic event, and that this procedure would prevent many more people from progressing to PTSD which requires specialized long-term treatment (Scott and Stradling, 1992).

The traumagenics model

Having established that psychological damage ranging from low emotional well-being, through postnatal depression to PTSD can result from childbirth, identifying which women will sustain psychological trauma from negative birth experiences remains a problem. Assistance in this regard may be obtained from describing the traumagenics model devised by Kendall-Tackett and Kaufman Kantor (1993) which they based on work

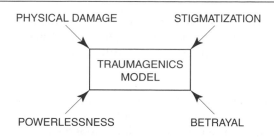

Figure 7.1 Traumagenics model of birth experiences (from Kendall-Tackett and Kaufman Kantor, 1993)

by Finkelhor (1987). They looked at the characteristics of traumatic births and identified that women may be affected by one factor or a variety of factors, and thus do not assume that trauma is caused by the same events for all women (Figure 7.1). Four main dynamics are identified: physical damage, stigmatization, betrayal and powerlessness.

Physical damage
Physical damage includes surgical incisions, e.g. episiotomy or caesarean section, and complications such as haemorrhage or infection. It is not the physical symptoms themselves that are trauma-producing, but the woman's interpretation of the injuries. If the woman feels wounded or damaged by the experience, then the physical damage is trauma-producing (Kendall-Tackett and Kaufman Kantor, 1993). Kitzinger (1975) suggested that even 'normal' body changes such as lochia, leaking breasts and flabby abdomen could result in traumatic feelings in some women. Women who undergo caesarean section may be concerned about their scars, and may also be more at risk of infection (Clement, 1992). Infection after delivery has been shown to contribute towards negative views of delivery (Tilden and Lipson, 1981). Perineal damage can be particularly trauma-inducing (Kitzinger, 1992), and many women report extreme pain from perineal sutures during the first week after delivery (Sleep, 1991). Dyspareunia is a common complication and women can feel 'ruined' even though they know that the perineum has healed (Kitzinger, 1992). Obvious reminders, such as scars and pain, can cause trauma in women by constantly reminding them of other trauma-producing events during childbirth.

Stigmatization
Finkelhor (1987) stated that stigmatization refers to the negative messages about the self experienced following trauma. Kendall-Tackett and Kaufman Kantor (1993) believed this occurs when a woman feels different from others because of some aspect of her labour experience. She may feel she is the only woman who did not have a wonderful birth experience, and if she verbalizes those concerns others may tell her she should be grateful she has a healthy baby, worth any pain or trauma. This can create isolation in that women feel they cannot share their experiences because they are not validated by others, or may upset others. She may feel that having an epidural, or pethidine, 'robbed' her of the 'real' experience of childbirth (Kitzinger, 1992). Shame and embarrassment may be felt by women if they screamed or swore, or were incontinent during labour (Konrad, 1987; Kitzinger, 1992). Others may feel embarrassed by 'strangers' seeing their most private parts, particularly if there is a multiplicity of carers during labour (Kitzinger,

1992). For some women embarrassment can become a trauma-producing event (Kendall-Tackett and Kaufman Kantor, 1993). Women who feel stigmatized need to have their responses validated and given support to cope with them (Scott and Stradling, 1992).

Betrayal
Kendall-Tackett and Kaufman Kantor (1993) considered that the dynamics of betrayal strongly affects women who had been very involved and interested in their pregnancies and had created careful birth plans, and thus developed strong ideas about the type of labour they would experience. If plans for a natural childbirth are disrupted by interventions, especially if they are not adequately explained, feelings of betrayal can result (Green, 1990; Hillan, 1992). Women can feel betrayed by their own bodies if they need an instrumental delivery (Martin, 1987), or if they develop a condition such as pre-eclampsia necessitating intervention. Perhaps even worse, women can feel betrayed by their carers, if the people the women relied on to provide care actually harm them. Kendall-Tackett and Kaufman Kantor (1993) cited Janoff-Bulman, who called this 'shattered assumptions' and commented that victims of trauma must redefine these shattered assumptions as part of the recovery process. Labouring women expect the support of staff and if sometimes they are treated roughly, rudely or with insensitivity this shatters their assumptions that 'hospitals are supposed to help people' (Kendall-Tackett and Kaufman Kantor, 1993). Further damage may occur when a woman turns to others for comfort following what to her was a trauma-producing experience: she expects to find a protective and supportive environment, yet if met with indifference or even harshness a second trauma may be produced. If told by professionals or family to 'pull herself together', the negative reactions of trusted individuals may be worse than the birth experience that originally produced the trauma (Kitzinger, 1992).

Powerlessness
Finkelhor (1987) considered the dynamics of powerlessness as having two main components: first the person's will, wishes and sense of efficacy are repeatedly overruled and frustrated; secondly, the person experiences the threat of injury or death. Feelings of powerlessness and lack of control over birth events may be one of the most important stressors leading to psychological trauma (Green et al, 1988; Green, 1990; Niven, 1992). Many publications preparing women for labour discuss the importance of power and control, as do women's accounts of their labours; yet power is what users of medical care, including women having babies, generally do not have (Oakley and Houd, 1990). Perception of control during labour is one of the most important and consistent predictors of a positive or negative birth experience (Green et al, 1988; Thune-Larsen and Misken-Pedersen, 1988). Green (1990) stated:

> *The sense of being in control, both of one's behaviour and body and of what staff were doing, was a constantly recurring theme.*   *(Green, 1990)*

Women who perceived themselves to be in control, whatever decisions were made, had higher emotional well-being scores, which increase a woman's ability to integrate her birth experience. Efforts should be made to empower women during their hospital stay, by individualizing care and avoiding the blanket use of routine procedures such as white hospital gowns, labour ward protocols and postnatal ward routines (Kendall-Tackett and Kaufman Kantor, 1993; Ball, 1995).

Powerlessness has been described as a dynamic for other victims of traumatic events. Figley (1986) found that traumatic events are troubling in that they are sudden, dangerous and overwhelming. Suddenness relates to the speed at which events happen, giving no time to prepare, devise an escape strategy or prevent the event occurring; all these can apply to women in labour, especially those who undergo caesarean section during labour (Kendall-Tackett and Kaufman Kantor, 1993).

The danger in the situations can be related to childbirth; some women undergoing emergency caesarean section in a study by Simkin (1991) perceived the situation to be life-threatening to themselves, their baby, or both. Fear of death affects all those who experience it, and can contribute to trauma (Figley, 1986).

The situation can be overwhelming, in that women can feel swept away by the labour and the hospital routines. If the woman is overwhelmed, it can lead to loss of control and a temporary helplessness. Affonso (1977) noted that some women experience the phenomenon of 'missing pieces', where they cannot remember important aspects of their labour, and found it linked to long labours with minimal information exchange between mothers and carers, or rapid labour where time to process the events was not available; in both scenarios women experienced sensory overload and were unable to process all the information, and were thus left with 'missing pieces', which may trouble them for years (Hillan, 1992; Charles and Curtis, 1994).

Before leaving the subject of trauma-producing labour events it is important to consider whether the event of caesarean section is always associated with psychological trauma. Kendall-Tackett and Kaufman Kantor (1993) concluded that negative reactions to the birth and baby are possible, and are more likely if general anaesthesia was used, a support person was lacking, or the operation was performed as an emergency. They also noted that women who received plenty of support following caesarean section, and who felt they had contributed to the decision-making process, were less likely to have a negative birth experience, proving that caesarean section *per se* is not necessarily trauma-producing. Kitzinger (1992) commented that a woman who has undergone an operative delivery may find it easier to accept feelings of disappointment and grief related to the process, because her emotions are validated by medical *facts*, which other people acknowledge.

Processing traumatic events

Horowitz (1974) described the common pattern of stress responses to a traumatic event. After the stressful event itself may come a time of denial and emotional numbing, followed by a period when women oscillate between this first response and episodes of intrusive ideas or images, attacks of emotion or compulsive behaviours, before hopefully reaching the final stage of working through the trauma, mood stabilization and acceptance of the meanings of the event (Horowitz, 1974). Denial may also explain why some women who may have been traumatized by the birth appear asymptomatic in the immediate postnatal period (Kitzinger, 1992), and an unwillingness to discuss the birth could be an indicator of problems (Konrad, 1987).

Intrusive thoughts are manifested through re-enactments of the event; these can be mental as in flashbacks or intrusive thoughts, or physical where women put themselves in positions where they can re-enact the event, i.e. become pregnant again or visit hospitals. Intrusiveness may also be characterized by hypervigilance, sleep and dream disorders, inability to concentrate on other topics, preoccupation and disorganization (Kendall-Tackett and Kaufman Kantor, 1993).

Affonso and Arizmendi (1984) noted that women having frequent and recurring thoughts about their birth experiences were less likely to adjust to motherhood smoothly. Affonso (1977) also noted that women experiencing the 'missing pieces' phenomenon have difficulty in integrating the birth experience; these women may ask people the same questions continually, experience dreams related to the birth, and be so preoccupied with the past experience that they cannot focus on the present, which can lead to poor mother–baby interaction (Ballard et al, 1995).

Parkinson (1993) suggested that there are four main tasks for midwives wishing to help women overcome trauma:

- helping women to accept the reality of their experiences and counteract the defence of denial (i.e. talk about them)
- encouraging women to feel the emotional pain and provide reassurance of the normality of their reactions (this also helps avoid denial)
- helping women adjust and adapt to the changes that have taken place
- helping women redirect their emotions (if appropriate) so they can move towards acceptance and healing

MIDWIVES' PERCEPTION OF LABOUR DEBRIEFING

The literature on negative birth experiences and debriefing provided no studies relating to midwives' views of labour debriefing. Having become interested in the subject, I undertook a research project to investigate midwives' perceptions using the qualitative research technique of focus groups (Krueger, 1994). The aims of the project were:

- to ascertain midwives' views in respect of labour debriefing: i.e. its importance or lack of it
- to identify midwives' concerns should a more 'formal' debriefing service be set up
- to plan to address identified needs and concerns should a debriefing service commence or be proposed
- to make recommendations for such a service.

The focus group discussions were tape-recorded and then transcribed; the data were analysed using the constant comparative method to identify concepts, categories and constructs (Strauss and Corbin, 1990). The questions used in the focus groups are listed in Box 7.2.

Advantages of labour debriefing

Midwives felt that almost all women want to discuss their birth experiences. This is an important aspect of motherhood, and one that should be encouraged. They considered that labour debriefing was of value both to the mother and midwife; this value being reflected by the advantages which were identified from questions 2 and 3, and are shown in Figures 7.2 and 7.3.

Midwives observed that women could experience memory loss of events in labour, for

Box 7.2 Focus group questions on debriefing

1. Do you feel women want to discuss their birth experiences?
2. What are the advantages/disadvantages of this discussion to the woman?
3. What are the advantages/disadvantages of this discussion to the midwife?
4. Who is the best person to initiate this discussion?
5. How many women (approximately) in this unit currently have a discussion about their labour?
6. Are women who experienced 'difficult' labours (e.g. caesarean section or forceps delivery) more likely to be given the opportunity?
7. Should all women be offered this opportunity?
8. Does this 'debriefing' discussion pose any concerns for the midwife?
9. If it became part of the 'routine care', how could we achieve this?
10. Do you think it should be documented anyway? If not, why not?
11. All things considered, are you in favour of offering a labour discussion opportunity to all women?

example owing to drugs or purely to the sensory overload that labour can precipitate; they were thus describing the phenomenon of 'missing pieces' and agreeing with Affonso (1977) that it was important to fill in these gaps. It was identified that sensory overload could occur in emergency situations, e.g. caesarean section during labour, thus concurring with Simkin (1991), and also during normal labour, agreeing with Charles and Curtis (1994). Midwives also felt that mothers should have any confusion dispelled, questions answered and explanations given for actions taken during the labour, even though explanations may have been given at the time – in this they were acknowledging that information is associated with positive psychological outcome, concurring with the study undertaken by Green et al (1988) which showed that women were happier about intervention if they felt 'the right thing was done'. The value to women of obtaining the truth was also highlighted, and this is certainly backed up by current research (Kirkham, 1993). Kirkham commented that the widespread medical fear of litigation can affect midwives and cause defensive attitudes, which may prevent midwives communicating

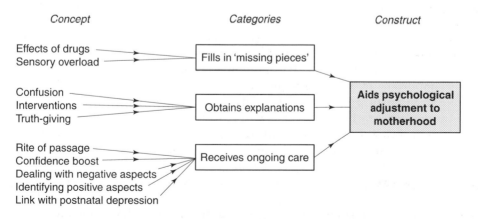

Figure 7.2 Advantages to mother of labour debriefing (Hammett, 1994)

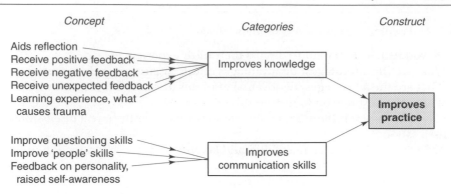

Figure 7.3   Advantages to midwife of labour debriefing (Hammett, 1994)

with women as equals. Research, however, has shown that truthful information is vital to mothers if anything has gone wrong (Jones, 1991, cited by Kirkham, 1993); truth followed by an apology is logical in the context of communication between equals, as well as being the first rule of risk management (Kent, 1991). Kirkham stated:

When defensive medicine is part of the context of our work, it is a comfort to midwives to know that legal research shows honesty is the best policy.   *(Kirkham, 1993)*

Midwives further demonstrated their awareness of women's psychological needs by identifying that childbirth is a rite of passage, and thus discussing it may aid integration (Raphael-Leff, 1991). Secondly, it was highlighted that discussing the labour can increase women's confidence in their ability to mother, and increase self-esteem which is known to decrease the likelihood of postnatal depression (Affonso and Arizmendi, 1984). Midwives were also aware of the fact that the labour experience itself has been linked with postnatal depression (Oakley, 1983; Kitzinger, 1992). Thirdly, some midwives revealed obvious counselling skills when they considered that debriefing was important so that women could begin to deal with the negative aspects and be helped to identify positive aspects of the experience.

Perhaps the most interesting reason given for its importance was that labour debriefing is a form of psychological care. Midwives felt strongly that a great deal of time was spent preparing women for the experience of labour, and thus to discuss that experience following delivery was a necessary part of postnatal care, agreeing with Ralph and Alexander (1994). The categories relating to maternal advantages of labour debriefing form the construct of 'aids psychological adjustment to motherhood' (Figure 7.2).

Midwives felt that receiving feedback, whether positive or negative or a mixture of the two, was important in improving their own knowledge. Feedback is indeed vitally important if midwives are to be able to verify their perceptions of who they really are. If there is a gap between how a midwife perceives herself and how others perceive her, confusion is likely to result. If the midwife does not seek feedback she may delude herself into an internal reality that does not match up to other people's experiences (Calvert et al, 1990). By being open to feedback, willing to examine themselves and honest with themselves, midwives will develop a greater self-awareness and thus enhance their practice.

Feedback was also important to midwives because sometimes it was unexpected, in that the midwife felt feedback would be negative but in fact it was positive, or vice versa. This type of feedback helps midwives understand women's perceptions better and creates learning experiences where trauma-producing incidents can be better identified, reflected on and handled more effectively in the future. Feedback may also contain comments related to the midwife's personality which may increase self-awareness and communication skills.

Midwives commented that debriefing women could improve their questioning skills. This is an important aspect, for if the midwife offers information and invites questions, women appreciate that communication is the midwife's aim and are likely to respond with questions. If the questions are answered clearly and quickly by the midwife the woman will feel encouraged to ask further, as the midwife's behaviour indicates that she believes the woman's knowledge and understanding to be important (Kirkham, 1993). It is important to invite questions as women may find it hard to ask questions of midwives unless encouraged (Read and Garcia, 1989); some women may find it hard to articulate what it is they want to know, and need help to identify questions (Perkins, 1991).

In talking to women about their deliveries, midwives felt they could improve their 'working with women' skills. Information gained could be used in the future to help in meeting the needs of other labouring women. Caution must be exercised here, as individualized care is very important and midwives must not use inappropriate stereotyping (Perkins, 1991).

Improved questioning and 'working with women' skills mean improved communication skills. Good communication is the cornerstone of good midwifery care and practice.

> *Communication is the vehicle by which all else is learnt and relationships are built. Communication cannot be separated from other areas of care because care is built on and of communication.*
>
> *(Kirkham, 1993, p. 2)*

Further evidence that midwives felt labour debriefing to be important was the fact that many midwives already undertook a postpartum discussion with as many as possible of the women they had delivered, usually giving up their own time to achieve this. Finally, midwives felt it to be an important aspect of the midwife's role and that all midwives should debrief women and thus gain the benefits. The categories of improved knowledge and improved communication skills lead to the construct of 'improves practice' (Figure 7.3).

Disadvantages of labour debriefing

Midwives felt there could also be disadvantages to labour debriefing (Figures 7.4 and 7.5). There was a concern that a midwife might strive less hard to give good care in labour if she felt the balance could be redressed by a labour debriefing. I believe it is more likely that some midwives do not appreciate the influence of their body language, or have failed to consider that, when reassuring an anxious woman, just saying 'Don't worry' is tantamount to saying, 'Shut up'. 'Don't worry, because...' (with an explanation) is what the woman needs (Kirkham, 1993). In many large maternity units the setting is still very medicalized and women 'patients' are expected to be passive. Kirkham (1989) showed that midwives tended to offer information to women who were unlikely to be disruptive, and withheld information from those they thought might use it to upset the smooth

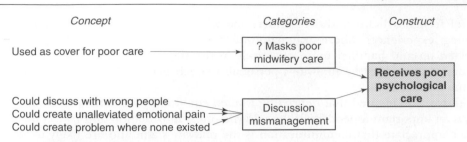

Figure 7.4 Disadvantages to mother of labour debriefing (Hammett, 1994)

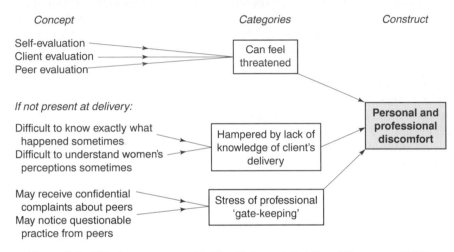

Figure 7.5 Disadvantages to midwife of labour debriefing (Hammett, 1994)

running of the ward. Kirkham does not believe that the midwives were unkind, merely that they had adapted to fit easily into a medically dominated and hierarchical system.

Another drawback voiced was that women might discuss birth experiences with people who were unable to assist them; this problem could be addressed by all women being offered an opportunity to talk to the midwife. The risk that debriefing could create unalleviated emotional pain or problems where none existed is perhaps a reflection of some midwives' anxieties about providing postnatal debriefing, when not all midwives possess the necessary skills. Failing to provide a debriefing or to develop the skills to perform the intervention effectively can also lead to the mother receiving poor psychological care, the construct cited for the disadvantages to mothers.

Concern was raised over the threats posed to some midwives from self, client and peer feedback. As Calvert et al (1990) pointed out, this may be because there seems to be some resistance in the British culture to self-understanding and awareness: many organizations do not encourage peer feedback; many individuals fear that 'feedback' is a polite word for criticism, judgment or blame. Feedback from colleagues should be constructive if points for improvement are identified and received in a supportive environment. Feedback from mothers is vital, and midwives should be aware that often women who have clearly received inadequate care express only mild criticism, or none at all, when asked to assess their satisfaction (Evans, 1987), and so if dissatisfaction is expressed, it should be taken seriously (Perkins, 1991).

It was felt that debriefing could be difficult if the midwife had not been present at delivery; this is often the case where continuity of carer schemes does not exist. A certain amount of discomfort also seems to be felt by midwives when peer assessment is mooted, whether they be in the role of assessor or assessed. It was thought that understanding a woman's perception of labour events could also be difficult if one had not been present; again leading to discomfort. Whether it provokes discomfort in the midwife or not, the only way to really understand a woman's perceptions of labour is to talk to her about them and listen carefully to her answers; that is, provide a debriefing opportunity.

Midwives were concerned about the stresses of professional gatekeeping, i.e. what would they do if they received a confidential complaint about a midwife or felt they had uncovered questionable practice. Issues of confidentiality and accountability are often difficult to deal with. With an issue of confidentiality, the midwife could discuss her dilemma with the woman, asking for permission for action, if thought necessary. Charles and Curtis (1994) writing about the 'Birth Afterthoughts' service recently set up in Winchester, said:

> We had to decide what we would do if we found evidence of bad midwifery or obstetric practice. We agreed that if we found any such incidents we should seek advice from a supervisor of midwives. Fortunately we have not found any such cases. *(Charles and Curtis, 1994)*

Accountability is a key feature of professionalism, by which a profession regulates itself and thus controls the professional activities of its members (Symon, 1994). These problems identified as disadvantages to midwives lead to the construct of 'personal and professional discomfort'.

Relationships between constructs

Four constructs were identified from the data relating to midwives' perceptions of the importance or otherwise of labour debriefing. The relationships between the constructs are explored diagrammatically in Figure 7.6.

If labour debriefing becomes the norm, then it could be postulated that some women would initially receive poor psychological care. However, some midwives adjusting to the practice of debriefing may suffer personal and professional discomfort due in part to listening to women and recognizing that the psychological care the women had received was poor; this discomfort, together with the benefits gained by the midwife from debriefing women, may lead to improved practice. This improved practice together with the benefits gained by women receiving a debriefing could aid psychological adjustment to motherhood.

Midwives' concerns related to a debriefing service

Concerns were raised regarding terminology. Resistance to the term 'debriefing' was often apparent, so I began to use the term 'post birth discussion' instead; equally, the word 'formal' was disliked and midwives expressed a desire for the discussion to be 'informal'– meaning the fact that a discussion had taken place should be recorded, not the discussion itself. Interestingly, in spite of disliking the term, midwives were keen to

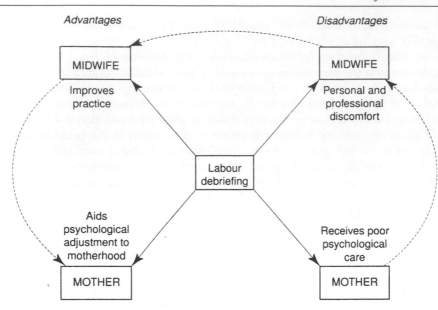

Figure 7.6 Relationships between constructs developed from data (Hammett, 1994)

develop debriefing skills, having appreciated that trauma could follow normal as well as abnormal deliveries. They were also keen to enhance and develop their communication and counselling skills and identified the need for personal support systems (Figure 7.7).

The amount of time that debriefing women might take was a concern frequently expressed; however, community midwives felt this was less of a problem, as they had more control over their time. A further issue was whether or not doctors should be involved in debriefing. This would need to be addressed through the combined obstetric and

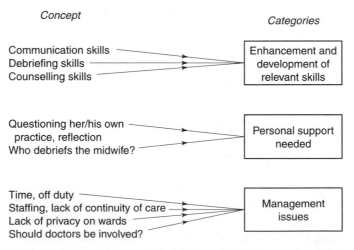

Figure 7.7 Midwives' concerns regarding a labour debriefing service (Hammett, 1994)

midwifery management team. Doctors should certainly be encouraged to consider the issue.

In the area where the data for this project was collected, major changes have occurred in the delivery of midwifery care in response to *Changing Childbirth* (DoH, 1993). Midwives now work in teams of six, each team carrying a caseload of 225 women per year. By working in small teams and visiting women wherever they are, midwives are freed from the constraints of a busy postnatal ward where they may look after 10 mothers and babies per shift, where expectations still exist that the morning shift midwives do almost all the day's work, and that sitting talking to mothers is not giving care (personal observation). Furthermore, more women are likely to be delivered at home or remain in hospital only briefly after delivery, thus the bulk of debriefing will take place in the home, allowing more privacy and partner involvement if desired. The team can provide a supportive environment to share both good and bad experiences; midwives can learn from each other, and support each other through the learning experience. The concerns raised about debriefing women one had not delivered will be reduced, as continuity of care will be greater.

Many midwives already possess the skills relevant to labour debriefing but perhaps wish to enhance them; others need to develop them – but 'training' is not always the correct approach. One midwife commented 'You can train people: it doesn't mean they improve', and Perkins (1991) wrote: 'Skills can always be further developed; the attitude that they matter is of primary importance'. Self-examination of knowledge skills and attitudes, i.e. self-awareness, is needed before the individual midwife can ascertain her personal needs in relation to debriefing. Thus, in Figure 7.8 the self-aware midwife is placed at the centre of the model, from whence she can identify her needs in relation to communication skills, support and education.

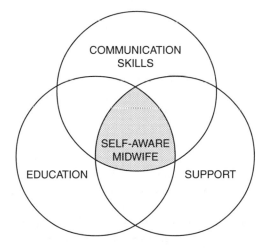

Figure 7.8 Conceptual model of midwife's needs in relation to labour debriefing (Hammett, 1994)

THE SELF-AWARE MIDWIFE

Burnard defined self-awareness as:

> *The gradual and continuous process of noticing and exploring aspects of the self, whether behavioural, psychological or physical, with the intention of developing personal and interpersonal understanding.*
>
> (Burnard, 1995)

Thus he considers that self-awareness is not pursued for its own sake, but because it is bound up with our relationships with others, and that it cannot be forced upon an individual, but actively sought by her. If the midwife is to understand the needs of women in her care, she has first to understand her own needs. Current nursing and midwifery curricula include this important subject area, and the development of good interpersonal skills is given considerable emphasis. Many midwives whose training did not include an interpersonal skills component will have excellent interpersonal skills, but it is possible that some would benefit from exploring their needs in relation to these issues. L. Jamieson and C. Hallworth (1995, personal communication) have described this difference between the 'old' midwifery training and current midwifery curricula in diagrammatic form (Figure 7.9).

Changes in nursing and midwifery curricula have occurred as a result of changes in the delivery of care: nurses and midwives are no longer expected to remain completely detached from the people in their care and have less opportunity to hide behind roles (Bond, 1986). By increasing self-awareness, midwives may explore the reasons behind their actions. I, for example, have taken years to move successfully away from the reductionist medical model of care; I am aware that vestiges of that model remain.

> *It is important to understand the dissonance that exists between the woman's experience and the culture of the medical system that defines the meaning of childbirth.*   (Kitzinger, 1992, p. 64)

It is not necessarily easy for midwives to migrate from hospital-based practice into the community; without self-awareness, they could take with themselves inappropriate aspects of hospital-based care (Cronk, 1995). Equally, midwives should consider their attitude in relation to 'control'. Midwives may well not wish there to be medical control of normal pregnancies and labours, but are they always happy to allow the mother to take all the initiative and share the available information and decision-making? Oakley and Houd (1990) considered that midwives are not trained to specialize in the interventions that remove the possibility of control from the mother, yet Kitzinger (1992) believed that interventions such as artificial rupture of the membranes, electronic fetal monitoring, enforced pushing in the second stage and episiotomy can cause feelings of trauma in women. Food for thought indeed! Thus times change and research-based knowledge grows, and so it is vital to remember that each practitioner does in good faith what that individual thinks is right at that time (Oakley and Houd, 1990).

Midwives need also to explore their own feelings in relation to the emotions a woman experiences during birth, particularly those of fear and pain. Some midwives close their minds to the experience of pain and prefer to offer the woman as much pain relief as possible, others acknowledge the pain and use their skills of distraction and support to help the woman through the labour (Oakley and Houd, 1990). Midwives may also adopt defence mechanisms to minimize the anxieties provoked by their frequent exposure to

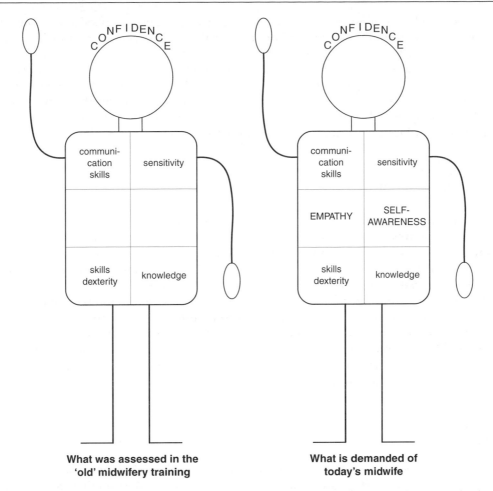

Figure 7.9 The old and the new (from L. Jamieson and C. Hallworth, personal communication)

the stress of caring for labouring women; these include denial, projection, rationalization and compensation (Oakley and Houd, 1990).

Self-awareness does not consist purely of introspection; feedback from others is also important. Self-evaluation and reflective practice are also intertwined, each complementing and enhancing the other. Reflection is often triggered by discomfort, and the midwife surprised by unexpected feedback may well alleviate the discomfort by reflecting and identifying a knowledge gap to be explored. Reflection turns experience into learning, and is therefore often not a comfortable process: it may mean living with uncertainty and keeping one's mind open to the possibility of being wrong (Burnard, 1995). Remaining open to reflection and remembering to reflect takes practice and discipline – it is sometimes easier and safer not to reflect, since we are not forced to confront the need to perhaps revise our ideas and practices (Burnard, 1995). Midwives may find it useful to keep reflective diaries (Price, 1994), although Hargreaves (1995) has questioned the ethics of using written records of interactions without the women's informed consent.

Increased self-awareness may promote empathy which can be described as the ability to imagine oneself in another's place and understand the other's feelings, desires, ideas and actions (Burnard, 1995). Empathy will assist the midwife to give non-judgmental, individualized care and is likely to lead to an increased ability to meet women's needs in relation to the birth experience. Midwives may find it much easier to demonstrate empathy 'with women' than with colleagues, managers, doctors and the institution in which they may be delivering care. For example, midwives who cope more easily with change may find it hard to empathize with those who appear to resist change.

Communication skills

Communication skills are best developed by working in small groups (Kirkham, 1993). Teams of midwives could be encouraged to incorporate 'team time' into their off-duty planning, perhaps 3 hours every week or two, when the whole team meets. This gives time for general communication and planning, and could also be an opportunity to utilize learning materials developed for small groups to aid communication skills. Kirkham (1993) cited learning materials developed by Eastcott and Farmer (1989), designed to be used over a period of time involving 12 sessions, nine of which require work-based learning to be documented between sessions and brought to the following one. I discussed the materials with one of the authors (B. Farmer, 1994, personal communication). He found that use of the materials had developed excellent group dynamics, providing a support base for group members.

Support

Niven (1992) commented that in order to provide good psychological care, midwives themselves need support. Midwives who seek self-awareness, reflect on their practice and actively seek feedback from mothers and peers need to be able to do so in a facilitative environment. No one particularly enjoys having their practice 'examined' (Oakley and Houd, 1990), and revelations that result from examining oneself and one's practice should be used positively in order to move practice forward.

Parkinson (1993) believes that 'debriefers' need to belong to a support group so that they in turn can be debriefed; for midwives working in teams, the team could form the ideal support base. Alternatively, if midwives work in pairs then the possibility of co-counselling or peer-counselling exists (Thomas, 1994). The two midwives meet for one hour; each spends half an hour as counsellor and half an hour as client. This gives an opportunity to discuss matters openly and in confidence, and may help to enhance practice and develop self-awareness in a supportive environment (Thomas, 1994).

Midwives are fortunate to have supervisors on call 24 hours a day to provide support if requested, and supervisors should be aware of a midwife's need to be 'debriefed' particularly in relation to incidents that may have caused the midwife trauma. Midwives would find it valuable to have easy access to a psychologist, to whom they could refer women causing them concern, and indeed for their own support if necessary.

Box 7.3. Suggested format for postnatal debriefing session (adapted from Dyregrov, 1989)

- Introduce yourself (if necessary)
- Issues of confidentiality
- Consider factors such as time, comfort, privacy
- Questions to ask:
  1. What did you expect to happen?
  2. What did happen?
  3. Do you understand why it happened?
  4. What were your thoughts at the time?
  5. What did you see, hear, smell, touch and taste?
  6. What was the worst about what happened?
  7. How did you react?
  8. How do you feel now?
- Normalization of feelings: it is normal to have difficult feelings about an experience as well as being happy about it
- Future:
    What other help might the woman need?
    Where does she get support from?
- Disengagement:
    Sum up and consider follow-up resources if applicable

Education

Workshops could be held to disseminate the knowledge related to the types and causes of psychological trauma related to childbirth. A psychologist could be invited to support these sessions and to facilitate understanding of the processing of traumatic incidents and the actual process of debriefing (Box 7.3). Hopefully, midwives will find this format useful in identifying women with problems who require further help. It is not anticipated that midwives will take responsibility for counselling women with PTSD or severe postnatal depression, but they may be able to identify such women early and refer them to a psychologist or full-time counsellor. The importance of encouraging mothers to talk about how they are feeling, and of listening constructively rather than making suggestions, will also be explored. Holden (1990) described the success that health visitors had in alleviating symptoms of postnatal depression by visiting depressed women weekly for 8 weeks and offering empathic listening. The health visitors had been given only a brief training in non-directive counselling, yet their visits led to twice as many women recovering compared with the control group.

CONCLUSION

Women can, and do, recover from psychological trauma; interventions to assist recovery should centre on helping women to acknowledge and accept their experiences, and on helping them regain self-esteem (Parkinson, 1993).

Midwives must be aware of the dynamics of the traumagenics model. They need to be alert for the symptoms of trauma, to teach women how trauma is processed, and support them through the process (Kendall-Tackett and Kaufman Kantor, 1993).

They have opportunities to prepare women psychologically for labour in a realistic manner, including the possibility of caesarean section. This will help to lessen the impact of unexpected events during labour, and should reduce anxiety and increase the woman's ability to take part in decision-making during labour (Elliott, 1989).

Midwives may provide emotional support during labour, and giving this support can often make the difference between a good and a bad labour experience (Oakley and Houd, 1990; Thomas, 1994). Support can be provided by communicating information, giving explanations, promoting relaxation and comfort, and keeping pain and discomfort within the woman's expectations (Niven, 1992; Kirkham, 1993).

In the immediate postnatal period, the midwife can discuss the labour with the woman, answering any questions the woman has about her labour and delivery and helping her to integrate the experience into her life. In order to debrief women the midwife needs to be self-aware, knowledgeable and able to communicate. Above all, she requires psychological support for herself, in order that her own needs which develop from being 'with woman', in this way are met.

IMPLICATIONS FOR PRACTICE

- A one-to-one debriefing opportunity should be offered to all women following delivery, preferably by the midwife who was present during labour and delivery. While it is accepted that some women do not always confront their caregivers with the truth (Evans, 1987), the use of a structured debriefing format will minimize this problem and allow feedback on practice. Parkinson (1993) believed that the debriefing should take place within 48 hours of the event and this should be borne in mind. However, for many reasons women may prefer to debrief in their own homes when the midwife visits; as many women transfer home before or around 48 hours after delivery, this should be possible.
- Women should be advised antenatally that a debriefing opportunity will be offered after delivery (Brant, 1971), and once the discussion has occurred the midwife will document this fact in the notes.
- It is strongly recommended that adequate support systems are in place, and that midwives receive adequate guidance before commencing 'formal' debriefing. If a midwife is concerned about a mother's reaction she must be able to seek guidance from peers, colleagues, or a psychologist or trained counsellor.

REFERENCES

Affonso DD (1977) 'Missing pieces'. A study of post-partum feelings. *Birth and the Family Journal* 4 (4): 159–164.
Affonso DD & Arizmendi TG (1984) Research on psychosocial factors and postpartum depression. A critique. *Birth* 11: 237–240.
Ball J (1995) *Reactions to Motherhood: The Role of Postnatal Care.* Cambridge University Press.

Ballard CG, Stanley AK & Brockington IF (1995) PTSD after childbirth. *British Journal of Psychiatry* **166**: 525–528.

Beech AB & Robinson J (1985) Nightmares following childbirth (letter). *British Journal of Psychiatry* **147**: 586.

Bond M (1986) *Stress and Self-awareness for Nurses.* London: Heinemann.

Brant M (1971) The post delivery interview. *Psychosomatic Medicine in Obstetrics and Gynaecology*, 3rd Internation Congress, London, 1971. Basel: Karger, pp. 290–292.

Burnard P (1995) *Learning Human Skills: An Experiential and Reflective Guide for Nurses,* 3rd edn. Oxford: Butterworth-Heinemann.

Calvert R, Durkin B, Grandi E & Martin K (1990) *First Find Your Hilltop.* London: Hutchinson.

Chalmers BE & Chalmers BM (1986) Postpartum depression. A revised perspective. *Journal of Psychosomatic Obstetrics and Gynaecology* **5**: 93–105.

Charles J & Curtis L (1994) Birth afterthoughts; setting up a listening service. *Midwives Chronicle* **107**: 266–268.

Clement S (1992) *The Caesarean Experience.* London: Pandora Press.

Compton J (1996) PTSD and childbirth. *British Journal of Midwifery* **4** (6): 290–293.

Cronk M (1995) Are midwives prepared for the home birth challenge? *British Journal of Midwifery* **3** (2): 105–106.

Crowe K & von Baeyer C (1989) Predictors of a positive childbirth experience. *Birth* **16** (2): 59–63.

[DoH] Department of Health (1993) *Changing Childbirth.* Report of the Expert Maternity Group. London: HMSO.

Dyregrov A (1989) Caring for helpers in disaster situations: psychological debriefing. *Disaster Management* **2** (1): 25–30.

Eastcott D & Farmer B (1989) *Communication Skills for Midwifery and Other Health Professions: Learning Methods.* Birmingham: West Midlands HA & Birmingham Polytechnic Learning Methods Unit.

Elliott SA (1989) Psychological strategies in the prevention and treatment of postnatal depression. *Baillière's Clinical Obstetrics and Gynaecology* **3** (4): 879–903.

Evans FB (1987) The Newcastle Community Care Project. In: Robinson S, Thomson AM (eds) *Midwives, Research and Childbirth*, vol 1. London: Chapman & Hall.

Figley CR (1986) Traumatic stress: the role of the family and social support system. In: Figley CR (ed.) *Trauma and its Wake*, vol. 2, pp. 39–54. New York: Bruner/Mazel.

Finkelhor D (1987) The trauma of child sexual abuse: two models. *Journal of Interpersonal Violence* **2**: 348–366.

Fisch RZ & Tadmore O (1989) Iatrogenic post-traumatic stress disorder. *Lancet* **2** (8676): 1397.

Green J (1990) Who is unhappy after childbirth? *Journal of Reproductive and Infant Psychology* **8**: 175–183.

Green J, Coupland V & Kitzinger J (1988) *'Great Expectations': A Prospective Study of Women's Expectations and Experiences of Childbirth.* Cambridge: Centre for Family Research.

Hammett P (1994) An investigation into the perceptions of midwifery practitioners on the subject of labour debriefing. BSc(Hons) thesis, University of Greenwich.

Hargreaves J (1995) Using patients: exploring the ethical dimension of reflective practice. *Nurse Education Tomorrow*, 6th Conference, Grey College. University of Durham.

Hillan E (1992) Issues in the delivery of midwifery care. *Journal of Advanced Nursing* **17**: 274–278.

Holden J (1990) Emotional problems associated with childbirth. In: Alexander J, Levy V, Roch S (eds) *Postnatal Care: A Research-based Approach.* London: Macmillan.

Horowitz M (1974) Stress response syndromes. *Archives of General Psychiatry* **31**: 768–781.

Kendall-Tackett KA & Kaufman Kantor G (1993) *Postpartum Depression: A Comprehensive Guide for Nurses.* London: Sage.

Kent P (1991) Letter to the Editor. *Health Service Journal* **101** (5244): 10.

Kirkham M (1989) Midwives and information-giving during labour. In: Robinson S, Thomson AM (eds) *Midwives, Research and Childbirth*, vol. 1. London: Chapman & Hall.

Kirkham M (1993) Communication in midwifery. In: Alexander J, Levy V, Roch S (eds) *Midwifery Practice: A Research-based Approach.* London: Macmillan.

Kitzinger S (1975) The fourth trimester? *Midwife, Health Visitor and Community Nurse* 11: 118–121.

Kitzinger S (1992) Birth and violence against women: generating hypotheses from women's accounts of unhappiness after childbirth. In: Roberts H (ed.) *Women's Health Matters* London: Routledge.

Konrad CJ (1987) Helping mothers integrate the birth experience. *Maternal and Child Nursing* 12: 268–269.

Krueger RA (1994) *Focus Groups: A Practical Guide for Applied Research.* London: Sage.

Levy V (1987) The maternity blues in postpartum and post-operative women. *British Journal of Psychiatry* 151: 368–372.

Martin E (1987) *The Woman in the Body: A Cultural Analysis of Reproduction.* Milton Keynes: Open University.

Moleman N, Van der Hart O & Van der Kolk BA (1992) The partus stress reaction: a neglected etiological factor in postpartum psychiatric disorders. *Journal of Nervous and Mental Disease* 180: 4271–4272.

Niven CA (1992) *Psychological Care for Families Before, During and After Birth.* Oxford: Butterworth-Heinemann.

O'Hara MW (1986) Social support, life events and depression during pregnancy and the puerperium. *Archives of General Psychiatry* 43: 569–573.

O'Hara MW, Neunaber DJ & Zekoski M (1984) A prospective study of postpartum depression: prevalence, course and predictive factors. *Journal of Abnormal Psychology* 93: 158–171.

Oakley A (1983) Social consequences of obstetric technology: the importance of measuring 'soft' outcomes. *Birth* 10: 99–108.

Oakley A & Houd S (1990) *Helpers in Childbirth: Midwifery Today.* WHO Regional Office for Europe. London: Hemisphere.

Parkinson F (1993) *Post-Trauma Stress.* London: Sheldon Press SPCK.

Perkins ER (1991) What do women want? Asking consumers' views. *Midwives Chronicle* 104 (1247): 347–354.

Price A (1994) Midwifery portfolios: making reflective records. *Modern Midwife* January: 35–38.

Ralph K & Alexander J (1994) Borne under stress. *Nursing Times* 90 (12): 28–30.

Raphael-Leff J (1991) *Psychological Processes of Childbearing.* London: Chapman & Hall.

Read M & Garcia J (1989) Women's views of care during pregnancy and childbirth. In: Enkin M, Keirse M, Chalmers I (eds) *Effective Care in Pregnancy and Childbirth* pp. 131–142. Oxford University Press.

Rubin R (1961) Basic maternal behaviour. *Nursing Outlook* 9: 683–686.

Samter J, Fitzgerald M, Brandaway C et al (1993) Debriefing, from military origin to therapeutic application. *Journal of Psychosocial Nursing* 31 (2): 23–27.

Scott MJ & Stradling SG (1992) *Counselling for Post Traumatic Stress Disorder.* London: Sage.

Simkin P (1991) Just another day in a woman's life? Women's long-term perceptions of their first birth experience. *Birth* 18 (4): 203–210.

Sleep J (1991) Perineal care: a series of five randomised controlled trials. In: Robinson S, Thomson AM (eds) *Midwives, Research and Childbirth*, vol 2. London: Chapman & Hall.

Stewart DE (1985) Possible relationship of postpartum psychiatric symptoms to childbirth education programmes. *Journal of Psychosomatic Obstetrics and Gynaecology* 4: 295–301.

Strauss A, Corbin J (1990) *Basics of Qualitative Research, Grounded Theory Procedures and Techniques.* London: Sage.

Symon A (1994) Midwives and litigation. 1: Accountability for midwives. *British Journal of Midwifery* 2 (3): 126–130.

Thomas P (1994) Accountable for what? New thoughts on the midwife/mother relationship. *AIMS Journal* 6 (3): 1–5.

Thune-Larsen KB & Misken-Pedersen K (1988) Childbirth experience and postpartum emotional disturbance. *Journal of Reproductive and Infant Psychology* **6**: 229–240.

Tilden VP & Lipson JG (1981) Caesarean childbirth: variables affecting psychological impact. *Western Journal of Nursing Research* **3**: 127–149.

Tylden E (1990) Post-traumatic stress disorder in obstetrics. *Fifth International Conference of the Marcé Society*, University of York.

Whiffen VE (1988) Vulnerability to postnatal depression. A prospective multivariate study. *Journal of Abnormal Psychology* **997**: 467–474.

Williams SL, Weir L & Waldmann C (1994) Post traumatic stress disorder in the ICU setting. *Care of the Critically Ill* **10** (2): 77–79.

8

Midwives coping: thinking about change

Elizabeth R. Perkins

Working for the UK National Health Service since the 1980s has been like riding a roller-coaster that accelerates. Some people enjoy fairground rides; others feel sick and wish the experience would come to an end. Both groups may become vague about the precise whereabouts of the ground. In the health service in the 1990s, there is no longer any option of avoiding the roller-coaster, or stopping it; organizational changes, professional changes and changes in practice proliferate. Maternity care is inevitably affected by the internal market and the shift to generic management, and by increasing budgetary difficulties which lead to reduced permanent staffing and an increasing reliance on agency staff to fill the gaps. Midwives have to find a way of coping.

The new climate can be seen as an opportunity to rethink practice creatively; if the service is in flux anyway, midwives can seize the opportunity to press for changes themselves. It is difficult to make a good case for the inefficient use of scarce resources, but pressure for efficiency alone, especially when exerted by managers who have no experience of midwifery practice, can pose a threat to midwifery values and client care. Rethinking practice needs to be done with a clear idea of where the professional central ground should be. It is difficult to rethink practice in the middle of a short-staffed ward; it can be easier in the short run to accept cost-cutting values and compromise – or even lose track of – one's own values.

These kinds of problems are common to many professional groups. Midwives have also been concerned for many years (e.g. Walker, 1976; Robinson, 1980, 1989) about their declining autonomy in practice, with the increasing concentration of births in hospitals, and the drift towards accepting, in practice if not in theory, a medical model of childbirth, normal only in retrospect. This is bad for morale in a profession which continues to assert the ideal of the midwife as independent practitioner, while recognizing the erosion of skills and confidence that results from the lack of opportunity to act alone. Midwives' sense of recognized value and capacity to influence their collective fate has not been improved by the arguments over the relationship between midwife and nurse education or by the clinical grading dispute.

These are changes that have been 'done to' midwives, rather than ones that they themselves have chosen. It is well established (Ford and Walsh, 1994) that it is easier to adjust to change of one's own making than to imposed change, and it is not surprising that midwives, in common with many others in the caring professions, can feel battered by the cumulative experience. However, there are also changes in midwifery practice which are midwife-led. The ideas set out in *Changing Childbirth* (DoH, 1993) (see Chapter 1) came from a convergence of the concerns of women's pressure groups about the quality of care received and the concerns of the midwifery profession about the quality of care given. Team midwifery schemes are one response to the dilution of professional skills and declining job satisfaction (see Chapters 1 and 2); the development of independent midwifery practice outside the NHS is another. Midwifery Development Units are a third type of initiative; they carry both status and a philosophy of practitioner-led change which can be set against the general experience of change in the NHS coming from the top down, and being unwelcome when it arrives. Change need not be treated as something to resist, circumvent or subvert; it could, in the right circumstances, be something to choose.

This chapter starts by looking at the costs of change, including the emotional costs which are frequently ignored by policy-makers. It explores the limited midwifery literature, which is mainly concerned with stress, before moving on to look at the experience of other professional groups, inside and outside the health service, and exploring the relevance of their solutions to midwives. A critical examination of management literature follows, focusing on its prescriptions about how to handle change and the extent to which business assumptions can be appropriately transferred to the health service in general and maternity care in particular. It finishes with a review of the more radical suggestions for innovation in large organizations, and a consideration of the implications of all these ideas for midwifery practice.

IMPLICATIONS OF CHANGE

A major omission from much of the official endorsement of change in the NHS, whether led by politicians, managers or midwives, is an explicit recognition of the cost. This includes financial cost – most new schemes these days are supposed to be implemented within existing resources. Yet new schemes require time to plan, to make mistakes in the early stages, to liaise with colleagues indirectly involved, to replan.... This time has to come from somewhere, and time costs money. Exhortations and instructions to change which ignore the reality inevitably imply either a reduction in level of service while the problems are sorted out, or an additional overload for existing staff, or both. It is not surprising that the emotional cost of change is rarely mentioned when these more straightforward costs are left out of account. Yet a failure to take these issues seriously can sink many schemes that look good on paper (Scott and Jaffe, 1990). Ford and Walsh (1994) commented on nursing behaviour as follows:

> *The reason nursing appears to resist change most of the time and yet be subject to sudden overnight changes is that they are usually imposed using the power-coercion top-down model. This gives the appearance of change taking place quickly, but in reality little has changed as people generally resent such approaches to change and largely carry on as before. The gulf that exists between NHS management and clinical nurses is such that management probably do not even realise that little change has occurred in practice.* (Ford and Walsh, 1994)

Given that most midwives were trained as nurses first, it would be surprising if midwives did not have the same weapon of passive resistance in the armoury and the same capacity to use it against imposed change, or change which causes more distress than they can handle.

The emotional costs of change

Why is change likely to be distressing? Some explanations have a built-in capacity to patronize the sufferers, or trivialize the problems they experience. An attachment to familiar routines does not weigh heavily in the balance against good patient care and efficient use of scarce resources, especially after the analysis offered by Walsh and Ford (1989) of nursing rituals, showing their limited connection with good care. Change, particularly imposed change, tends to damage the sense of control of one's work – but many people are uncomfortable with the idea of claiming control as a right, and this may be particularly true for midwives in the climate of *Changing Childbirth*, and the current slogan of 'choice, continuity and control' for women. Yet the distress caused by change is real, and should be taken seriously by all innovators, whether they are politicians, managers or practitioners. One framework which makes this easier is to see change in terms of loss (Marris, 1974).

Firstly, even if everyone agrees that the change will be for the best, the old ways were well known and had the security which goes with familiarity. They also, for professionals, represent patterns of work with patients or clients, and it can be uncomfortable to face the possibility that one's past practice was, perhaps, not the best possible. Secondly, it is often not possible to be sure that the new ways *will* be better. When change is linked to a cost-cutting exercise, and many changes in the NHS over the years have had that link present or suspected (e.g. general management, Harrison et al, 1992), it is entirely reasonable for practitioners to suspect that change will at best maintain levels of care and may worsen it. Professionals thus risk losing their sense of doing a good job for those in their care. Thirdly, change may damage the networks within which people work. It is easier to work with familiar colleagues whose strengths and weaknesses are known; this is probably particularly true for those, like midwives, whose work involves periodic emergencies. Difficulties of this type are not confined to changes in one's immediate colleagues. It can also be important to be able to ring up other departments and know that requests will be easily understood and treated with intelligence. Change can even mean the loss of the familiar enemy – the manager you love to hate, or the department that can always be blamed when things go wrong. The more rapid or more persistent the change, the greater the insecurity generated.

Loss is distressing in itself; pretending that no loss is involved in change deprives people of the right to be sad. Marris (1974) extended the idea of bereavement to cover, for example, communities' reactions to slum clearance. Robinson (1991) built on his work in an examination of resistance to Project 2000 among nurse educators (see Box 8.1). Massey (1991) used a bereavement model in his assessment of the reactions of staff of a psychiatric hospital to its closure, as did James and Dewhurst (1995) exploring difficulties experienced by staff in a new joint-agency home for frail older people. Smaller changes than these should not be overlooked; change in the caring professions has been frequent and cumulative.

One bereavement symptom is anxiety. Psychologists studying health-care professionals (e.g. Menzies, 1970; Miller, 1979; Payne and Firth-Cozens, 1987; Obholzer and Roberts, 1994) emphasize that these jobs in normal times involve more anxiety than most. Health-care workers are dealing with people in physical and emotional crises, which is distressing in itself, and they have immense power to do harm as well as to help. While midwifery is apparently one of the happier health professions, in that midwives deal with a process that is likely to produce a healthy mother, a healthy baby and a joyful family, they also know full well that things can go wrong and that their vigilance and skill is a major factor in seeing that all ends well. Parents know this too, and often confide their anxieties in their midwives. Change which causes anxiety in itself, and which threatens confidence that care will be at least as good as it was before, can only increase the emotional strain of absorbing the anxieties inherent in the job.

All this argues for a cautious attitude to change, and a recognition that it has definite non-financial costs. It is also worth bearing in mind that emotional costs to staff eventually turn into financial costs to the service, through, for example, stress-related illness, high staff turnover, poor communication and poor decision-making. There has been evidence of this in both the business world and the caring professions since the 1970s, and preventive programmes have been developed in the private sector to counter the damaging effects of stress at work on company performance (e.g. Quick and Quick, 1984; Cooper et al, 1988). A recent study of the mental health of the NHS workforce confirms the continued existence of this problem, with 26.8% of their sample identified as probable cases of minor psychiatric disorder, compared with 17.8% in the general working population. The highest scoring groups in the NHS sample were managers, nurses and doctors (Borrill et al, 1996). The production of a prevention manual for the NHS, through the Health Education Authority's Health at Work in the NHS team (OPUS, 1996) is clearly very timely; there needs to be less empty rhetoric about the value of NHS staff, and more practical concern for their welfare. For those involved in planning or implementing change, Marris offers helpful warnings:

> So whenever we impose disruptive changes on ourselves or on others, we need to allow some kind of moratorium on other business, so that people can give their minds to repairing the thread of continuity in their attachments; and we should not burden ourselves with so many simultaneous changes that our emotional resilience becomes exhausted. There is some evidence that an accumulation of personal changes, even if they are all desired, can provoke a breakdown in health. For the same reason, familiar features of the social environment may be worth preserving, even if they have no other value.
>
> *(Marris, 1974)*

Stress in midwifery

The relevant midwifery literature is concerned with stress rather than change, and stress can arise from the multiplication of familiar demands as well as from changes in their nature. Wheeler and Riding (1994) compared midwifery and nursing stress, and found that the three main sources of stress for both groups were staff shortages, excess paperwork and insufficient time to complete tasks properly. Nurses reported higher stress than midwives resulting from management, relationships and facilities. Carlisle et al (1994) found that their (hospital) midwives felt significantly less involved with their work than their nursing colleagues, and perceived themselves as receiving less support, being less autonomous, experiencing greater pressure at work, and having less clarity in their roles. Both these studies are comparatively small and more work is needed; helping midwives to develop good coping strategies will be made easier by a fuller understanding of the problems as they are perceived in the field. While feelings of overload are one of the most common stressors among health professionals (Payne and Firth-Cozens, 1987), the detailed studies show that midwives do not see their world in quite the same way as nurses. They may not use the same coping strategies either. For example, Sacker (1990) found that her sample of midwives smoked significantly less than the national average for their socioeconomic group, while the nurses smoked significantly more. The use of social support is one alternative coping strategy, and different work environments may make this easier or more difficult. For example, labour wards have busy periods and slack times in which colleagues may be able to share problems and experiences, whereas other wards may have a more even flow of work which does not facilitate group support in the same way.

The literature also includes attempts to address stress for midwives more directly, in the context of problems with the job. Mander (1994) writes sensitively on the problems raised for midwives, as well as for the families they care for, by loss and bereavement in childbearing; her book grapples with the problem of how to face up to imperfect outcomes. Santangeli (1988), a midwifery tutor, recognized the need to address the problem of 'how midwives of the future can be prepared to cope with and perform effectively in a non-ideal world'. The logic of initial client assessment using risk factors is that some will receive less care than others. She hoped that low obstetric risk would coincide with limited need for other aspects of midwifery care, such as emotional support, and suggested reclassifying women during pregnancy where this does not work. As staffing restrictions bite deeper, the hope that good care can continue to be provided in an increasingly imperfect world may seem a somewhat hollow one.

LOOKING FOR SOLUTIONS: PROFESSIONAL INSIGHTS FROM OUTSIDE MIDWIFERY

The lack of an extensive midwifery literature on change has already led us to look at the experience of other professions and at more general academic theories. While it is rarely appropriate to transfer experience wholesale, it can often be useful to realize that problems are shared.

Common ground with other caring professions

Wheeler and Riding (1994), in their small-scale study of midwives and nurses, found that both groups identified their major sources of stress as staff shortages, excess paperwork and insufficient time to complete tasks properly. Many professional groups would make similar complaints. Lipsky, an American political scientist, examined a wide range of groups, including teachers, police officers, social workers, doctors and judges, and found a number of common features in the way they saw their work problems and the way in which their managers and political masters shaped their difficulties. Despite the differences in culture, this complex study, *Street-level Bureaucracy* (Lipsky, 1980), has much to say to the caring professions in Britain today. A common feature of all his groups is the considerable discretion which all the workers have in the way they do their work – many have professional status and all have responsibility delegated to them. This is not only for the way in which they do their job with individuals, important though this is; they also have a responsibility for classes of people, where they have to balance the needs of one client against those of another. Do they do an excellent job with one, at the cost of neglecting the rest of the group, the crowded waiting room, the unsolved crimes elsewhere? Or do they spread themselves so thin that they achieve little personal contact with anyone and go home at night with a sense of failure, both personal and professional, because they are not living up to the ideals with which they started the job?

This is the dilemma Santangeli (1988) raised, and hoped could be solved by a mixture of risk assessment, flexibility and client-regulated demand. Lipsky recognized this strategy, but saw it as limited in its effectiveness and permanently liable to breakdown. Many managers of professionals are developing their equivalent of risk assessment, to routinize the process of selecting those who will receive more attention and those who will receive less, and distance the process of rejection from the professional–client relationship. In theory, this could be helpful; in practice, most individual professionals dislike it, because it limits their discretion and damages their ability to make untrammelled relationships with their clients. They therefore tend to subvert guidelines or protocols that attempt to limit care, always in the direction of providing more care not less. (It is worth noting that the flexibility Santangeli advised also seemed only to be exercised in this direction.) Overload is therefore normal; this is naturally a chronic strain on staff, who handle it in part by distancing themselves from their clients and thus reducing the personal quality of the care they give, one of the signs of 'burn-out' (Maslach, 1976; Maslach and Schaufeli, 1993).

Workers do this to conserve their own resources. They need to manage their involvement with clients, both to give themselves some control over their work, and to prevent themselves from being swamped by emotional demands they cannot meet. A midwifery example is Methven's study of booking interviews (Methven, 1989), where she found the process was dominated by the midwife's agenda, as represented by the booking form, to the detriment of discovering important health needs of many of the women interviewed. Most of these interviews were undertaken by the 'least experienced, non-permanent clinic staff'; Methven said that 'they were unsure if they would see the woman again and so deliberately tried not to get involved with her during the interview'. Lipsky's point is that this kind of process is built in to a system that runs on chronic overload, not the result of the personal failings of particular individuals. Staff act to protect themselves, and then feel guilty, since this is not what they believe they should be doing, and complain to managers that they are short-staffed and that the quality of care is suffering as a result. This may well be true – many consumer groups protesting about a variety of health, education and welfare services complain about shortage of time spent with each individual client, a lack of individual concern, and stereotyping. The lay agenda which contributed to *Changing Childbirth* is a good example of this (see Chapters 1 and 2).

Lipsky (1980) also explored the policy-makers' contribution: 'Street-level bureaucrats characteristically work in jobs with conflicting or ambiguous goals'. Midwives who have recognized their dilemma so far may feel they part company from his theory at this point, for surely there *is* a straightforward aim for midwifery practice – a happy, healthy mother and a happy, healthy baby? This may be a straightforward *professional* aim, but most midwives work for institutions and institutions have other goals as well, such as the efficient use of resources, the protection of the institution against complaint or legal action, and the collection of data to prove its virtues. Policies are made to further these goals, and staff are expected to implement them as well as to care for clients. These should not automatically be dismissed as inferior goals; John Ovretveit, an eminent management researcher and trainer, commented on the difficulty of convincing clinicians 'that efficiency is also important to caring and that inefficiency is unethical' (Ovretveit, 1996). When a scarcity of resources means that poor use of funds in one area effectively results in depriving patients in other areas, he has a point. However, efficiency must be pursued with understanding. Bed occupancy rates that suit administrators' overall targets may not be appropriate for maternity units whose flow of patients is unpredictable. Holding down permanent staffing and filling gaps by bank or agency staff may leave wards short-staffed at crucial times, since casual labour is not guaranteed to be available on demand. Complaints about the amount of time spent on paperwork are endemic. There is a tension between the needs of the institution and the needs of the client – and the needs of the worker, for the needs of the client and the needs of the worker are not identical, as we saw earlier.

How does this analysis help? To start with, it is useful to avoid unrealistic assumptions that it will all come right in the next reorganization, or when the current manager moves on. Resources are limited, and will continue to be so. Extra resources for development are only likely to become available from redistribution, either within services or between them. It is therefore desirable to avoid what Lipsky described as the natural tendency to circumvent management guidelines for appropriate care by endlessly revising them upwards in practice, and then finding that the burden is too much to carry. Instead, there needs to be dialogue between managers and practitioners, making use of research findings where available, about what can be achieved with the resources available. For example, there is already research suggesting that much antenatal care for low-risk women serves no useful purpose (e.g. Hall et al, 1980). If systems are designed to take account of this, and staff are willing to make them work because they believe that the reduced care can actually be good care, this would free resources for use elsewhere. This could involve a major change of attitude, however, since it can be difficult for professionals to believe that in certain circumstances their absence could be more beneficial than their presence. Managers can play a helpful role here, in encouraging practitioners to consider what is better – or at least acceptable – left undone.

At the same time, midwives will need to be self-protective. New systems of care should be examined to see how they handle the overload problem. Team midwifery schemes without caseloads, for example (Wraight et al, 1993) or with very high caseloads – 30–40 women per full-time midwife is recommended (Ball et al, 1995) – will simply change the labels. What is needed are approaches that will help midwives to find more acceptable compromises between the needs of clients, the needs of the institution, and their own needs for a reasonable degree of professional satisfaction and a personal life which is not mainly taken up with recovering from the work. These approaches will not emerge easily either from entrenched positions or from an uncritical acceptance of one point of view.

Lipsky's theory also has implications for the gap between theory and practice, a problem found outside nursing and midwifery but which is of particular concern to educators within these professions. Lipsky implies that this gap is inevitable – care is bound to fall short of the standards taught in training. Educators who accept this could then focus on the problem of defining 'good enough' practice (cf. Speck, 1994, on care of the dying) and on helping students to learn to live with their own and others' imperfections, while resisting tendencies to drift into unacceptable error.

Lipsky's own recommendations for changing this unsatisfactory situation are appropriately rooted in the American political context from which his theory is developed, and do not transfer easily outside it. It is interesting, however, that included in his suggestions are peer review and group caseloads, to increase the support available to practitioners and reduce the temptation to drift into bad practice which is strong for those working alone under pressure. He also commended the passing of responsibility for planning work down to practitioner level, thus capitalizing on the discretion which is part of the job. There is common ground here with team midwifery and group practice (see Chapter 1), with the encouragement of Midwifery Development Units (e.g. McGinley, 1993; Turnbull et al, 1995; Walker et al, 1995) and the promotion of reflective practice (see Chapter 7). To balance the alternative risk of groups of practitioners drifting together into unacceptable attitudes and practice, and protecting one another from outside criticism, Lipsky recommended more client involvement in planning services at street level. This has echoes in the midwifery profession's increasing willingness to work with client groups like the National Childbirth Trust, La Leche League and the Association for Improvements in the Maternity Services, rather than reject them as interfering busy-bodies who do not really understand. The genesis of *Changing Childbirth* shows that alliances between mothers and midwives can work to set out a vision which politicians and managers will share and promote, and obstetricians can accept; the document itself recommends that women should be involved in the monitoring and planning of maternity services. It could be worth exploring the potential for further co-operation in the daunting task of making the vision live.

Nursing and change

Lipsky's analysis is rational. It points up the tendency of caring professionals both to cling to and complain about their workloads, and suggests ways of easing the strain. It recognizes that this will not be easy, but it keeps the discussion of difficulties on the level of social and political obstacles – as, indeed, is reasonable for a political scientist. This level of analysis is becoming increasingly familiar in assessing the difficulties of changing health service practice; the well-publicized problems of putting research into practice make that clear:

> *The hope that if individual nurses could be educated to read research they could change their practice accordingly seems, on the basis of this study, to be simplistic. If changes in practice are warranted it is not sufficient to inform staff and leave ward sisters or qualified practice staff to be autonomously responsible for making the changes. As has been demonstrated, changing inappropriate organisational contexts and resources and negotiating with a range of other disciplines are generally beyond the capacity of any one individual.* (Hunt, 1987)

For midwives wishing to improve their coping strategies when faced with stress, overload and imposed change, and to contemplate new approaches to their work of their own devising, it may be helpful to try another way of looking at the world as well. Some of the studies of change in the health services take a psychodynamic approach, looking for the emotional reasons why apparently unreasonable and unhelpful practices persist. It is becoming increasingly obvious that it is not enough to make a rational case for change, or even to look at the social and political forces within an institution which cause some groups to have an interest in supporting a particular change and others to oppose it. One of the earliest studies that made this point was undertaken by Isabel Menzies (1970), called in to investigate problems of nurse training and retention in the 1960s. She found much concern, intelligence and sincere sympathy for the difficulties of student nurses expressed by senior nursing staff, and a complete inability to undertake any radical reform of a system which was clearly seen to be damaging to individuals and working badly for the institution. She stressed that this should not be seen as the fault of a particularly obtuse or indecisive bunch of senior staff, but as a pointer to the kind of problem under consideration:

> *Recommendations or plans for change that seem highly appropriate from a rational point of view are ignored or do not work in practice. One difficulty seems to be that they do not take sufficiently into account the common anxieties and the social defences in the institution concerned, nor provide for the therapeutic handling of the situation as change takes place... The nursing system presents these difficulties to a high degree since the anxieties are already very acute [by the nature of the work]. (Menzies, 1970)*

Working within the same tradition, but this time on a study of change on psychogeriatric wards in the 1970s, Miller (1979) showed how the problems inherent in the work – 'the insoluble problems of aging, death and bereavement' – lead to a heavy burden of dependency for nurses, and the need to be dependent in one's turn. This kind of work arouses fears of sharing the fate of those for whom one cares, and such anxieties cannot be reasoned away. Nurses use routines and authority structures to encourage a feeling of security, but this does not produce the best possible care for individuals, and thus intensifies anxiety rather than solving the problem. Miller sees the consultant as 'the linch-pin of the defensive dependency structure', absorbing anxieties from other staff. The multitude of organizational changes since Miller wrote have not necessarily been paralleled by emotional changes of the same magnitude, and consultants may still be 'carrying' much of this anxiety. Within a self-contained system, change becomes difficult to sustain; Miller recommended support from outside the system, coupled with an opening up of the system to contact with the outside world. In midwifery, the combination of greater autonomy for midwives with the crossing of boundaries between hospital and community work has striking parallels – but what kind of additional support will midwives have to handle the multiple anxieties aroused by change itself, by the increased responsibility they carry compared to the reality of much familiar hospital practice, and by the inevitable tangling of work and personal agendas?

Nurses and midwives have traditionally tried to handle this last problem by a taboo on 'getting involved with the patient'. This is now less fashionable; every patient is supposed to have a 'named' nurse or midwife, and this is intended to encourage a more personal approach to care, with greater possibility for the nurse to 'get involved'. Abolishing the taboo in theory does not abolish the problem in practice, however; Ford and Walsh (1994), in a critical review of primary nursing, commented that:

> *The danger is that unprepared nurses may go from one extreme to the other, from fragmentation and distancing the patient to enveloping and internalizing all the individual's problems. A nurse should neither have Teflon skin nor become an enormous sponge, soaking up all 'his' or 'her' patients' problems. This will create an intolerable burden for the nurse to carry.*   *(Ford and Walsh, 1994)*

Midwives face different problems from nurses, and at first sight they would seem to be at less risk; after all, midwifery is basically assisting a healthy process to produce life, not trying to resist a disease process which may result in death. However, pregnant women may have problems, and if so, they are encouraged to confide in their midwives. They may be very anxious about the well-being of the child they carry. They may have social or relationship problems which complicate their pregnancy and their hopes of a happy family life for their child. The birth of a first child is a major transition which creates anxiety even when all is well. Midwives, like other caring professionals, have to learn to leave such problems at work, and to manage their involvement with mothers intelligently. This can be hard, particularly if the client's problem has some connection with a midwife's own experience. What about midwives who have difficulty with their own childbearing? What about those who have to defer their own families, for whatever reason? Dr Wendy Savage had the courage to make this point about women obstetricians to the Winterton Committee:

> *For women the long training period before appointment to consultant position is particularly difficult to reconcile with having children or deferring childbearing while delivering other women.*
>
> *(Winterton, 1992)*

Cohn (1994), writing about her work as a psychotherapist with staff of a special care baby unit, described the difficulties experienced by a member of staff undergoing infertility treatment. Her colleagues had encouraged her to believe that being with babies would be good for her, but she was finding it increasingly distressing. She realized, with the support of the psychotherapist, that she was increasingly envious and angry, and that she would be caring for the babies as well as for herself in arranging some time off and a transfer to other work.

Special care work is recognized as being particularly stressful (Winterton, 1992; Mander, 1994) and thus particularly likely to break down carefully constructed barriers between personal life and work, but it is unlikely to be the only situation that would do this. Mander (1994) researched responses of staff as well as parents to the loss of a baby, including loss by adoption, and writes sensitively and perceptively about the range of different ways in which midwives cope with their work in this area. It is clear that staff are often unclear about what to do, dissatisfied with their practice, and hampered by mixed feelings about the propriety of 'getting involved'. Mander stressed the importance of support, from peers, from managers, and from staff support groups; support needs to be appropriate to the individual concerned, allowing space for feelings aroused by the work to be explored. Miller (1979) made the same point in the context of psychogeriatric care. The more midwives move outside routines, and dispense with the protective barriers between themselves and their clients, the more likely they are to find that the barriers between personal problems and work problems dissolve (see Chapter 5 for a discussion of this in relation to doulas). With appropriate support and personal insight, this may lead to the provision of better care, not worse – but to assume that these difficulties will not arise is naive, and likely to lead to the reimposition of routines as the only way in which staff can protect themselves.

Barriers, routines and resistance to change have a function; they protect us from problems we do not know how to face. Robinson (1991), analysing resistance to change in nurse education during the implementation of Project 2000, saw the resistance as providing time – to make the crucial links between the old order and the new, to tease out what was valuable in the old system and carry it forward to the future, 'to re-establish a sense of meaning and cohesiveness in what teachers do'. Teachers in her survey asked for time to meet together to reflect, 'abreact and exchange views and opinions' – the familiar suggestion that group support in this process can be helpful. Midwives facing wholesale change may need to do the same.

The importance of understanding

Change may bring improvements, for midwives and the women for whom they care. Alternatively, it may hold service provision at an acceptable level, but at an increasingly personal and professional cost to midwives. It may even reduce the quality of care, either through ignorance or misjudgment on the part of those who plan it or through the diversion of resources to other priority areas. Since much change comes gift-wrapped with rhetoric about providing better care with fewer resources, midwives need to examine the packages carefully. It is also important that they consider the effect that the changes will have on themselves – midwives are, after all, one of the main resources in the maternity services, and it is not good for the service if resources are allowed to deteriorate. A useful framework for this purpose has been developed by Antonovsky (1987), who reversed the pattern of much work on stress and disease by seeking to identify factors that promote health, rather than those that tend to cause illness. He suggested that individuals cope better with major trauma if they have a strong *sense of coherence*, made up of three main components:

- comprehensibility
- manageability
- meaningfulness

Individuals with a strong sense of *comprehensibility* expect that their world will be predictable – or where there are surprises, that they will be explicable and able to be ordered. Those who are strong on *manageability* tend to see events in life as challenges that can be met – they expect to have resources, either of their own or under the control of reliable others, to deal with new situations. People with a strong sense of *meaningfulness* see the demands of life as worthy of commitment and engagement. Antonovsky found that the most crucial of these three components was that of meaningfulness – people facing trauma which seemed incomprehensible or unmanageable were keen to identify explanations or resources if they believed that the challenges were important and worthy of personal commitment. Without a strong sense of meaningfulness, it could seem not worthwhile to seek and use resources to cope.

How could this be applied to change in midwifery? Midwives start with an advantage in the nature of their jobs. The case of pregnant women and the delivery of babies is readily seen as meaningful by most people. Caroline Flint (1995) suggested that a midwife delivering a women she has cared for under a group practice programme will find that the involvement will carry her through the odd sleepless night, in the same way that being in love makes it possible to do without sleep from time to time! It is interesting that Carlisle et al (1994) found midwives were less, not more, involved with their work than nurses – a finding that surprised the researchers, and which they tentatively explained as the result of the fragmented care offered in many hospitals, leading to fragmentation for the midwives as well. Team midwifery has enjoyed such a vogue because it offers the possibility of greater continuity for midwives, and thus greater involvement with their work; the implications of this and a range of models of midwifery care are discussed more fully in Chapter 1.

This is not, however, to be read as an argument for the indefinite extension of dedication to cover all manner of change, on the grounds that midwives will put up with anything for the sake of patients. Long-term personal relationships do not work for most of the time at the heady level of first love, and in the same way services should not be planned to rely for all their activities on a parallel level of commitment from their staff, even if they are willing to pull out the stops from time to time. On the contrary, midwives could use Antonovsky's approach to assess projected changes to see whether they can be expected to increase or decrease their sense of comprehensibility and manageability. These two are linked:

> *Living in a world one thinks is chaotic and unpredictable makes it most difficult to think that one can manage well.* (Antonovsky, 1987)

It is for this reason that detailed accounts of team midwifery practice, like those by Campbell and Bailey (1995), Flint (1995) and Leap (1996) are so valuable. Those who have done the job this way and survived to tell the tale have found ways of limiting its demands on their personal lives – that is, limited the extent to which their world becomes unpredictable. In the same way, midwives faced with demands for change should also make a shrewd assessment of what will happen to their resources. The most obvious resource is time – is it going to be reduced by more staff cuts or yet more paperwork? However, it is important not to neglect resources under the control of trusted others – who will help midwives as they do their daily work, and will the changes affect contact with them? For team midwifery schemes in the community, for example, one would need to look at the effects on relationships with general practitioners and health visitors. Midwives are likely to know far more about these kinds of issues than non-midwifery managers, and could raise problems before they happen, thus protecting their own welfare as well as that of others.

LOOKING FOR SOLUTIONS: INSIGHTS FROM MANAGEMENT STUDIES

Another good place to look for ideas on surviving change, or generating desirable changes, is the management literature. After all, health service managers are charged with the responsibility of taking forward the health service reforms which have generated so much change for so many people, and these were intended to inject some business efficiency into the health service. The specialist management sections of bookshops are full of books with titles like *Thriving on Chaos* (Peters, 1988) and *The Change Masters* (Kanter, 1983). 'Management of Change' courses now abound in the NHS, and simple guides to facilitating change are now found in slim volumes aimed at first-line management course students (e.g. Rumbold, 1995) and ordinary nurses (Wright, 1989). Scott and Jaffe (1990) defined the stages of change, as summarized in Box 8.1.

The simple guides and courses make use of well-established psychological theories on how groups work best, and these transfer reasonably well from one setting to another. The broader theories of management, however, are more problematic. It is important to check whether the models of organizations, of workers and management, and of policy-making, actually fit with the realities of the health service in Britain in the 1990s before applying their approaches to its current problems. This section reviews the snags in transferring various types of management theory from the business world to the public sector, and considers how far ideas from this source can safely be used there.

Box 8.1   The stages of change (Scott and Jaffe, 1990)

Scott and Jaffe (1990) see people – and teams – going through the following stages in adjusting to a change:

'• **Denial**   You are likely to see: withdrawal, 'business as usual', attention turned to the past. There is activity but not much is accomplished.
• **Resistance**   You will see: anger, blame, anxiety, depression and even a downing of tools: 'What's the difference, this company doesn't care any more'.
• **Exploration**   You will recognize: overpreparation, confusion, chaos, energy. 'Let's try this and this, and what about this...?' Lots of energy and ideas but a lack of coherence.
• **Commitment**   This occurs when employees begin working together. There is co-operation, and better co-ordination: 'How could we work on this?' Those who are committed are looking for the next challenge.'

Some move quickly, others can get stuck. There can also be shifting about between the various stages – this is not a simple progression. Scott and Jaffe offer advice to managers on how to help individuals and groups move on, for example:

'• **During resistance**   Listen, acknowledge feelings, respond empathetically, encourage support. Don't try to talk people out of their feelings, or tell them to change or pull together. If you accept their response, they will continue to tell you how they are feeling. This will help you to respond to some of the concerns.'

Managerialism in the public sector

Christopher Pollitt, a professor of public policy with experience in the civil service, has produced a sophisticated analysis of the limitations of managerialism in the public sector (Pollitt, 1993). He sees managerialism as an ideology, and this is well supported by the almost religious tone of some of the 'how to manage better' books which are found in the management sections of serious bookshops as well as in station bookstalls. They are crammed with advice on how to transform your (working) life, coupled with instructive anecdotes featuring firms, managers or workers who have done that very thing. Some of the advice may well apply anywhere – most staff would approve of a manager who took advice to 'become obsessed with listening' (Peters, 1988), particularly since Peters intends this to be applied to both staff and customers! Other facets of the approach may suit industry but be incompatible with the different constraints which apply in the public sector.

   Pollitt argues that one difficulty with managerialism as it is manifested in the public sector in Britain is its considerable debt to the ideas of F. W. Taylor. He published *The Principles of Scientific Management* in 1911, and was a pioneer of time and motion studies. His approach became enormously influential, and is still alive and well in many big organizations today. His model of the worker is set out as follows:

> *Hardly a competent workman can be found who does not devote a considerable amount of time to studying just how slowly he can work and still convince this employer that he is going at a good pace.*

> *Under our system a worker is told just what he is to do and how he is to do it. Any improvement he makes*
> *upon the orders given to him is fatal to his success.* (*F. W. Taylor, quoted by Pascale, 1991*)

Taylor's views are still important enough in modern industry to be worth attacking in management literature in the 1990s (e.g. Pascale, 1991). When Taylorite approaches are transferred to the NHS, an organization with an explicit caring ethic and a staff including large numbers of professionals and semiprofessionals who expect to control their own work processes anyway, it seems so inappropriate as to be bizarre. How did this happen?

Pollitt suggests that Taylorite managerialism fits well with the increasing political concern during the 1970s and 1980s, both in the USA and the UK, about the cost of state provision and 'bureaucracy'. It was, however, politically unacceptable to cut services. Increasing control would therefore be needed to hold down costs; there is increasing emphasis on results, performance and outcomes. The previous, deplored, condition, developed in the absence of active management. The answer to the problem was therefore seen to be managers, exercising positive control and active leadership, drawing on the assumed greater efficiency to be found in the business world. Neo-Taylorism came to the public sector. Economy, efficiency and effectiveness became the watchwords; managers were supposed to deliver these benefits. There has been much concern in the public sector about the effects of this new approach on professional practice: a useful statement of the case for care ('Love is not a marketable commodity') is found in Wilkinson (1995).

The limitations of the business model

The Griffiths report (DHSS, 1983) is a useful marker for the start of this process. It rests on a set of assumptions about the similarities between business and the public sector:

> *We have been told that the NHS is different from business in management terms, not least because the*
> *NHS is not concerned with the profit motive and must be judged by social standards which cannot be*
> *measured. These differences can be greatly exaggerated. The clear similarities between NHS manage-*
> *ment and business management are much more important.* (*DHSS, 1983*)

As Pollitt (1993) pointed out, however, this statement is highly debatable and the issue of profit is certainly not the only point of difference. One of the major difficulties is embedded in the policy-making process; public sector managers have to take far more notice of politicians than do their private sector counterparts. Politicians are reluctant to say they are cutting services, even when they do want to cut costs, and tend to be responsive to the cries of pain from particular constituents when services are demonstrably reduced. Health service managers can produce a string of large and small examples of political obstruction of their efforts to rationalize services. Reducing services in a prosperous area in order to concentrate them on a more deprived one where greater effectiveness could be expected, making lists of ineffective treatments which will no longer be available, closing clinics or hospitals in order to concentrate resources and save money – all these tend to be unpopular with constituents and generate political protest. High-level commitment to the generation of Charters also indicates politicians' ambivalence; they demand a caring and respectful service, responsive to the needs of individuals, while also wanting a tightly controlled service to ensure the efficient and economical delivery of effective services. As Lipsky (1980) pointed out, it is not possible to abolish the discretion of 'street-level bureaucrats' without wrecking their ability to deliver the kind of service required of them.

Pollitt (1993) stressed that the production of ill-defined, fuzzy policy statements is an inevitable part of the political process – the politicians' job is to contain as many different subgroups as possible within their political fold, and therefore they need to produce statements that will satisfy as many subgroups as possible. This naturally means that the statements will provide bad guides to managers trying to do something definite based on the latest policy. No wonder they have to spend so long on the latest circulars.

> *The very essence of leadership is that you have to have a vision. It's got to be a vision you articulate clearly and forcefully on every occasion. You can't blow an uncertain trumpet.*
> *(Father Theodore Hesburg, Former President, Notre Dame University, quoted in Peters, 1988)*

In the public sector it is difficult for managers to deliver this clear leadership, based on a clear vision of how the service should be, if they have to base this on a series of ambiguous policy statements written by someone else. There is scope here for finding support for one's own preferred path within the confusions of central guidelines, but this is a somewhat risky strategy and has not commended itself to all.

Another way in which the transfer of concepts from commerce to the public sector runs into trouble is concerned with the effects of demand. If you deliver a good service in business, you expect demand for it to increase. Indeed, this is one of the reasons why you are aiming to ensure the quality of your products. In the NHS, the delivery of a good service may well achieve the same results – people will come back and talk more about their problems to a midwife who has been sympathetic the first time, and this is one of the informal ways in which field staff get confirmation that they are doing a good job. On an organizational scale, it is expected that general practitioners will refer more patients to hospitals that perform better. In the commercial world, successful firms make money, take on more staff, and carry on with a glow of success. In the NHS, successful staff and institutions cannot expand; they end up with more work than they can fund. The result can be temporary ward closures as a 'reward' for good practice. The multitude of difficulties inherent in 'money following the patient' have not been solved, and may never be solved at the level of the individual field worker.

In business, it is good practice to identify a sector of the market and specialize (e.g. Ohmae, 1982; Peters, 1988). Sir Roy Griffiths said:

> *No company would ever get itself into the position of the health service of trying to be all things to all men and to be increasingly expected to meet every possible demand.* (quoted in Pollitt, 1993)

Certainly, niche markets could be identified in midwifery: how about a maternity unit aiming to provide the best possible care for highly educated middle-class women, ignoring the needs of others? Certainly it would be easier to do a good job with a tightly defined group of clients; facilities, appointments and information could be tailor-made to suit. But, as Pollitt points out, the NHS is obliged by public statute to provide a 'comprehensive' service, and specialized units catering only for a segment of the population can be justified in terms of clinical need, but not market advantage. Furthermore, this is seen as a fundamental principle of the NHS, and there are outcries over suggestions that fund-holding general practitioners may be rejecting patients with complex and expensive treatment needs.

In short, treating the NHS like a business with a few odd quirks is inappropriate – the differences are major and need to be taken seriously. This means that the case for neo-Taylorism needs to be made afresh (and will not, it should be clear, be made by me!) and that other ideas from the world of commerce and industry should be treated with reserve. Their appeal may dissolve on inspection.

Radical approaches to change

One major theme in the literature of business management is coping with change. Unstable economic conditions and rapid technological change have made the business world uncomfortably aware that stability is not an option – it is only a recipe for failure. Handy (1991) argued that change is now happening so fast that we are now facing a new kind of change, where looking for continuity with the past is pointless – radical, discontinuous change. Taylorite approaches are useless here; to cope with it, the gurus recommend:

- openness to change as learning (Handy, 1991); the learning organization
- managers should balance reduced stability in the wider environment with stability of the purpose of the work – 'vision, values and stability based on trust' (Peters, 1988)
- organizational flexibility, with small, autonomous work groups; reducing the permanent staff and using agency workers or short-term contract staff (Handy, 1991)

These ideas, and the way in which they are presented, can look much more appealing than neo-Taylorite management control. However, caution is still needed in transferring them to the NHS. The work of Marris (1974), briefly discussed above, suggested that it is pointless to try to dispense with continuity, but rooting a sense of continuity in values rather than institutional forms sounds a promising strategy for professionals. It may be necessary, however, for them to do much of this themselves through their own professional bodies; we have seen in the previous section how difficult it is in the health service for managers to deliver a clear vision. Midwives will need to find their own ways of maintaining the principles of good midwifery in a world of change.

This may combine well with the second suggestion, for more autonomous work groups. Autonomy needs defining in practice, for it can mean many different things – what level of decision-making is the group responsible for? Midwifery Development Units, group practice and team midwifery (see Chapters 1 and 2) all fit this kind of approach, and one of the spurs to team midwifery has been the de-skilling of midwives trained to be autonomous practitioners but working under medical supervision (Robinson, 1989). The transition is not easy, but there are enthusiasts who have survived to share their enthusiasm with others (e.g. Page, 1995). Managing autonomous work groups is not easy either; Peters, a dedicated exponent of 'really letting go', tells a rueful story of a project he was managing when he had a severe car accident which put him out of action for two or three months, and left his team to cope:

> *Rather than behave decently (as I would have put it then) and cancel the numerous engagement that I had booked, every single activity had been taken on by a team member. And while, a decade later, I still harbour the suspicion that I might have done any one activity 2 per cent better than they, the reality is that a dozen people caught fire – all at once.* (Peters, 1988)

The development of autonomous work groups, furthermore, is directly opposed to the neo-Taylorite philosophy which has seeped into the health service through political pressure for cost controls and identifiable outcomes. They will not be simple to achieve.

Autonomy gives scope for innovation, although it does not guarantee it. Michael West, professor of work and organizational psychology, has studied innovations in a range of health service settings; he found innovation was common among health visitors, one of the more autonomous nursing groups in the health service (West, 1989). The types of innovations included change in objectives, changes in working methods, changes in relationships, new skills, new visiting practices, professional liaison, and new clerical practices. Social support and good leadership relationships were, as predicted, related to high levels of innovation; so, to West's surprise, was high workload. He suggested that either professionals may innovate because they have high workloads, as a coping strategy, or that innovation attempts lead to higher workloads. West and Wallace (1991) examined team innovativeness in primary health care teams; their work suggested that the innovativeness of teams was not strongly associated with individual characteristics or tendency to innovate. Instead, they found that:

> *Innovative teams tend to legitimate controlled experimentation, be tolerant of a diversity of approaches and support the initiation and development of ideas... furthermore, innovation is associated with high levels of team commitment – i.e. a desire to maintain membership, a belief in and acceptance of the values and goals of the team and a willingness to exert effort for the team. The results also suggest that open communication, information sharing, mutual trust and a tendency to resolve conflict by group consensus are characteristic of innovative teams.* (West and Wallace, 1991)

Autonomous work groups are the acceptable, indeed the exciting, face of organizational flexibility. The other side is represented by cuts in the permanent workforce, and increasing reliance on part-time and agency staff. Women can be short-term beneficiaries of any development that encourages institutions to develop more flexible employment patterns, since conventional full-time jobs rarely combine easily with child care. This trend does, however, need watching; will the non-permanent workforce be appropriately valued? There are obvious issues around pay, and less obvious ones around the provision and design of training, and the value placed on non-standard experience for promotion (Davies, 1990). Patient care, as well as professional development, will be affected by the way in which these issues are handled.

The idea that change is best seen as an opportunity to learn something new, and to be changed thereby, represents the optimist's view of the excitement of change, and is none the worse for that (Handy, 1991). Most people who have chosen to be involved in a process of developmental change will remember the excitement and the learning as well as the stress involved. Efforts to extend this approach beyond the individual or small group to the vision of a 'learning organization' take rather more effort to maintain. Bennett and Ferlie (1994), reviewing the literature in the light of their own research on HIV and AIDS, characterized the NHS as a 'forgetting organization'. If transfer of learning from one area to another is difficult in the NHS, as their work suggests, why might this be?

Organizational cultures

The NHS is a very large organization. Within it there are many different organizational cultures, defined by Charles Handy as:

Different sets of assumptions about the basis of power and influence, about what motivates people, how they think and learn, how things can be changed. These assumptions result in quite different styles of management, structures, procedures and reward systems. Each will work well in certain situations... Different cultures... are needed for different tasks. Cultures, too will need to change over time, as the tasks change, as the organisation grows, or as people change. Much of the trouble in organisations comes from the attempt to go on doing things as they used to be done, from a reluctance to change the culture when it needs to be changed. (Handy, 1995)

Cultures are well established and resistant to change; it is a mistake to expect rapid change to result from official fiat or the leadership of a new and dynamically different leader (Pollitt, 1993). Some may be better at learning than others. There are many different approaches to cultural analysis (see Hampden-Turner, 1994, for an introduction). One which may be useful to midwives is that of Handy (1993, 1995), who built on the work of Harrison (1972) to develop a typology of organizational cultures which can be used to explain the differences between occupational groups and the various difficulties they have with change (Box 8.2).

Many people see the NHS as a whole as bureaucratic, a role culture where paperwork and procedure take precedence over creativity. Most, if not all, organizations have bureaucratic elements, and Handy, like other theorists discussed earlier, sees a crisis developing for big organizations which will force them to change in the direction of smaller, more flexible, more autonomous work groups. Midwives could be seen as a subgroup within the wider organization, but in fact they themselves are divided; wards vary, both in their tasks (labour wards need to differ in culture from antenatal clinics or postnatal wards) and in the personalities of senior staff. Community midwives will have a different culture from hospital midwives, and team midwives crossing hospital and community boundaries may be different again. It can be helpful to work out which culture you work in and how suitable it is for you personally; Handy (1995) provides a questionnaire for this purpose. It can also be useful for teams experiencing problems with change to do this as a group; the questions themselves can promote discussion of buried issues, and the group responses may explain a number of difficulties which had been obscure before (Perkins and Lovelock, 1996).

One of these difficulties, which Nursing and Midwifery Development Units may find familiar, can be the relationship between a small, innovative work group and the wider organization where there are different attitudes to change in general or to the changes the small group wishes to pursue. Maintaining links is crucial for the protection of innovation but may be difficult to achieve in practice (Towell and Harries, 1979; Boyd et al, 1995). If the NHS as a whole is, as Bennett and Ferlie (1994) suggested, a 'forgetting' organization, it becomes even more important for those who want to manage change to share strategies with other innovative teams. This will help staff to maintain morale, share reasons for successes and failures, and recognize that their difficulties are not unique. The Nursing and Midwifery Development Unit network has experience of the value of this; it could be sensible for those engaged in developing team midwifery or group practice to consider a similar approach.

Box 8.2   Organizational cultures (Handy, 1993, 1995)

Handy makes it clear that no organization, not even a subgroup, will fit one pure type; all are mixtures with one or two dominant features. He lists four cultural types:

- power culture
- role culture
- task culture
- person culture

Power culture is found in small organizations or subgroups centred on a charismatic leader. This leader makes all the decisions and recruits staff who are personally congenial; the group depends on trust and empathy for its effectiveness and it is important that subordinates should be able to work out what the boss would like done if they cannot ask for instructions. Organizations like this work well when they are small; they can move fast in pursuit of opportunities or when under threat. They start to falter when they get too big to run on personal relationships and need systems instead; their natural employees ignore or subvert systems as a time-wasting drag on their initiative. They also decline when the boss loses his or her touch – 'a web without a spider has no strength' (Handy, 1993).

Role culture is based on rules and procedures. The role is often more important than the person who fills it; individuals are chosen because they can do a particular job to specification, not with the expectation that they will exercise initiative and develop a new approach. They offer security, the opportunity to develop specific expertise, and a well-defined career structure to an individual prepared to conform. Role cultures work well if work and responsibilities are allocated rationally, and if the environment in which they operate stays reasonably stable. In crisis they are slow to see the need for change, and slow to respond even when the need is identified.

Task cultures are oriented towards particular tasks. They operate in shifting groups, bringing in some people and releasing others according to the needs of a particular job. Leadership, similarly, shifts according to the needs of the task. They are very flexible and creative, but have little capacity to maintain their innovations – workers tend to prefer to move on to the next challenge. Although they value expertise, the shifting nature of the task tends to limit the depth to which this can be developed. They have problems in times of limited resources, since they respond badly to competition, which wrecks the co-operative work culture, or to management control, which is viewed as a threat to creativity.

Person cultures are centred on individuals. They tend to be professional firms or subgroups of professionals within a wider organization. They see organization as there to serve the development of the work of that individual, and having no purpose beyond this – the staff of a solicitor's office is one example from outside the health service.

IMPLICATIONS FOR MIDWIFERY PRACTICE

Change is happening anyway, and will continue to happen. Midwives need strategies to protect themselves from the damage that ill-managed change can cause, and may wish to support changes of their own devising. There are no completely reliable prescriptions from the literature reviewed here, but a number of ideas emerge which can be developed by midwives themselves.

- Threads of continuity between past and future are important; midwives should retain their own vision, and not allow it to be obscured by others' new enthusiasms. For example, the ideals of continuity of care and carer promulgated in *Changing Childbirth* (see Chapters 1 and 2) were not invented by the Expert Maternity Group which prepared the report, or even by the Winterton Committee (Winterton, 1992) whose deliberations inspired it; community midwives have been offering a more limited form of continuity for years. Valuing the past need not be done in opposition to the present; if Marris (1974) is right, it is a way of supporting the present and thus building the future more effectively.
- Limited resources are a reality faced by midwives and managers alike. There needs to be a dialogue about how change can be implemented without simply asking staff to work harder, a strategy that will not work in the long term or even the medium term. This will mean deciding what aspects of present practice should be reduced or abandoned, as well as what should be developed or enhanced.
- It is necessary, when working within an institution, to recognize organizational demands. However, these should not be treated as having unlimited authority – both because they should be balanced with concern for patients and staff, and because they are liable to change as government policies change. The old saying can be updated: 'Never run after a man, a bus or a management idea – there'll be another one along soon!'
- Theories from other disciplines should be taken with several pinches of salt; midwives should treat them critically, make use of what fits their situation, and develop their own approaches.
- Change is likely to be less damaging if you are involved with it, rather than a passive victim. Midwives should not therefore be put off generating their own changes by the side-effects of those that have been imposed on them. Furthermore, some of the changes brought forward by midwives, like team midwifery and group practice (see Chapters 1 and 2), debriefing, reflective practice and self-awareness (see Chapters 7 and 9), and the policies set out in *Changing Childbirth*, fit well with ideas that have emerged from several different sources in this chapter. Small, autonomous, supportive work groups, balanced by the importance of listening to clients, and possibly involving them in planning, will sound familiar and desirable to many midwives.

Change can be exciting. It can offer real possibilities of better care and more professional satisfaction to midwives and the women for whom they care. However, it does not come free. Those who wish to push it forward should plan to avoid casualties, and this means accepting that staff as well as patients have needs – for support, for time to reflect, and for scope to have some control over what is happening to them.

REFERENCES

Antonovsky A (1987) *Unravelling the Mystery of Health: How People Manage Stress and Stay Well.* San Francisco: Jossey-Bass.

Ball JA, Garvey M, Jackson-Baker A, Flint C & Page L (1995) Who's left holding the baby? Meeting the challenge of the Winterton report. In: Page L (ed.) *Effective Group Practice in Midwifery: Working with Women.* Oxford: Blackwell Scientific.

Bennett C & Ferlie E (1994) *Managing Crisis and Change in Health Care.* Buckingham: Open University Press.

Borrill CS, Wall TD, West MA et al (1996) *Mental Health of the Workforce in NHS Trusts,* Phase 1 final report. Sheffield University Institute of Work Psychology.

Boyd M, Marley L & Perkins ER (1995) *Poverty and Health Needs: How Can Health Visiting Respond?* Nottingham Community Health Trust, Strelley Nursing Development Unit.

Campbell M & Bailey V (1995) Seeking effective practice: the work of the clinical leader. In: Page L (ed.) *Effective Group Practice in Midwifery: Working with Women.* Oxford: Blackwell Scientific.

Carlisle C, Baker GA, Riley M & Dewey M (1994) Stress in midwifery: a comparison between midwives and nurses using the Work Environment Scale. *British Journal of Nursing Studies* **31**(1): 13–22.

Cohn N (1994) Attending to emotional issues on a special care baby unit. In: Obholzer A, Roberts VZ (eds) *The Unconscious at Work: Individual and Organisational Stress in the Human Services.* London: Routledge.

Cooper CL, Cooper RD & Eaker LH (1988) *Living with Stress.* Harmondsworth: Penguin.

Davies C (1990) *The Collapse of the Conventional Career; the Future of Work and its Relevance for Post-Registration Education in Nursing, Midwifery and Health Visiting.* Project Paper 1, English National Board for Nursing Midwifery and Health Visiting.

[DoH] Department of Health (1993) *Changing Childbirth.* Report of the Expert Maternity Group. London: HMSO.

[DHSS] Department of Health and Social Security (1983) NHS Management Enquiry (the Griffiths report). London: DHSS.

Flint C (1995) Being and becoming the named midwife. In: Page L (ed.) *Effective Group Practice in Midwifery: Working with Women.* Oxford: Blackwell Scientific.

Ford P & Walsh M (1994) *New Rituals for Old: Nursing Through the Looking Glass.* Oxford: Butterworth-Heinemann.

Hall M, Chng P & MacGillivray I (1980) Is routine antenatal care worthwhile? *Lancet* **ii**: 78–80.

Hampden-Turner C (1994) *Corporate Culture.* London: Piatkus.

Handy C (1991) *The Age of Unreason* 2nd edn. London: Arrow.

Handy C (1993) *Understanding Organisations,* 4th edn. Harmondsworth: Penguin.

Handy C (1995) *Gods of Management,* 3rd edn. London: Arrow.

Harrison R (1972) Understanding your organisation's character. *Harvard Business Review* May–June: 119–128.

Harrison S, Hunter DJ, Marnoch G & Pollitt C (1992) *Just Managing: Power and Culture in the National Health Service.* London: Macmillan.

Hunt M (1987) The process of translating research findings into nursing practice. *Journal of Advanced Nursing* **12**: 101–110.

James J & Dewhurst J (1985) Death in service. *Health Service Journal* 18 May: 26.

Kanter RM (1983) *The Change Masters: Corporate Entrepreneurs at Work.* London: Allen & Unwin.

Leap N (1996) Caseload practice: a recipe for burn out? *British Journal of Midwifery* **4**(6): 329.

Lipsky M (1980) *Street-level Bureaucracy: Dilemmas of the Individual in Public Services.* New York: Russell-Sage.

Mander R (1994) *Loss and Bereavement in Childbearing.* Oxford: Blackwell Scientific.

Marris P (1974) *Loss and Change.* London: Routledge & Kegan Paul.

Maslach C (1976) Burned out. *Human Behavior* September: 16–22.

Maslach C & Schaufeli WB (1993) Historical and conceptual development of burnout. In: Schaufeli WB, Maslach C, Marek T (eds) *Professional Burnout: Recent Developments in Theory and Research.* Washington: Taylor & Francis.

Massey P (1991) Institutional loss: an examination of a bereavement reaction in 22 mental nurses losing their institution and moving into the community. *Journal of Advanced Nursing* **16**: 537–583.

McGinley M (1993) 1990s: commitment to change. *Midwives Chronicle and Nursing Notes* February: 42–44.

Menzies IEP (1970) *The Functioning of Social Systems as a Defence Against Anxiety.* London: Tavistock.

Methven R (1989) Recording an obstetric history or relating to a pregnant woman? A study of the antenatal booking interview. In: Robinson S, Thomson A (eds) *Midwives, Research and Childbirth*, vol. 1. London: Chapman & Hall.

Miller E (1979) Autonomy, dependency and organisational change. In: Towell D, Harries C (eds) *Innovation in Patient Care: An Action Research Study of Change in a Psychiatric Hospital.* London: Croom Helm.

Obholzer A & Roberts VZ, eds (1994) *The Unconscious at Work: Individual and Organisational Stress in the Human Services.* London: Routledge.

Ohmae K (1982) *The Mind of the Strategist: The Art of Japanese Business.* New York: McGraw Hill.

OPUS (1996) *Organisational Stress: Planning and Implementing a Programme to Address Organisational Stress in the NHS.* London: Health Education Authority.

Ovretveit J (1996) Ethics: a counsel of perfection? *IHSM Network* **3** (13): 4–5.

Page L, ed. (1995) *Effective Group Practice in Midwifery: Working with Women.* Oxford: Blackwell Scientific.

Pascale R (1991) *Managing on the Edge: How Successful Companies use Conflict to Stay Ahead.* Harmondsworth: Penguin.

Payne R & Firth-Cozens J, eds (1987) *Stress in Health Professionals.* Chichester: John Wiley.

Perkins ER & Lovelock C (1996) *The Change Process.* In: Final Report of Sheffield Nursing Development Unit. Sheffield City Council Occupational Health Division.

Peters T (1988) *Thriving on Chaos: Handbook for a Management Revolution.* London: Macmillan.

Pollitt C (1993) *Managerialism and the Public Services*, 2nd edn. Oxford: Blackwell.

Quick JC & Quick JD (1984) *Organizational Stress and Preventive Management.* New York: McGraw Hill.

Robinson J (1991) Project 2000: the role of resistance in the process of professional growth. *Journal of Advanced Nursing* **16**: 820–824.

Robinson S (1980) *The Midwifery Project: A Preliminary Report.* London: Nursing Education Research Unit, Chelsea College.

Robinson S (1989) Caring for childbearing women: the interrelationship between midwifery and medical responsibilities. In: Robinson S, Thomson A (eds) *Midwives, Research and Childbirth*, vol 1. London: Chapman & Hall.

Robinson S & Thomson A, eds (1989) *Midwives, Research and Childbirth*, vol 1. London: Chapman & Hall.

Rumbold GC (1995) *Management Skills for Community Nurses.* Dinton: Mark Allen Publishing.

Sacker A (1990) Smoking habits of nurses and midwives. *Journal of Advanced Nursing* **15**: 1341–1346.

Santangeli B (1988) Coming to terms with stress at work. *Senior Nurse* **8** (7/8): 11–13.

Scott CD & Jaffe DT (1990) *Managing Organisational Change: A Guide for Managers.* London: Kogan Page.

Speck P (1994) Working with dying people; on being good enough. In: Obholzer A, Roberts VZ (eds) *The Unconscious at Work: Individual and Organisational Stress in the Human Services.* London: Routledge.

Taylor FW (1911) *The Principles of Scientific Management.* New York: Harper.

Towell D & Harries C, eds (1979) *Innovation in Patient Care: An Action Research Study of Change in a Psychiatric Hospital.* London: Croom Helm.

Turnbull D, Reid D, McGinley M & Sheilds NR (1995) Changes in midwives' attitudes to their professional role following the implementation of the midwifery development unit. *Midwifery* **11**: 110–119.

Walker JF (1976) Midwife or obstetric nurse? Some perceptions of midwives and obstetricians of the role of the midwife. *Journal of Advanced Nursing* **1**: 129–138.

Walker JM, Hall S & Thomas M (1995) The experience of labour: a perspective from those receiving care in a midwife-led unit. *Midwifery* **11**: 120–129.

Walsh M & Ford P (1989) *Nursing Rituals, Research and Rational Action*. Oxford: Butterworth-Heinemann.

West MA (1989) Innovation amongst health care professionals. *Social Behaviour* **4**: 173–184.

West MA & Wallace M (1991) Innovation in health care teams. *European Journal of Social Psychology* **21**: 303–315.

Wheeler H & Riding R (1994) Occupational stress in general nurses and midwives. *British Journal of Nursing* **3**(10): 527–534.

Wilkinson MJ (1995) Love is not a marketable commodity; new public management in the British National Health Service. *Journal of Advanced Nursing* **21**: 980–987.

Winterton NC (1992) *Maternity Services*, vol. 1. Second Report of the House of Commons Health Committee (Winterton report). London: HMSO.

Wraight A, Ball J, Secombe I & Stock J (1993) *Mapping Team Midwifery*. IMS Report 242. Brighton: Institute of Management Studies.

Wright S (1989) *Changing Nursing Practice*. London: Edward Arnold.

9

Stories and childbirth

Mavis J. Kirkham

The universe, somebody said, and I know now it is true, is made of stories, not particles; they are the wave functions of our existence. If they constitute the event horizon of our particular black hole they are also our only means of escape.

(Brink, 1996)

Our life experience is constructed as a myriad of linked stories. The construction of these stories renders our experience coherent and gives it meaning.

As children we absorb the structures of our social world through stories, and as adults we demonstrate and consolidate our value systems as we build the stories of our lives. Our stories express our selves and in their telling we convey our sense of self and negotiate it with others (Linde, 1993). Most of this is done without conscious consideration of all that is transmitted. Efforts to change values through stories, as in recent writing of feminist fairy stories or Plato's more ambitious plans (*The Republic*, Book 3) serve as tribute to the social power of stories.

A story tells more than its tale. It speaks of context and of values. Listeners absorb the story through the web of their own view of the world and by links with their own stories. The tellers reinforce different aspects of their own values in each unique story-telling. The meanings of stories may be multiple and their embodied social constructs many-layered. This is true in several dimensions. I seek to examine individual and collective birth stories and fiction concerning birth. Cultural values and personal experience pervade all these stories. Tess Cosslett (1994) demonstrated how medical discourses have pervaded the literature of 'natural childbirth'. It is also relevant that several women have told me that, when reading Cosslett's analysis of fictional accounts of childbirth, they were sure of the nature of Cosslett's own birth experiences long before she revealed them in the last chapter.

Stories reveal important aspects of midwives' work and their careful examination may open up new dimensions in which we can usefully be with women.

Women's writings about birth do not reveal a common or universal experience, but they often demonstrate a dazzling ability to interweave memory, fantasy, theory, myth, ideology and science, and they may show us a way to turn the reproductive revolution to women's advantage.

(Adams, 1994, p. xi)

As midwives our scope is even wider, for we work with the spoken as well as the written story.

STORIES OF BIRTH AND LIFE AS WOMEN

Women who have given birth construct a birth story which they will tell for the rest of their lives though the context of the telling and therefore the significance of the story will change.

VIGNETTE

My mother told the story of her first birth to nurses in the hospice shortly before her death. A practical woman, she chose to praise the hospice nurses for their kindness and gentleness by recounting the harshness and hurt she experienced at the hands of midwives:

> *... and in the morning [after my mother had laboured through the night alone, hearing bombs fall nearby and fearing they fell on her husband] this lady came round. She said 'How are you?' and put her hand on the bedcover. I reached out for her hand and she pulled it away then tapped me on the back of my hand and said, 'I am the Matron'.*

This had been told for 50 years as a tale of hurt and humiliation at a time of great vulnerability. When told to the matron of the hospice, who sat by her bed, held her hand and listened, it turned into a song of praise for hospice care. The teller, though vulnerable again as she approached her death, could now smile at the shortcomings of a wartime matron.

The entrance of a new member into a society and a woman's transition to motherhood provide rich material for stories. These stories have a special intensity. In describing the letters she received at the Patients Association, Jean Robinson reported:

> *Letters about birth were different. They had an immediacy and clarity of expression which made them leap off the page. Even if the writer was poorly educated descriptions of labour and birth were incredibly vivid. Women had intensity of recall for birth experiences which was different from other memories.*
>
> (Robinson, 1995)

Stories of birth create bonds between women as they recount their common though unique experiences. Birth is a rite of passage in which much is revealed. A woman recently turned to me after a strong contraction and said, 'Now I know what my mother went through'. It is interesting that 'Women for the most part, undergo initiation through their natural processes' (Lambert, 1993) rather than through constructed rituals. There is much ritual around childbirth but in this society little of that is constructed by childbearing women, which makes women's stories even more important. The sense that an experience is held in common is strengthening. As Sorel wrote in the introduction to her anthology of personal reflections on childbirth:

> *Never mind, I told myself – it was the same for Cleopatra, for Maria de Medici, for Anna Magdalena Bach and Sophia Tolstoy and Sophia Loren – and Eve.*   (Sorel 1984)

It was also at the same time different, and birth stories can shed light on the similarities and the differences.

Particular common experience can be immensely strengthening, as can be seen in the poignant stories in the newsletters of self-help groups such as the Miscarriage Association. These newsletters give testimony to how common experience makes support possible. Stories with which we may identify can also help us to understand our own situation as individuals and as mothers. In Adams' view, 'the closest we can come to reconstructing our origins is to ask our mothers to tell us their stories' (Adams, 1994). Other women's birth stories can shed light on our own childbearing. They can help prepare pregnant women for labour and motherhood and they can certainly deepen midwives' understanding.

Stories also affect the teller, and birth stories crystallize out as a woman takes on the responsibilities of parenthood; just when she needs support and reinforcement as to her ability to cope with such responsibilities. Yet so often women's birth stories have experts as central, active figures and the woman's part in her own story is personally undermining and profoundly disempowering. As a fictional heroine observed, 'They do the doing, I do the suffering (patient means that)' (Bowder, 1983). The tap on the hand embodied in the vignette above can go on wounding, more subtle undermining may go on disempowering.

Old wives' tales

Professionals acknowledge the power of the recounted birth story in warning pregnant women against 'old wives' tales'. Bourne's book *Pregnancy* is described on its cover as 'The Pregnancy Bible' and has been in print since 1972. It states:

> *The majority of old wives' tales are essentially destructive or demoralising. ... Probably more is done by wicked women with their malicious lying tongues to harm the confidence and happiness of pregnant women than by any other single factor.* (Bourne, 1996)

The language used in early editions of *Active Management of Labour* suggests that O'Driscoll and colleagues saw the recounted experience of multiparous women as a real threat to their view of pregnancy (O'Driscoll and Meagher, 1980). The current edition still sees these women as in need of 'an exercise in rehabilitation' (O'Driscoll and Meagher, 1993), which must be kept separate from antenatal education of first time mothers who must learn 'correct attitudes' (Bourne, 1996) from medical experts, not from experienced mothers.

Rapid technological and social change together with increasing emphasis on the experts' version of events now inhibits mothers from telling their daughters the story of their birth. It often surprises me in taking antenatal histories how many young women know little about the labour that preceded their own birth.

Thus the voices of women are muted by the voices of experts, though only women experience birth. The derogatory meaning which the term 'old wives' tales' has taken on has hastened this muting process and 'fosters the process of self-silencing' (Astbury, 1996).

The official story

The official story of a woman's childbearing is contained in the record of her maternity care. The structure of 'the notes' is a medical construct and their repeated use reinforces for all readers the values there embodied. Ironically the majority of readers are midwives, and now the readers include clients holding their own records.

The language of the official record is that of obstetrics; doctors and midwives are accustomed to that language, and experience 'the comforts and rewards that come with the embrace of certain magical verbal constructs' (Coles, 1989). As student midwives we learnt what was acceptable to write by looking at past entries. Thus unlikely phrases such as 'slept well' and 'comfortable day' appeared often in inpatient records. Records are now held by those they describe, but still consist of professionals' 'magical verbal constructs' abbreviated from Latin and Greek. Professionals feel at home with their story in their language. Indeed, student midwives who are already nurses have been found to shield themselves from the discomforts of their new setting by attending overclosely to providing the data for this official record (Davies and Atkinson, 1991). In the focused technical data collection of 'doing the obs' they felt safe, surrounded by the uncertainty of women who sought to tell and to understand their own stories.

The official record sees childbearing from the medical perspective. This is the same process that Kleinman (1988) described whereby illness (as experienced) is reduced to disease (a professional concept).

> *Illness complaints are what patients and their families bring to the practitioner. ... Disease is what the practitioner creates in the recasting of illness in terms of theories of disorder. ... In the narrow biological terms of the biomedical model, this means that disease is reconfigured only as an alteration in biological structure or functioning.*   *(Kleinman, 1988)*

This reconfiguration takes place in the production of medical records even when the subject is a normal process and the woman is well. In this recasting something essential to the woman's experience is lost. 'It is not legitimate as a subject of clinical concern, nor does it receive an intervention' (Kleinman, 1988, p. 6) – it is discounted.

In this process labels are given and categorizations are made. In the pressures towards economies of time and resources we inevitably develop shorthand. Yet through 'over-wrought language and overwrought theory' we can 'explain people away'. There is therefore a real danger that obstetric records do not do their subjects justice (Kleinman, 1988). In William Carlos Williams' lucid words:

> *Who's against shorthand? No one I know. Who wants to be short-changed? No one I know.*
>   *(quoted by Coles, 1989)*

While the professional story will be different from the woman's story since it serves another purpose, there is a real danger of reductionism and missing the essence of the matter. Robinson looked at academic medical writing as well as the treatment of individual patients around induction of labour in the 1970s and concluded:

> *The obstetricians wrote nothing about the possibility that induced labour might be more painful or emotionally distressing. Either they did not see it, which says little for their powers of observation, or they saw it and did not report it, which says little for their ethical and scientific standards.* *(Robinson, 1995)*

This may be the result of a view of maternity care which concentrates on separate clinical problems. Issues that cannot be addressed or are not currently under consideration then become unimportant. This separation of clinical problems from distressing experience may also serve doctors as a defence mechanism. In Hemingway's story 'The Indian Camp', the doctor tells his young son that the screams of the 'Indian lady' in labour 'are not important. I don't hear them because they are not important' (Hemingway, 1925), as he proceeds to perform a caesarean section with his jack-knife. Reductionism echoes on. Distress later became a further medical problem to be solved with epidural analgesia, a move which is in itself reductionist, for pain is only part of distress.

Antenatal screening is an area where stories diverge markedly. The medical story is of progress in screening techniques and refining risk assessment, leading to choice for parents and improved outcomes. Women, including those who ultimately provide the good outcomes, often tell stories of 'backing into testing' and 'draconian decisions'. After the detection of fetal anomalies, Sandelowski and Jones (1996) found parents 'constructed subtly different accounts of pregnancies continued or terminated that located the moral agency for effecting these pregnancy outcomes either in themselves or elsewhere'. These findings show 'the importance of appraising how people story the adverse events in their lives' in order to help them best 'restory' those events. Helen Stapleton gives a good example of this process after a fetal death (Chapter 3). In order to support such 'restorying' very subtle record-keeping is required, and concepts such as 'choice' lack subtlety.

The data required for monitoring the fetal and maternal condition antenatally and in labour are now largely gained by direct technological means such as ultrasonography or biochemical analysis. There is therefore a real sense in which the mother's story is irrelevant to her technical care. It is possible to see this situation as one where skilled help is needed to bridge the gap between technical and experiential knowledge, for the benefit of all concerned. Yet such bridging is a low-status activity. There is a strong pressure on those of us who become owners of professional power and a professional vocabulary towards 'moral thoughtlessness' and 'moral drift' (Coles, 1989). This is particularly worrying at a time when society is highly medicalized and the cultural authority of medicine is growing,

The Midwives Rules (UKCC, 1993) require a midwife to:

> *Keep as contemporaneously as is reasonable detailed records of observations, care given and medicines or other forms of pain relief administered by her …* *(Rule 42)*

While this is a basic requirement, it in no way limits the records a midwife may keep. When things go wrong, as in the cases of suboptimal care identified in the Confidential Enquiry into Stillbirths and Deaths in Infancy (CESDI, 1996) where midwives were felt to be partially responsible for family practices such as 'prop' feeding or exposure of the baby to cigarette smoke, midwives are seen as responsible because they 'failed to give advice to women about these issues or, if they had done, had not recorded the advice'. It therefore appears to be in the midwife's interests to keep records which are more detailed than many we see in practice and which are easily intelligible to the client. We may learn here from independent midwives whose records tend to be more detailed than those kept by NHS midwives.

Changing Childbirth (DoH, 1993) recommended that 'all women should be entitled to carry their own notes'. For this to have meaning, the carrying of notes must be seen as a first step towards a real sharing of their content. We can learn here from other professions. Around the introduction of client-held health visiting records, Jackson (1991) described 'painful work' on 'attitudes to clients, control and how to let go', and concluded:

> *The greatest challenge for the health visitors has been learning how to record information so that clients can understand and use it.*   *(Jackson, 1991)*

She records a breakthrough for one health visitor when,

> *... an Asian client wrote in the record in her own language, Gujerati. But what that meant for us was that we needed an interpreter – not her.*   *(Jackson, 1991)*

Another area, entirely in our control, where such efforts are needed is that of care plans. It is difficult to see how effective care plans can be developed with women and then written in official language, yet jargon has grown here too. Nurses are working in this area; Harvey recommended:

> *... a phenomenological approach based on my understanding of each woman's lived experience of her situation, gained from listening to her story, helps me to work with the woman to develop her care plan.*
> *(Harvey, 1993)*

Sharing the official story is possible, with all the sharing of power thus symbolized, and we can learn from those who share this aim.

MIDWIVES AND STORIES

Midwives bring support and technical skill to women in their care. In recent years the technical skills needed by midwives have greatly increased and the proliferation of technical and organizational tasks has lessened the time and priority given to supporting clients. At the same time, the increase in status which came with identification with medical advances has also led midwives towards medical habits of thought as well as record-keeping. Nevertheless, the midwife's fundamental job remains to provide safe care for mothers and babies. Research (MIDIRS, 1996) as well as government documents (e.g. DoH, 1993) have also stressed the importance of support and the relationship between the childbearing woman and her carer. This can put added stress upon the midwife whose relationship with the narrow technical focus of obstetric practice and with obstetric language may be strained when she seeks to support women in all of the many ways in which support may be needed.

Midwives and birth stories

Midwives are closely linked into all the many strands of 'their' women's childbearing stories. Indeed these stories, and the midwife's own stories of caregiving, are woven into the material with which the midwife works with each successive client. Jordan's research as an anthropologist leads her to state that, in a traditional setting:

> *To acquire a store of appropriate stories, and, even more importantly, to know what are appropriate occasions for telling them, is part of what it means to become a midwife.*   *(Jordan, 1993)*

In such a setting her growing skill in the use of childbearing stories is important in defining the point at which an apprentice comes to be seen as a midwife. In any culture, as a midwife's own story grows richer, she gains in repertoire and skill in effective storytelling.

A growing wealth of clinical experience as a midwife affects our practice in a number of ways. With real experience we recognize the clues to the unexpected in physiology and in behaviour. Previous experience alerts us in a way theoretical knowledge cannot. With growing expertise we learn to recognize patterns in increasingly sophisticated ways and the practice of real experts has a subtlety which theoreticians strive in vain to capture.

A community midwife with much experience of home birth without the use of ergometrine (Syntometrine) recently gave me an example of this. 'When the placenta is about to deliver you usually see a little shiver. You can see it in her shoulders, you don't need to be intrusive'. Observation at my next delivery showed this to be the case. Thus a small and practical gift has been added to my body of clinical knowledge.

Sometimes our stories, if we assemble rather than suppress them, challenge our textbook knowledge and can be complex, as shown in the following vignette.

VIGNETTE

Some years ago I helped Rose arrange a home birth in a situation where this was difficult. She asked me to be with her in labour as her friend. When she rang to say she was in labour I went to her and we spent some time pottering around the house preparing for the birth. Her contractions became stronger and she asked me to examine her, which I did and found her cervix to be 6 cm dilated. We therefore called the community midwife. Shortly afterwards two community midwives and a student midwife arrived, all strangers to Rose, plus her general practitioner and her husband returned with friends. The community midwife examined Rose and found her cervix to be 2 cm dilated. After this she doggedly coped with a long labour and delivered normally at home.

I pondered the change in Rose's cervix for the rest of her labour and many years after. I felt I understood when her divorce revealed the dominance of her husband, whom she feared. She still maintains that her cervix 'shrank when officialdom arrived'.

Textbooks describe cervical dilation in labour. Never have I seen one mention cervical contraction, as in this vignette. But, as William Carlos Williams (1983) observed:

> *Dissonance*
> *(if you are interested)*
> *leads to discovery.*

This dissonance served to 'open the doors of perception' (Powell, 1993) for me. Thinking about Rose's contracting cervix and other similar circumstances made me aware that the cervix can contract in labour, and less dramatically but more frequently it can fail to dilate, when a woman feels threatened (there may, of course, be other reasons). Often she may feel threatened by someone in the room. Sometimes she may feel threatened by a parallel in her past experience, thus a woman's reactions to care in labour may give crucial clues to past trauma such as sexual abuse. The relationship between a woman's past life, her present labour and cervical dilation is complex, and is illustrated in the second vignette. Midwives' awareness of such parallels in the stories of which we are a part can be one factor in our endeavours to give more sensitive care.

VIGNETTE

Leah and Gordon came to book and consult with me at 39 weeks. This was their second pregnancy, the first had resulted in the normal birth in hospital of a little boy, James, who died of congenital abnormalities at 8 days. They clearly had very bitter memories and felt antagonistic towards the hospital and its staff, though it was known to me as a friendly and progressive establishment. Three days later Leah called me in early labour. They coped well with a slow and tedious labour, unlike the first which had progressed easily. Eventually her cervix was fully dilated; Leah wanted to push, was apparently pushing and the vertex was visible. Half an hour of good contractions passed without progress. She tried hands and knees, my birth stool, left lateral and the supported squat she had used in her first labour without progress. She was finding pushing very painful, but couldn't stop. We changed position again to all fours, more good contractions, I had a good look at the perineum and vulval area and checked the position. It was definitely LOA, well flexed and not a very big baby. As I looked and felt she had a contraction, tried to push and to my surprise I observed the perineal muscles and the introitus in spasm and tightening. I had seen this before but only in women whom I knew, or subsequently discovered, had been sexually abused. Leah had no vaginismus when I examined her and, while one never knows, I thought it unlikely that she had been abused and she had an easy normal birth with the first baby.

I said, 'Are these the positions you tried when you had James?'

'Yes,' she yelled, as again she tried to push and screamed with pain.

'I think your body is afraid, and isn't letting you have this baby. Your body seems to be remembering what happened last time,' I said. 'I want you to do something totally different … on your bed and on your back.' Gordon and I got her onto her bed and onto her back, and helped her hold her legs. She pushed. It was quite different, up came the head. With the next contraction Roger was born, and we all wept.

The experienced, independent midwife who told me the story in the vignette above said, 'I really don't know what caused the penny to drop'. She laughingly said she never used the 'trussed chicken' or 'stranded beetle position', but it worked on this occasion. Aware of the dissonance between the favourable factors and the lack of progress, she knew that parallels with previous threatening experience could stop progress and felt that the threat could be the fear of facing again the terrible discovery at James's birth. So she changed the birth position away from that used in the progressive hospital which was so deeply associated, for Leah, with loss and fear of further loss. During the next few days the midwife helped the couple grieve for James as they hugged Roger, and Leah confirmed that, despite all the tests, she had been terrified this baby would be abnormal and could not face the possibility of another loss.

It must be said that not all midwives learn in this way from their past experience, however long they may have been practising. Indeed, the power of medical orthodoxy serves to suppress awareness of dissonance and thus keeps the doors of perception shut. When such knowledge is recounted, it is as stories of past experience with common threads. Some midwives appear particularly skilled in gaining expertise from situated knowledge rather than from theory. It must, however, be said that this is the point where qualitative research and the ability to learn from stories come very close together (Clarke, 1995).

Situated knowledge

Lave and Wenger (1991) discussed 'participation as a way of learning – of both absorbing and being absorbed in the culture of practice'. When involved in the 'culture of practice', learning and socialization are part of the same process by which apprentices extend their competence. 'There is very little observable teaching: the more basic phenomena is learning.' In the view of Lave and Wenger, 'a learning curriculum is essentially situated' in the reality of the practice which is to be learned.

> *Thus, participation in the cultural practice in which any knowledge exists is an epistemological principle of learning. The social structure of this practice, its power relations, and its conditions for legitimacy define possibilities for learning …. Conflict is experienced and worked out through a shared everyday practice in which differing viewpoints and common stakes are in interplay.   (Lave and Wenger, 1991)*

The learner's 'identity in relation to practice', her life story to date, is part of this process of situated learning. This interaction between the individual and the social setting of practice

> *… helps to account for the common observation that knowers come in a range of types from clones to heretics.   (Lave and Wenger, 1991)*

'Learning how to talk (and be silent) in the manner of full participants is crucial.' Here where teaching may seem to be invisible, stories are the currency by which knowledge is transmitted. They may be official stories as contained in medical records, or personal accounts of childbearing women.

Jordan's initial frustration with traditional Maya midwives answering theoretical questions with stories (Jordan, 1993) changed in the light of the wide range of stories these midwives called upon. Thus, while their thinking was concrete, they were very aware of the complex variables of practice, an issue often overlooked in conceptual analysis. In decision-making during labours, she described the 'most impressive' way in which stories function:

> *As difficulties of one kind or another develop, stories of similar cases are offered up by the attendants, all of whom, it should be remembered, are experienced birth-givers sharing a collective expertise. In the ways in which these stories are treated – elaborated, ignored, taken up as themes, characterized as typical and so on – the collaborative work of deciding on the present case is done.   (Jordan, 1993)*

This is an impressive example of shared decision-making, in which the apprentice and the labouring woman can play a part. Experience is pooled, evaluated and examined as to its relevance. Such experience, in the form of stories reveals 'packages of situated knowledge, knowledge that is not available abstractly'. Because it is thus situated it is intelligible to all participants and it is relevant because it is 'called up as the characteristics of the situation require'.

Since it does not involve the generalizations of applied theory, situated learning also enables the learner to appreciate many interacting factors:

> *Women are now recognised as having multiple dimensions of difference – gender, class, colour, race, age and culture … Each of these differences is infused with hierarchies of power and they intersect in each specific context.   (Nelson and Wright, 1995)*

There is a real sense in which situated knowledge is more complex and more relevant to the care of individuals than conceptual teaching.

While decision-making is more complex when it also involves policies, procedures, clinical guidelines and the many issues associated with evidence and research-based practice, there is still much we can learn from the processes Jordan described. Whatever the theoretical educational input, these issues of situated knowledge are still important because midwifery remains a practical activity. Examination of situated learning and the role of stories casts light on how decision-making can be shared; stories also give an empowering degree of control to the learner in selecting what is to be learnt. Dissonance between stories is highlighted, which is rarely the case where an accepted body of theoretical knowledge is seen as true. Study of these issues may suggest solutions to some dilemmas such as the theory–practice gap and the empowerment of childbearing women and midwives.

These issues are of practical relevance in antenatal care. Medical studies have shown that 'agreement between physician and patient about the nature of the presenting problem is closely linked to a good outcome' (Brody, 1994). In such a situation 'where narratives are jointly constructed, power is shared . . . and the sharing of power constitutes an important ethical safeguard within the relationship'. If this is so in medicine it is likely to be even more so in midwifery care, given all that we know about the links between women's perceptions of control and positive outcomes (e.g. Green et al, 1989). Yet, when taking an antenatal history for instance, the pressure on midwives is to translate the woman's experience into an official medical record, not to build a 'jointly constructed narrative' where concerns are shared.

Old professionals' tales

Stories of past experience can act as a conservative pressure on current practice. We all know midwives or doctors whose practice is marked by a past negative experience. The fact that the experience was rare and research evidence shows that it cannot be generalized, does not weigh as heavily with the individual as the scars from one bad personal experience. Thus some practitioners are opposed to home births, vaginal breech births or whatever they generalize from an experience of disaster. Midwives and doctors are scarred by their pasts, and sometimes I think these scars may be contagious: as stories of past disasters are recounted, they can also slip into institutional policies. Old professionals' tales have a wider and more powerful influence than old wives' tales. The ability to generalize from negative experience is sometimes very great and we all know settings where every suggestion for innovation is met with the response, 'We tried that before and it doesn't work'. These negative aspects of learning from experience merit closer attention. Perhaps they are symptoms of incipient burnout. Perhaps such scars lead to defence mechanisms as a result of a lack of professional support or the absence of opportunities for professional debriefing. Certainly these negative stories go on being told. (These issues are considered further by Elizabeth Perkins in Chapter 8.)

The midwife's tale

Before the twentieth century most midwives were illiterate members of the working class or agricultural communities which they served. They could not leave us their story and we inherit descriptions of 'meddlesome midwives' written by male practitioners who were often competing with them for trade. There are notable exceptions such as the diaries of Martha Ballard, a midwife in Maine 1785–1812 (Ulrich, 1991). More recent historical research also gives us insights (e.g. Gelis, 1991; Marland, 1993). In

Britain medical dominance was profound, and where the midwife's story is told it is in the context of medical innovation and reforming zeal for the new, as in *The Midwife: Her Book* (Gregory, 1923). The unwritten work of older practitioners and bona fide midwives can occasionally be glimpsed in other writings. Llewelyn Davies (1977) gives a brief description of Mrs Layton, a bona fide midwife who petitioned parliament for maternity benefit to be included in the first National Insurance Bill. We are left wondering how many other working-class midwives buttressed the labour movement earlier this century rather than identifying with the movement to professionalize midwifery.

For more recent times, Leap and Hunter's work on the oral history of midwifery brings us something of the stories of ordinary midwives (Leap and Hunter, 1993). Yet this is little compared with the literature on developments in obstetrics, and some books claiming to give a history of midwifery simply recount the achievements of great medical men (e.g. Rhodes, 1995).

As Brooke Heagerty demonstrates in Chapter 4, the 1902 Midwives Act was constructed with due deference to the male medical establishment of that time. The ladies of the Midwives Institute, while seeking to raise midwifery to the status of a profession, did so with the skills of deference and working through powerful men which were so highly developed in reforming Victorian ladies.

Modern midwifery in Britain was very much defined by the more powerful profession of medicine and there is clear evidence that midwives internalized the values of that profession (see Chapter 4 and Kirkham, 1996a). Midwives therefore fit the definition of an oppressed group (Roberts, 1983) as one 'which is controlled by societal forces that have determined its leadership behaviour'. The analysis of Freire (1972) gives us insight into how, in the process of internalizing the values of the masters, the original characteristics of the subordinate group come to be negatively valued. This creates a situation where the midwife's tale cannot be told except as one that is being transformed by medicine. The insights of the midwife's tale are therefore muted or denied, with damaging effects for those who thereby reject all value in their own identity and tradition. The resulting low self-esteem is highly self-destructive, especially as it is held in counter-point with submission to the powerful profession. The tension thus produced was seen by Fanon (1963) as released in 'horizontal violence': conflict within the oppressed group especially towards those seen as slightly deviant, which in turn reinforced the status quo. A secondary process is fear of change. How often I have seen both these processes acted out in midwifery.

In countries where midwifery was not 'co-opted' (Weitz and Sullivan, 1985) by medicine, the situation was different for the midwives who practised, often outside the law, were aware of their difference from medical practice and did not internalize its values. American texts for midwives (as distinct from nurse/midwives who had another orthodoxy), such as Elizabeth Davis's *Hearts and Hands* (Davis, 1983) and Ina May Gaskin's *Spiritual Midwifery* (Gaskin, 1977) are structured around women's birth stories and are still eagerly read by student midwives in Britain. The American journal *Midwifery Today* is similarly grounded in the stories of mothers and midwives which are distilled out in its 'tricks of the trade' page. It is significant that the anthology of stories and poems *Life of a Midwife: A Celebration of Midwifery* is published by *Midwifery Today* (1995), and has no equivalent in Britain.

Stories and professional development

Pressures to medicalize and professionalize midwifery, together with the move of midwifery education into universities, have served to legitimize conceptual learning. This has tended to squeeze out true dialogue with the woman's experience, where power is shared (Freire, 1972). There is an acknowledged, small place for the use of vignettes in research (Sapsford and Abbot, 1992). Otherwise, stories of practice only appear in the narrow structured contexts of reflective practice, critical incidents or case studies, with all their attendant jargon. So the directness and simplicity of story-telling is lost, as is the freedom for the hearers to learn what they find appropriate from a story not truncated or constricted into a conceptual mould. It is ironic that the literature on reflection is often 'complex and abstract' (Atkins and Murphy, 1993) and there are considerable problems in reaching insight rather than professional narcissism by means of reflection (Kirkham, 1997). Our history leads us to reflection proofed against insight:

> *In the process of 'story telling', midwives are able to construct a rational, caring depiction of midwifery and to contrast this with a non-rational, inhumane, representation of other occupational groups: the 'bogey man' is characterised, categorised and coped with.*   *(Curtis, 1992)*

There is little written on the actual skills that might overcome the dilemmas inherent in reflection.

If we can overcome narcissism there is a large place for 'storytelling as a professional development tool' (Bowles, 1995). Insight from women's experience may provide the catalyst we need to improve our skills in being with women. The use of 'simulated case scenarios' in preparing midwives for caseload management (Wise, 1996) is a cheering move in this direction.

Peer review can also be a useful tool for practitioners seeking insight into their own practice and development of their repertoire of stories. This has been recognized for some time in some areas of medicine (e.g. Brody, 1987) and is now being explored in midwifery (e.g. Page, 1995).

Writing: fictional and reflective

In seeking the catalyst that gives us insight into the experience of those we serve, there is also a place for fictional stories (Rowland, 1995). 'Writing fiction as inquiry into professional practice' (Rowland (Rowland now Bolton) et al, 1990) can be very fruitful for midwives, general practitioners and other health workers. In a group this is a safe activity.

> *By sharing fictional accounts related to our practice we are representing to the group the values, fears and hopes which underlay our work. However, since the events portrayed would not actually have taken place, criticism from others would be relatively unthreatening. We may be prepared to tackle the risk of revealing ourselves and exploring new strategies and perspectives on our work when these are related directly to the fictional characters we have invented, rather than to our own selves.*
> *(Rowland et al, 1990)*

It is therefore possible to look from many viewpoints, to write the story of the same events as told by another actor in those events, and to use the many viewpoints in the writing group. Thus 'the character who was initially the hero of our story may emerge as the villain, once his or her actions have been the subject of the group's scrutiny'. We may thereby through fiction gain insight into the limitations of our own professional system of thought. Ted Hughes observed 'The progress of any writer is marked by those moments when he managed to outwit his own inner police system' (Cope, 1986, quoted by Rowland et al, 1990). We have to overcome the problem that fiction writing has become an activity as specialized as obstetrics before we can not only outwit our 'inner police system' but map that system and become aware of its shortcomings in terms of midwifery practice. Such writing groups, whether concerned with fiction or stories of practice, provide learning opportunities at many levels.

> *The support of group members is vital, for allowing habitual mental structures to be temporarily*
> *suspended can be an uncomfortable process.*   *(Rowland et al, 1990)*

Though free from the uncertainties of clinical practice, having the 'courage to come into this kind of contact with our own creativity is powerful and revealing'. It can therefore be threatening, and learning to accept and request support in coping in these circumstances can prove another area of learning relevant to practice as a midwife. The 'therapeutic space' created in such a writing group can give us insight into our own needs as well as those of clients and, most importantly, insight where those needs come together.

> *Writers end up writing about their obsessions. Things that hurt them; things that they can't forget; stories*
> *they carry in their bodies waiting to be released.*   *(Goldberg (1986) quoted by Bolton, 1995)*

Such 'self-educative and releasing' experience enables us to move forward in our practice.

Writers' workshops have provided similar opportunities for many people. A considerable number of these groups have enabled mothers to tell 'the real story' (OLDP, 1996) of their experience of motherhood, and gain much in its telling.

Debriefing

Pauleene Hammett provides a clear example in Chapter 7 of how, in debriefing the woman after childbirth, the midwife gains access to the woman's birth story. In the light of this she can reassess the care she gave that woman.

As well as providing fuel for professional reflection, debriefing is an example of skilled work with stories. Debriefing after childbirth raises issues that are not part of the literature on debriefing after trauma. Birth may be traumatic, but there are issues beyond recovery from trauma in the start of a new life and new family relationships. The birth story goes on as part of parenting. The midwife, therefore, in debriefing has access to this powerful story while it is still plastic. In debriefing from the labour notes the midwife can help the woman to understand and fill in gaps in her birth story. Filling in gaps in time is important, and we are a very time-oriented society.

Time is, however, not the only dimension here. Astbury asks:

> *Can the fragments [in the patient's memory] only form one fixed shape, in the same way as the pieces of a*
> *child's puzzle can only form a rabbit or a cat, or are they more like the fragments in a kaleidoscope*
> *which a shift of angle, a turn or rotation will produce an entirely new configuration?*   *(Astbury, 1995)*

If the latter is true, midwives are in a powerful position, for they can produce a shift in the angle from which the woman sees her own story. By careful choice of words the midwife can help the woman to build a story which is empowering, though the experience itself may have been disempowering. This involves careful listening to the feelings expressed by the woman as she pieces together her story. Helping her to acknowledge her feelings and then expressing how she coped with them helps greatly here. Comments such as, 'That must have been frightening. You were so brave', or a comment to the partner such as, 'You must be so proud of how she coped with all she had to go through', can give the couple permission to see themselves as strong and enduring rather than just passive. Sometimes we have to move responsibility back onto professional shoulders if a woman is carrying a weight of self-blame into the future in her birth story. We may have to help a woman acknowledge that we could have acted better. Openings such as 'it must have been even more frightening for you since things were not explained' or 'it must have been terrible waiting alone in the corridor outside theatre', addressed to a father, can be the start of this aspect of building a useful story. This is almost the opposite of the official story, for feelings are of paramount importance.

Debriefing is a subtle skill and midwives must be aware of the power they have in this process. 'Stories... can often not be easily told, and they are always embedded in the political flow' (Plummer, 1995). The political flow in hospitals favours the institution's powerholders rather than the client. Plummer raises a series of issues which midwives can usefully consider in the context of debriefing.

The nature of stories

> *Which kinds of narratives work to empower people and which degrade, control and dominate? Some stories may work to pathologise voices or turn them into victims … other stories give the voice a power to transform and empower.*
> (Plummer, 1995)

What is the relationship between the story of the expert who delivered the baby, supported by her written word, and the story of the woman? These are crucial questions, which I have not heard asked in midwifery practice or midwifery education.

The making of stories

What strategies enable stories to be told? Plummer (1995) described the role such as a midwife takes as that of 'coaxer' to the story. The coaxer has great power. 'Does a coaxer, for example, facilitate stories (enabling new voices to be heard) or entrap stories, into a wider story of his or her own?' There must be a parallel here between the way midwives may block conversation so that a woman's concerns are not addressed (Kirkham, 1989) and the way in which women's stories may be entrapped. We need a high level of self-awareness in order to work well. 'The way they nod their head, fidget, or look at the patient influences how the patient tells the … story' (Kleinman, 1988), as do the values of our language. The 'normal' delivery, for example, may be experienced as highly traumatic and very far from the woman's expectation of normality.

Close relationships lead to a deep mutual effect upon the personal stories of those concerned. It is interesting to listen to couples rewriting each other's life stories, and this continuing process is part of what it means to claim each other as a couple in our society. The midwife can have a brief but not dissimilar effect upon the short part of a mother's story with which she is concerned. Because the role is professional and therefore limited in extent and in time, this effect upon the story must be approached consciously, lest the midwife's approach marks the mother's story with the midwife's own perspective.

The consuming of stories

Who has access to stories? This is an issue with the spoken and written story. How staff respond to the telling of the story can have a real effect while the story is still plastic. We are all aware of personal details in medical notes becoming common knowledge amongst staff. Stories are by definition very personal.

As the writing of a birth plan can help a woman to become clear in her mind as to how she sees her future labour and birth, it may be that there is therapeutic value in her writing a birth story after debriefing to clarify what happened, how she feels about those events and how those feelings may affect her in the future. I have cared for women who later asked each person who was present during the labour to write their story of it and the bringing together of those stories was mutually enlightening for carers and family (e.g. Nolan, 1996). Many years ago at such a gathering after a home birth I remember the general practitioner remarking, 'We each wrote the story as though we were the star'. Subsequent thought on that observation and our roles as carers and supporters has changed my view of my practice as a midwife, and his view of his practice as a GP. Such stories play an important role in helping me evolve my philosophy of practice.

I feel that good midwifery practice is essentially silent in that it helps a woman towards achievements which she rightly sees as hers and not her midwife's. If the professional is the star in the mother's story this is worrying, not least because of the links between lack of perceived control in childbearing and impaired postnatal emotional outcomes (Green et al, 1988). In order to facilitate the mother's active role, midwives need experience of the facilitation they endeavour to offer the mother. This raises issues of where midwives experience support and facilitation, and where they learn to tell their story and to understand the role of 'coaxer' in story-telling. Clearly the provision of debriefing for midwives is important here on several levels.

Antenatal education

Story-telling can play a powerful part in antenatal education. Midwives know that the words, 'I once looked after a woman who . . .' will claim the attention of an antenatal group because what follows will certainly be seen as relevant to them, as well as demonstrating the skills of the teller.

Bringing new parents back to tell their stories has a very real effect upon a group of women and their partners. The group identifies with the new parents. They have a real authority for having recently passed through the experience of labour that looms so large for the group. They laboured in the setting in which the women in the group will labour, and they can speak of the reality of that setting. The experience of spending time with new parents with their babies also serves to focus the group's thoughts on the early days of parenthood as experienced by these current experts on that subject. In contrast, when groups are addressed by midwives it is extremely difficult to get them to think beyond the labour which seems to stand like a wall between them and parenthood. These new parents are evidence that the wall can be – and for the group soon will be – scaled, and the new parents' baby is here and has to be given attention.

Most importantly, the use of parents in antenatal groups whether as breast-feeding mothers or parents describing their labours, reinforces the philosophy of active parents rather than expert midwives. The story being told in these circumstances must be the parents' story, not the official story or that of the professionals. Such feedback on our workplace and colleagues can be chastening for us as midwives, but as Freire (1972) observed 'dialogue cannot exist without humility'. The whole activity serves to professionally legitimize story-telling and to demonstrate that we are willing to listen.

There is also, I think, a place for other stories in antenatal education. I have always felt I lacked the ability to answer clearly the questions most frequently asked by pregnant women such as, 'What do contractions feel like?' It was a breakthrough to me when I first read to an antenatal group an excerpt from Enid Bagnold's novel *The Squire* (Bagnold, 1938), in answer to this perennial question. I am aware that this is very much a novel of its time, deeply influenced by the thought of Grantly Dick-Read (1933) as is demonstrated by Cosslett (1994). Yet that novel was right for that hospital, its clientele, its late 1980s classes and for me. It started me on a long and pleasurable search for writers and artists whose answers to the perennial questions are more eloquent than mine and fit within all manner of social settings. Maybe one day there will be midwife artists we can quote.

Language

Language is tremendously powerful. 'Transformed into words, the inconceivable, the overwhelming becomes manageable' (Adams, 1994). Only with language can we collect information and be prepared for events. While it makes communication possible, language also structures our experience. This is most obvious in the written word. Not only were working-class and mainly illiterate midwives affected for centuries by the way their history was written by rival male practitioners, but Dickens' fictional character Sairey Gamp in *Martin Chuzzlewit* (Hughes, 1990) was distorted and long and effectively used to discredit working-class midwives.

In English, men and women use language rather differently (Tannen, 1991). As Tannen observed:

> *Even though both styles are equally valid and logical in themselves, styles common amongst women often put them at a disadvantage in the workplace as it is currently run, according to styles more common amongst men.*
> *(Tannen, 1995)*

Added to this is the problem midwives have in working with the language of obstetrics, which is designed to measure and to set norms for what is being measured in pregnancy and labour. Obstetric language does not seek to describe the experience of the childbearing woman. A lay language has developed which includes terms such as the 'transition' between the first and second stages of labour, which is likely to be experienced as unique by the woman but is not physiologically measurable. Yet if a midwife (or a doula – see Chapter 5) seeks to prepare a woman for labour and support her through it, an appropriate language is necessary. Such a language can only be developed from the accounts of women who have had the experience for which we seek to prepare others. Yet the most powerful pressures in the midwives' working lives are usually organizational and medical, setting priorities in a very different language.

Women's different use of language and the authority of the expert language of obstetrics both affect the stories around birth. Plummer suggested:

Women's stories may actually be told in a different way – and have a different outcome. They may 'stumble' more, be told with less assuredness and boldness, be more qualified and hesitant, and hence (initially) sound less convincing. Women may generally find it harder to consider their stories as possessing 'authority', harder to express themselves in public, harder to believe that others will respect their story. There is almost certainly a massive gender skew to sexual story telling. (Plummer 1995)

Thus, around birth, mothers and midwives become a 'muted group' (Hardman, 1973):

… whose members become muted or are relatively less articulate compared with the dominant group because they have to express themselves through the structures and idioms of that group. It is not that muted groups can't speak but that they can't be heard. (Astbury, 1996)

In this hierarchy of language reflecting the professional hierarchy, stories are not a professionally acceptable form of communication and the knowledge within them is devalued. Such 'subjugated knowledges' (Foucault, 1976, quoted by Astbury, 1996) are devalued:

… as inadequate to their task or insufficiently elaborated: naive knowledges, located low down on the hierarchy, beneath the required level of cognition or scientificity. (Astbury, 1996)

Midwifery's acceptance of the language and values of obstetrics here obscures the difference between the 'task' of midwifery and that of obstetrics. Midwifery, as concerned with care around normal childbirth which is done by the woman, is primarily concerned with supporting and enhancing that woman's childbearing and continuing that care when the midwife is also called upon to assist the obstetrician. Obstetrics is concerned with the abnormal, with medical technology to detect or treat abnormality and with needed medical interventions. With the development of medical monitoring and surveillance of healthy childbearing women and the general level of self-monitoring of health in the community, it can be argued that normality is no longer a useful concept (Arney, 1982). Nevertheless this concept, enshrined in the 1902 Midwives Act, is useful in highlighting how midwifery and obstetrics spring from different bodies of knowledge and skill. While midwives have learnt much from the increasing body of obstetric knowledge, the traditional knowledge of midwifery has been muted or lost in this process of scientific dominance. The knowledge thus muted or devalued is knowledge of the area where mothers' and midwives' stories come together; each can learn from the other, and midwives can draw on women's birth stories to prepare the mothers of the future. It is therefore not surprising that this knowledge is not heard, and if this is the case for midwives and relatively articulate women, it is likely to be even more true for Black and working-class women.

Sadly, we pay a price for not being heard. The frustrating experiences of a muted group and their attempts to articulate their concerns in a language which tends to denigrate female concerns 'actively fosters the process of self-silencing' (Astbury, 1996). Jack's research highlighted the importance of self-silencing in the development of depression (Jack, 1991). Brown et al (1994) concluded from their large Australian study:

Motherhood often brought with it a sense that what one was doing or feeling was being dismissed as trivial, disregarded as unimportant, or even not heard at all. This is accentuated in this study by the fact that more than half of the women interviewed had been depressed, so that the darker shades of women's experiences as mothers are given full weight, rather than being discounted. (Brown et al, 1994)

Could it be that silenced individuals become depressed, while silenced professional groups become oppressed? The symptoms of these two afflictions are frighteningly similar.

WEAVING THE STORIES TOGETHER: IMPLICATIONS FOR PRACTICE

- Before any changes are possible we must listen to each other. Otherwise we cannot cross the 'reality gap' between 'the one-dimensional approach' (Leap, 1996) based on the official story, and women's experience. Brown et al (1994) concluded from their research that what women wanted most was the recognition that someone was listening. Sensitive midwives have always known that listening to women is a very clear way of stating that they are worth hearing. Such a demonstration of worth boosts women's self-esteem. This is equally true of midwives.
- Significant changes are now taking place. Efforts to increase continuity of carer are strengthening the bond between midwives and mothers. Research evaluating such projects suggests that the midwives involved are experiencing the profound discomfort of a change in primary allegiance from employing institution to clients (Brodie, 1996). Changes in the organization of midwifery care to facilitate such changes in practice could also have profound effects upon allegiances and power structures (e.g. Page, 1995; Warwick, 1996) as power is devolved downwards to the clinical midwife and the mother working together. An increasing attention to support, supervision and relationships amongst midwives (Kirkham, 1996b), together with the beginnings of services aimed to meet the emotional needs of women (e.g. Menage, 1996) should make more powerful the relationships between mothers and midwives and their need to hand on their mutually linked stories.
- It can be said that in the recent past 'birth was kept a mystery by medical men who sought to control it', whereas:

    Today women are reclaiming their birthing rights, and it is our hope that in sharing their birth stories, women will further understand the process and their individual power to take control.

    (Wellish and Root, 1987)

This 'individual power' comes in a social context, and 'control' is a word now used, together with 'choice' and 'continuity of care', to describe what the service should offer to the childbearing woman. This implies great political change and it is real progress that we can openly work towards this. To do so we must change the story of midwifery:

Oppressed people resist by identifying themselves as subjects, by defining their reality, shaping their new identity, naming their history, telling their story.   *(hooks, 1989)*

In such redefining the stories of mothers and midwives come together, as do our needs around story-telling.

- The present climate is such that we have a real opportunity for change, but constructive change is deeply political. Tales can be told to different effects. Stories can raise collective consciousness, bring dissonance to light and be a spur for real organizational change. Yet we also have a culture where personal stories are increasingly told as confessions. While such stories make their subjects an issue of public concern:

> ... *it is in the very nature of the self help culture not to make them political. Instead a central organising idea of the therapeutic culture is the individualisation of problems.* (*Plummer, 1995*)

This can easily lead to personal self-blame which weakens individuals and thereby undermines any possibility of collective action. We can learn here from the struggles of Black women, where in bell hooks' view 'our collective struggle is often undermined by all that has not been dealt with emotionally' (hooks, 1993). Emotional issues can be addressed in ways that are collectively strengthening, but in doing this control of the emotional story is crucial. We can see this in the medicalization and inevitable personal isolation of postnatal depression, which is now beginning to be retold as postnatal distress (Barclay and Lloyd, 1996), and in research on social aspects of postnatal depression, not least the muting referred to above (Brown et al, 1994).

● Within midwifery we repeatedly find that the defence mechanisms we built to enable us to cope with the alienation of the past prevent us from moving into new ways of working. For instance:

> *Many senior midwives and medical staff opposed the change [to team midwifery] since the need to devolve responsibility, for total care of the woman, down to the team midwife caused them anxiety.* (*Wraight et al, 1993*)

More recently the response of midwives working around new team midwifery schemes has been found in a number of settings to be threatening to those schemes and evidence of a profound wish for them to fail, because the midwives in the core staff themselves felt threatened by such change (Brodie, 1996; M. Kirkham, work in progress). It is essential that we address these issues, or the scars we bear from our past will undo our efforts to move forward.

If 'stories can be told when they can be heard' (Plummer, 1995), then the political climate is such that our time has now come, even if ironically a conservative, individualistic political context made this possible. Midwives and mothers must plan together how our personal sufferings can become collective participation and how medicalized language can be turned to be empowering for women. There are moves in this direction such as the Listen With Mother conferences (Dodds et al, 1996). For other social groups, 'stories of private pathological pain have become stories of public, political participation' (Plummer, 1995). This must be possible here, for stories of birth affect us all.

REFERENCES

Adams AE (1994) *Reproducing the Womb: Images of Childbirth in Science, Feminist Theory and Literature.* Ithaca: Cornell University Press.
Arney WR (1982) *Power and the Profession of Obstetrics.* University of Chicago Press.
Astbury J (1996) *Crazy for You: The Making of Women's Madness.* Oxford University Press.
Atkins S & Murphy K (1993) Reflection: a review of the literature. *Journal of Advanced Nursing* **18**: 1188–1192.
Bagnold E (1938) *The Squire.* London: Virago (republished 1987).

Barclay LM & Lloyd B (1996) The misery of motherhood: alternative approaches to maternal distress. *Midwifery* **12**(3): 136–139.

Bolton G (1994) Stories at work – critical writing as a means of professional development. *British Educational Research Journal* **20**(1): 55–68.

Bolton G (1995) Taking the thinking out of it: writing – a therapeutic space. *Counselling* August: 215–218.

Bolton G, Rowland S & Winter R (1990) Writing fiction as enquiry into professional practice. *Journal of Curriculum Studies* **22**(3): 291–293.

Bourne G (1996) *Pregnancy.* London: Pan.

Bowder C (1983) *Birth Rites.* Brighton: Harvester.

Bowles N (1995) Story telling: a search for meaning within nursing practice. *Nurse Education Today* **15**(5): 365–369.

Brink A (1996) *Imaginings of Sand.* London: Secker & Warburg.

Brodie P (1996) *Australian Team Midwives in Transition.* International Confederation of Midwives 24th Triennial Congress, Oslo.

Brody H (1987) *Stories of Sickness.* New Haven: Yale University Press.

Brody H (1994) My story is broken; can you help me fix it? Medical ethics and the joint construction of narrative. *Literature and Medicine* **13**(1): 79–92.

Brown S, Lumley J, Small R & Astbury J (1994) *Missing Voices: The Experience of Motherhood.* Oxford University Press.

[CESDI] Confidential Enquiry into Stillbirths and Deaths in Infancy (1996) *Third Annual Report: 1 Jan–31 Dec 1994.* London: Department of Health.

Clarke L (1995) Nursing research: science, visions and telling stories. *Journal of Advanced Nursing* **21**: 584–593.

Coles R (1989) *The Call of Stories.* Boston: Houghton Mifflin.

Cope W (1986) *Making Cocoa for Kingsley Amis.* London: Faber.

Cosslett T (1994) *Women Writing Childbirth: Modern Discourses of Motherhood.* Manchester University Press.

Curtis P (1992) Supervision in clinical midwifery practice. In: Butterworth T, Faugier J (eds) *Clinical Supervision and Mentorship in Nursing.* London: Chapman & Hall.

Davies RM & Atkinson P (1991) Students of midwifery: 'doing the obs' and other coping strategies. *Midwifery* **7**: 113–121.

Davis E (1983) *A Guide to Midwifery: Hearts and Hands.* New York: Bantam.

Dick-Read G (1933) *Natural Childbirth.* London: Heinemann.

Dodds R, Goodman M & Tyler S (1996) *Listen With Mother: Consulting Users of the Maternity Services.* Hale, Cheshire: Books for Midwives.

[DoH] Department of Health (1993) *Changing Childbirth.* Report of the Expert Maternity Group. London: HMSO.

Fanon F (1963) *The Wretched of the Earth.* New York: Grove Press.

Foucault M (1992) Lecture 1: 7 January 1976. In: Gordon C (ed.) *Power/Knowledge: Selected Interviews and Other Writings 1972–77.* New York: Pantheon.

Freire P (1972) *Pedagogy of the Oppressed.* Harmondsworth: Penguin.

Gaskin IM (1977) *Spiritual Midwifery.* Summertown, TN: Book Publishing.

Gelis J (1991) *History of Childbirth: Fertility, Pregnancy and Birth in Early Modern Europe.* Oxford: Polity Press.

Goldberg N (1986) *Writing down the Bones: Freeing the Writer Within.* Boston, MA: Shambhala.

Green JM, Coupland VA & Kitzinger JV (1988) *'Great Expectations': A Prospective Study of Women's Expectations and Experiences of Childbirth.* Cambridge Child Care and Development Unit.

Gregory A, ed. (1923) *The Midwife: Her Book.* London: Frowde/Hodder & Stoughton.

Hardman C (1973) Can there be an anthropology of children? *Journal of the Anthropological Society of Oxford* **4**: 85–99.

Harvey S (1993) The genesis of a phenomenological approach to advanced nursing practice. *Journal of Advanced Nursing* **18**(4): 526–530.

Hemingway E (1925) The Indian Camp. In: *In Our Time.* New York: Scribners.

hooks bell (1989) *Talking Back: Thinking Feminist, Thinking Black.* Boston, MA: South End Press.

hooks bell (1993) *Sisters of the Yam: Black Women and Self Recovery.* Boston, MA: South End Press.

Hughes D (1990) Sarah Gamp – Midwife. *Midwifery Matters* **46**: 12.

Jack DC (1991) *Silencing the Self: Women and Depression.* Cambridge, MA: Harvard University Press.

Jackson C (1991) Power to the parent. *Health Visitor* **64**(10): 340–342.

Jordan B (1993) *Birth in Four Cultures*, 4th edn Prospect Heights, IL: Waveland.

Kirkham M (1989) Midwives and information-giving during labour. In: Robinson S, Thomson AM (eds.) *Midwives, Research and Childbirth* vol. 1. London: Chapman & Hall.

Kirkham M (1996a) Professionalisation past and present: with women or with the powers that be? In: Kroll D (ed.) *Midwifery Care for the Future.* London: Bailliere Tindall.

Kirkham M, ed. (1996b) *Supervision of Midwives.* Hale, Cheshire: Books for Midwives.

Kirkham M (1997) Reflection in midwifery: professional narcissism or seeing with women? *British Journal of Midwifery* **5**: 5.

Kleinman A (1988) *The Illness Narratives: Suffering, Healing and the Human Condition.* New York: Basic Books.

Lambert J, ed (1993) *Wise Women of the Dreamtime: Aboriginal Tales of the Ancestral Powers* (collected by Langloh Parker K). Rochester, Vt: Inner Traditions.

Lave J & Wenger E (1991) *Situated Learning: Legitimate Peripheral Participation.* Cambridge University Press.

Leap N (1996) *A Midwifery Perspective on Pain in Labour.* Unpublished MSc dissertation, South Bank University, London.

Leap N & Hunter B (1993) *The Midwife's Tale: An Oral History from Handywoman to Professional Midwife.* London: Scarlett Press.

Linde C (1993) *Life Stories: The Creation of Coherence.* Oxford University Press.

Llewelyn Davies M, ed. (1977) *Life As We Have Known It: By Co-operative Working Women.* London: Virago.

Marland H, ed. (1993) *The Art of Midwifery: Early Modern Midwives in Europe.* London: Routledge.

Menage J (1996) Post-traumatic stress disorder following obstetric/gynaecological procedures. *British Journal of Midwifery* **4**(10): 532–533.

MIDIRS and the NHS Centre for Reviews and Dissemination (1996) *Informed Choice for Professionals: Support in Labour.* Bristol: MIDIRS.

Midwifery Today (1995) *Life of a Midwife: a Celebration of Midwifery.* Eugene, OR: Midwifery Today.

Nelson N & Wright S (1995) *Power and Participatory Development.* London: Intermediate Technology.

Nolan M (1996) One labour: two very different experiences. *Modern Midwife* Feb: 6–9.

O'Driscoll K & Meagher D (1980) *Active Management of Labour.* London: WB Saunders.

O'Driscoll K & Meagher D (1993) *Active Management of Labour*, 3rd edn. London: Mosby.

[OLDP] Oldham Literature Development Programme (1996) *The Real Story: Young Motherhood from the Fifties to the Nineties.* Oldham Education and Leisure Services Arts and Heritage Publications.

Page L, ed. (1995) *Effective Group Practice in Midwifery.* Oxford: Blackwell.

Plato. *The Republic.* Harmondsworth: Penguin, 1987.

Plummer K (1995) *Telling Sexual Stories.* London: Routledge.

Powell J, transl. (1993) *Sappho: A Garland.* New York: Farrar Straus Giroux.

Rhodes P (1995) *A Short History of Midwifery.* Hale, Cheshire: Books for Midwives.

Roberts SJ (1983) Oppressed group behaviour: implications for nursing. *Advances in Nursing Science* July: 21–30.

Robinson J (1995) Why mothers fought obstetricians. *British Journal of Midwifery* **3**(10): 557–558.

Sandelowski M & Jones LC (1996) 'Healing fictions': stories of choosing in the aftermath of the detection of fetal anomalies. *Social Science and Medicine* **42**(3): 353–361.

Sapsford R & Abbott P (1992) *Research Methods for Nurses and the Caring Professions.* Buckingham: Open University Press.

Sorel NC (1984) *Ever Since Eve.* London: Michael Joseph.

Tannen D (1991) *You Just Don't Understand: Women and Men in Conversation.* London: Virago.

Tannen D (1995) *Talking From 9 to 5: Women and Men at Work: Language, Sex and Power.* London: Virago.

[UKCC] United Kingdom Central Council for Nursing, Midwifery and Health Visiting (1993) *Midwives Rules.* London: UKCC.

Ulrich LT (1991) *A Midwife's Tale: The Life of Martha Ballard Based on her Diary 1785–1812.* New York: Vintage Books.

Warwick C (1996) Leadership in midwifery care. *British Journal of Midwifery.* 4(5): 229.

Weitz R & Sullivan D (1985) Licensed lay midwifery and the medical model of childbirth. *Sociology of Health and Illness* 7(1): 36–54.

Wellish P & Root S (1987) *Hearts Open Wide: Midwives and Births.* Berkeley, CA: Wingbow.

Williams WC (1983) *Paterson.* Harmondsworth: Penguin.

Wise J (1996) Preparation for caseload management. *Modern Midwife* Jan: 15–17.

Wraight A, Ball J, Seccombe I & Stock J (1993) *Mapping Team Midwifery.* A report to the Department of Health. Brighton: Institute of Manpower Studies.

Index